Managing Cardiovascular Complications in Diabetes

EDITED BY

D. John Betteridge BSc, MBBS, PhD, MD, FRCP, FAHA

Consultant Physician
University College London Hospital;
Dean
Royal Society of Medicine
London, UK

Stephen Nicholls MBBS, PhD, FRACP, FACC, FESC, FAHA, FCSANZ

SAHMRI Heart Foundation Heart Disease Team Leader
South Australian Health & Medical Research Institute;
Professor of Cardiology, University of Adelaide;
Consultant Cardiologist, Royal Adelaide Hospital
Adelaide, SA, Australia

WILEY Blackwell

This edition first published 2014 © 2014 by John Wiley & Sons Ltd.

Registered office: John Wiley & Sons, Ltd, The Atrium, Southern Gate, Chichester, West Sussex, PO19 8SQ, UK

Editorial offices: 9600 Garsington Road, Oxford, OX4 2DQ, UK
   The Atrium, Southern Gate, Chichester, West Sussex, PO19 8SQ, UK
   111 River Street, Hoboken, NJ 07030-5774, USA

For details of our global editorial offices, for customer services and for information about how to apply for permission to reuse the copyright material in this book please see our website at www.wiley.com/wiley-blackwell

Library of Congress Cataloging-in-Publication Data

Managing cardiovascular complications in diabetes / edited by D. John Betteridge, Stephen Nicholls.
   p. ; cm.
   Includes bibliographical references and index.
   ISBN 978-0-470-65949-6 (pbk.)
   I. Betteridge, John, editor of compilation. II. Nicholls, Stephen J., editor of compilation.
   [DNLM: 1. Cardiovascular Diseases – etiology. 2. Diabetes Complications. 3. Cardiovascular Diseases – therapy. WK 835]
   RC660.4
   616.4'62 – dc23
                              2013049546

A catalogue record for this book is available from the British Library.

Wiley also publishes its books in a variety of electronic formats. Some content that appears in print may not be available in electronic books.

Cover image: iStock - File #21522822 © janulla
Cover design by Steve Thompson

Typeset in 9.5/13pt MeridienLTStd by Laserwords Private Limited, Chennai, India
Printed in Singapore by Ho Printing Singapore Pte Ltd

1   2014

Contents

List of Contributors

R.A. Ajjan MRCP, MMedSci, PhD
Associate Professor and Consultant in Diabetes
and Endocrinology
Division of Diabetes and Cardiovascular
Research
Leeds Institute of Genetics, Health and
Therapeutics
Multidisciplinary Cardiovascular Research
Centre
University of Leeds
Leeds, UK

Jordan Andrews BS
South Australian Health & Medical Research
Institute
Adelaide, SA, Australia

Stephen C. Bain MA, MD, FRCP
Professor of Medicine (Diabetes)
Honorary Consultant Physician
Swansea University College of Medicine
Swansea, UK

**D. John Betteridge BSc, MBBS, PhD,
MD, FRCP, FAHA**
Consultant Physician
University College London Hospital;
Dean
Royal Society of Medicine
London, UK

Sujay Chandran MRCP
SpR Cardiology
Department of Cardiology
St Georges Hospital
London, UK

Elizabeth Ellins BSc(hons), MA
Senior Vascular Scientist
Swansea University College of Medicine
Swansea, UK

José A. García-Donaire MD
Nephrologist
Hypertension Unit
Hospital 12 de Octobre
Madrid, Spain

Peter J. Grant MD, FRCP, FMedSci
Professor of Medicine
Honorary Consultant Physician
University of Leeds and Leeds Teaching
Hospitals NHS Trust;
Division of Cardiovascular and Diabetes
Research
The LIGHT Laboratories
Leeds, UK

Julian Halcox MA, MD, FRCP
Professor of Cardiology
Director, Cardiovascular Research Group Cymru
Swansea University College of Medicine
Swansea, UK

Christopher M. Huff MD
Cardiology Fellow
Heart and Vascular Institute
Cleveland Clinic
Cleveland, OH, USA

Meg Jardine MBBS, PHD, FRACP
Senior Research Fellow
Renal & Metabolic Division
The George Institute for Global Health;
Consultant Nephrologist
Concord Repatriation General Hospital
Sydney, NSW, Australia

Andrew Lansdown MBChB, MRCP
Clinical Research Fellow
Institute of Molecular and Experimental
Medicine
Cardiff University School of Medicine
Cardiff, UK

Alice H. Lichtenstein DSc
Stanley N. Gershoff Professor
Friedman School of Nutrition Science
and Policy
Director and Senior Scientist, Cardiovascular
Nutrition Laboratory
Jean Mayer USDA Human Nutrition Research
Center on Aging
Tufts University
Boston, MA, USA

A. Michael Lincoff MD
Professor of Medicine
Cleveland Clinic Lerner College of Medicine
Case Western Reserve University;
Vice Chairman, Heart & Vascular Institute
Cleveland Clinic
Cleveland, OH, USA

Akhila Mallipedhi MBBS, MRCP
Specialist Registrar in Diabetes & Endocrinology
Department of Diabetes & Endocrinology
Morriston Hospital, ABM University Health
Board
Swansea, UK

**Stephen Nicholls MBBS, PhD, FRACP,
FACC, FESC, FAHA, FCSANZ**
SAHMRI Heart Foundation Heart Disease Team
Leader
South Australian Health & Medical Research
Institute;
Professor of Cardiology, University of Adelaide;
Consultant Cardiologist, Royal Adelaide
Hospital
Adelaide, SA, Australia

Hitesh Patel MBBS, BSc
Cardiology Registrar
Department of Cardiology
St George's Hospital
London, UK

**Vlado Perkovic MBBS, PhD, FRACP,
FASN**
Executive Director
The George Institute for Global Health;
Professor of Medicine
University of Sydney
Sydney, NSW, Australia

**Kausik K. Ray BSc (Hons), MBChB,
MD, FRCP, MPhil (Cantab), FACC,
FESC, FAHA**
Professor of Cardiovascular Disease Prevention
Cardiac and Vascular Sciences
St George's University of London
London, UK

Luis M. Ruilope MD, PhD
Professor
Hospital 12 de Octobre
Madrid, Spain

Gerit-Holger Schernthaner MD
University Professor of Medicine
Department of Medicine II
Division of Angiology
Medical University of Vienna
Vienna, Austria

Guntram Schernthaner MD
Professor and Head
Department of Medicine I
Rudolfstiftung Hospital Vienna
Vienna, Austria

Rüdiger-Egbert Schernthaner MD
Department of Radiology
Division of Cardiovascular and Interventional
Radiology
Medical University of Vienna
Vienna, Austria

**Jeffrey W. Stephens BSc, MBBS, PhD,
FRCP**
Professor of Medicine (Diabetes & Metabolism)
Honorary Consultant Physician
Swansea University College of Medicine
Swansea, UK

Kiyoko Uno MD
Departments of Cardiovascular Medicine and
Cell Biology
Cleveland Clinic
Cleveland, OH, USA

Amanda Y. Wang MBBS, MSc, FRACP
Medical Fellow
Renal & Metabolic Division
The George Institute for Global Health;
Consultant Nephrologist
Sydney Adventist Hospital
Sydney, NSW, Australia

Introduction

The International Diabetes Federation produced a very important publication over a decade ago entitled "Diabetes and Cardiovascular Disease: Time to Act". In his introduction the then President of IDF, Prof Sir George Alberti stated "With the rising tide of diabetes around the globe, the double jeopardy of diabetes and cardiovascular disease is set to result in an explosion of these and other complications unless preventive action is taken [1]. Indeed the care of people with diabetes costs two to three fold more than those without the disease and can amount to up to 15% of national health care budgets [2].

There is no doubt that diabetes is a significant contributor to the global burden of chronic non-communicable disease which accounts for over 36 million (63%) of deaths worldwide. Importantly, 80% of these deaths occur in low and middle income countries. Even in areas of the world where deaths from infectious disease are higher such as the Africa Region, the prevalence of NCDs is rising rapidly [3].

The projected increases in the prevalence of diabetes worldwide are simply staggering. In an important contribution from the Global Burden of Metabolic Risk Factor of Chronic Disease Collaborating Group [4] national, regional and global trends in fasting plasma glucose and diabetes prevalence since 1980 were studied in a systematic analysis of health examination surveys involving over two and a half million participants and 370 country-years observations. They estimated that the number of people with diabetes increased from 153 (95% uncertainty interval 127–182) million in 1980 to 347 (314382) million in 2008 [4]. Global projections produced by IDF are shown in Figure 1. The projections are from 2013 to 2035. The percentage increases are most dramatic in Africa, the Middle East, North Africa, South East Asia and South and Central America [5]. Clearly, primary prevention of diabetes should be high on public health agendas throughout the world with polices to reduce overweight and increase activity.

As emphasized by Alberti [1] the increasing prevalence of diabetes brings with it the added burden of cardiovascular disease (CVD). Disease in all vascular beds is increased and post mortem studies have demonstrated a particularly aggressive form of atherosclerosis characterised not only by increased plaque burden but also increased necrotic core and macrophage and T cell infiltration [6]. The importance of diabetes as a CVD risk factor

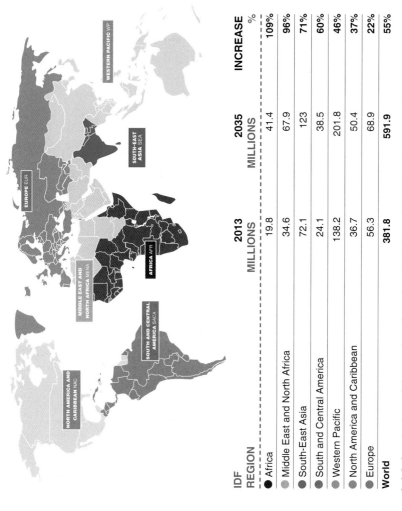

IDF REGION	2013 MILLIONS	2035 MILLIONS	INCREASE %
● Africa	19.8	41.4	109%
● Middle East and North Africa	34.6	67.9	96%
● South-East Asia	72.1	123	71%
● South and Central America	24.1	38.5	60%
● Western Pacific	138.2	201.8	46%
● North America and Caribbean	36.7	50.4	37%
● Europe	56.3	68.9	22%
World	**381.8**	**591.9**	**55%**

Figure 1 IDF Regions and global projections of the number of people with diabetes (20–79 years), 2013 and 2035. (Source: International Diabetes Federation [5]. Reproduced with permission of the International Diabetes Federation (IDF)).

Table 1 Diabetes mellitus, fasting blood glucose concentration, and risk of vascular disease: a collaborative meta-analysis of 102 prospective studies. (Source: Emerging Risk Factors Collaboration [9]. Reproduced with permission of Elsevier.)

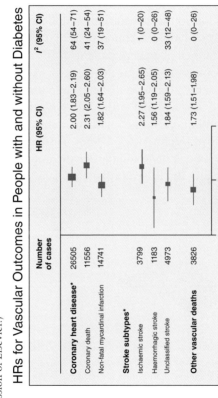

HRs for Vascular Outcomes in People with and without Diabetes

	Number of cases	HR (95% CI)	I^2 (95% CI)
Coronary heart disease*	26505	2.00 (1.83–2.19)	64 (54–71)
Coronary death	11556	2.31 (2.05–2.60)	41 (24–54)
Non-fatal mycardinal infarction	14741	1.82 (1.64–2.03)	37 (19–51)
Stroke subtypes*			
Ischaemic stroke	3799	2.27 (1.95–2.65)	1 (0–20)
Haemorrhagic stroke	1183	1.56 (1.19–2.05)	0 (0–26)
Unclassified stroke	4973	1.84 (1.59–2.13)	33 (12–48)
Other vascular deaths	3826	1.73 (1.51–1.98)	0 (0–26)

698,782 people in 102 prospective studies with 52,765 CVD outcomes

The Emerging Risk Factors Collaboration*

was acknowledged by the formation of a joint Task Force on Diabetes and Cardiovascular Diseases by the European Society of Cardiology (ESC) and the European Association for the Study of Diabetes (EASD) which published its evidenced based guidelines on prevention and management in 2007 [7]. The guidelines have recently been updated [8].

The massive data base of the Emerging Risk Factor Collaboration, a collaborative meta-analysis of 102 prospective studies including data from almost 700,000 individuals has provided further robust evidence relating diabetes to CVD risk after adjusting for age, smoking status, BMI and systolic blood pressure [9]. The hazard ratios for coronary heart disease, stroke and other vascular deaths are shown in Table 1. In addition to increased risk of CVD patients with diabetes and established vascular disease have a poorer outcome than those without diabetes [7, 8]. Peripheral arterial disease is increased 2-4 fold in the diabetic population and lower limb amputations are at least 10 fold more common such that half of non-traumatic amputations are performed in diabetic patients [3, 7, 8].

The focus of this book is to assist the physician or surgeon in preventing and managing CVD and CVD risk in diabetic patients. We have been fortunate that respected international authorities have agreed to contribute "state of the art" contributions in their particular area of expertise. We are grateful to our publishers, John Wiley & Sons, Ltd, for their patience and encouragement. If this book helps to improve the outcome of the individual patient and so reduce the huge burden of CVD in diabetes then it will have achieved its goal.

D. John Betteridge
Stephen Nicholls

References

1 International Diabetes Federation. Diabetes and Cardiovascular Disease: Time to Act. IDF 2001.
2 Zhang P, Zhang X, Brown J et al. Global healthcare expenditure on diabetes for 2010 and 2030. *Diabetes Research and Clinical Practice* 2010; 87: 293-301.
3 World Health Organization in collaboration with the World Heart Foundation and the World Stroke Organization. *Global Atlas on Cardiovascular Disease Prevention and Control* (Eds, Mendis S, Puska P, Norving B) World Health Organization Geneva 2011.
4 Danaei G, Finucane MM, Yuan L et al. National, regional and global trends in fasting plasma glucose and diabetes prevalence since 1980: systematic analysis of health examination surveys and epidemiological studies with 370 country-years and 2.7 million participants. *Lancet* 2011; 87: 293-301.
5 International Diabetes Federation. IDF Diabetes Atlas 6th edition. IDF 2013.
6 Burke AP, Kolodgie FD, Zieske A et al. Morphologic findings of coronary atherosclerotic plaques in diabetics: a post-mortem study. *Arterioscler Thromb Vasc Biol* 2004; 24: 1266-71.

7 The Task Force on diabetes, pre-diabetes and cardiovascular disease of the European Society of Cardiology and of the European Association for the Study of Diabetes.Guidelines on diabetes, pre-diabetes and cardiovascular diseases. *European Heart Journal* 2007; 9: suppl C, C1-74.

8 The Task Force on diabetes, pre-diabetes and cardiovascular disease of the European Society of Cardiology and developed in collaboration with the European Association for the Study of Diabetes. ESC guidelines on diabetes, pre-diabetes and cardiovascular diseases in collaboration with the EASD. *European Heart Journal* 2013; 34: 3035–87.

9 Emerging Risk Factors Collaboration. Diabetes, fasting blood glucose concentration and risk of vascular disease: a collaborative meta-analysis of 102 prospective studies. *Lancet* 2010; 375: 2215–22.

CHAPTER 1

The Vascular Endothelium in Diabetes

Andrew Lansdown[1], Elizabeth Ellins[2] and Julian Halcox[2]
[1] *Cardiff University School of Medicine, Cardiff, UK*
[2] *Swansea University College of Medicine, Swansea, UK*

Key Points

- The endothelium is a key participant in the homeostasis of the vessel wall.
- Nitric oxide (NO) plays a key role in regulating healthy vascular function.
- Reduced local NO bioavailability is a characteristic hallmark of vascular endothelial dysfunction.
- Endothelial dysfunction is chiefly driven by oxidative stress and inflammation.
- A number of techniques for assessing endothelial function are available; flow-mediated dilatation (FMD) is the current noninvasive 'gold-standard' methodology.
- A number of circulating markers are also helpful in assessment of endothelial dysfunction.
- Hyperglycemia, insulin resistance, and dyslipidemia are all important contributors to endothelial dysfunction.
- Endothelial dysfunction in diabetes is associated with adverse micro- and macrovascular complications.
- Drug therapies, including statins, insulin sensitizers, and ACE inhibitors, have been shown to improve endothelial dysfunction in diabetes.

Introduction

The vascular endothelium, the monolayer of thin cells lining the arteries and veins, serves as the key regulator of arterial homeostasis. It plays a vital role in regulating vascular tone, cellular adhesion, platelet activity, vessel wall inflammation, angiogenesis, and vascular smooth muscle cell proliferation. In order to regulate these functions, a number of important vasoactive molecules, including nitric oxide (NO), endothelium-derived hyperpolarizing factor (EDHF), prostacyclin (PGI2), and endothelin (ET-1), are produced and released by the endothelial cells [1, 2].

Managing Cardiovascular Complications in Diabetes, First Edition.
Edited by D. John Betteridge and Stephen Nicholls.

Normal Endothelial Cell Function

The arterial endothelium is composed of a layer of spindle-shaped endothelial cells that are bound together by tight junctions and communicate directly with each other and the underlying smooth muscle cells via gap junctions. This forms a protective barrier between the blood and the rest of the vessel wall that is relatively impermeable to low-density lipoprotein (the core component of atherosclerotic lesions), able to sense molecular cues and interact with cellular components of the circulating blood.

Furchgott and Zawadzki first demonstrated in 1980 that endothelial cells are essential in order for underlying smooth muscle relaxation to occur in response to acetylcholine administration in the rabbit aorta [3] and NO was subsequently identified as this endothelium-derived relaxing factor [4]. A healthy endothelium is able to secrete NO, a diatomic molecule generated from L-arginine, by the action of the enzyme endothelial NO synthase (eNOS) in the presence of cofactors such as tetrahydrobiopterin [5]. NO exerts its action by diffusing into vascular smooth muscle cells where it activates G-protein-bound guanylate cyclase, resulting in c-GMP generation, smooth muscle relaxation, and vasodilatation [1] (Figure 1.1). eNOS, in normal physiology, is activated by shear stress from blood flow through the vessels and also by molecules such as adenosine, bradykinin, serotonin (in response to platelet aggregation), and vascular endothelial growth factor (induced by hypoxia; Figure 1.1) [6, 7, 8].

In addition, NO has antiplatelet effects and can down-regulate inflammatory pathways and also decrease the generation of ET-1, a potent vasoconstrictor polypeptide, which also possesses pro-inflammatory, pro-oxidant, and pro-proliferative activity [9].

Other endothelial-derived vasodilators exist and act independently of NO to maintain vasodilator tone. PGI2, produced from the cyclooxygenase system, and EDHF are such molecules, with the latter able to compensate for the loss of NO-mediated vasodilator tone when NO bioavailability is reduced [10, 11]. Normal health and physiological functioning of the vascular endothelium are maintained by a balanced release of endothelial-derived relaxing factors, such as NO and prostacyclin (PGI2), and vasoconstricting factors like ET-1 and angiotensin II. The dysequilibrium of their production, release, and action is the chief characteristic of endothelial dysfunction [12].

Beyond its function in regulating vessel tone, the vascular endothelium also serves to play an important role in both mediating and responding to inflammatory pathways. In addition to its constrictor effects, angiotensin II generated by the endothelium has effects on vascular smooth muscle cell contraction, growth, proliferation, and differentiation. A range of selectins and adhesion molecules are produced, resulting in the binding and

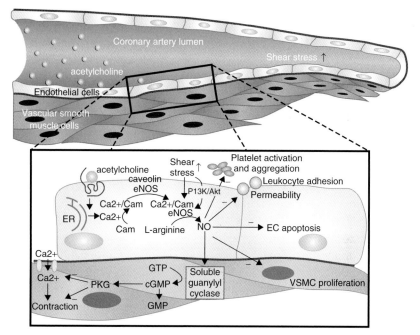

Figure 1.1 Illustration of the stimulation of endothelial NO synthase by acetylcholine and shear stress leading to increased nitric oxide (NO) production in endothelial cells by receptor and nonreceptor and calcium-dependent and noncalcium-dependent pathways. (Source: Herrmann J et al. 2010 [8]. Reproduced with permission of Oxford University Press.) (Color plate 1.1).

transendothelial migration of inflammatory cells [13, 14]. Furthermore, the endothelium is directly involved in the balance between coagulation and fibrinolysis, which is mediated by its synthesis of both tissue-type plasminogen activator (t-PA) and its inhibitor, plasminogen activator inhibitor-1 (PAI-1) [12, 15].

Measuring Endothelial Function

Following the in vitro work of Furchgott and Zawadzki, Ludmer et al. demonstrated for the first time in humans that locally administered acetylcholine caused vasoconstriction of atherosclerotic coronary arteries and vasodilatation in normal coronary vessels in subjects undergoing cardiac catheterization [16]. Subsequently, a noninvasive method was developed for assessing endothelial function in the conduit arteries of the peripheral circulation. This method used a period of forearm ischemia followed by reactive hyperemia to increase blood flow through the brachial artery, increasing local shear stress, mediating NO release and brachial artery dilatation [17]. Peripheral endothelial vasodilator function correlates with coronary endothelial function and cardiovascular risk factors, including smoking, dyslipidemia, and diabetes, and can predict incident cardiovascular events in older adults [18, 19, 20, 21].

Various techniques have been developed that use pharmacologic agents to act on the endothelium or that measure the vasodilator response to increased shear stress. No one test has been shown to be ideal and indeed a combination may be required to evaluate fully the various aspects of vascular endothelial biology (Figure 1.2).

Invasive methods for assessing endothelial function include venous occlusion plethysmography and quantitative coronary angiography with Doppler flow wire to assess coronary diameter and blood flow.

The original tests of endothelial function used the latter techniques to assess coronary circulatory physiology. Pharmacologic agents, such as acetylcholine, are used to induce an endothelium-dependent vasomotor response, measuring changes in the epicardial and microvascular circulation. At the doses traditionally used, a vasodilator response is usually observed in normal coronary vessels, but in the presence of endothelial dysfunction, where NO bioavailability is reduced, the action of acetylcholine on smooth muscle muscarinic receptors predominates, resulting in vasoconstriction [22]. This method of measuring endothelial function is limited to patients with more advanced and established arterial disease who warrant cardiac catheterization, but is helpful in quantifying the response to potential beneficial therapeutic agents, such as statins, on endothelial function [23].

A further invasive technique for evaluation of forearm microcirculation and resistance is by measuring changes in forearm blood flow (FBF) using venous occlusion strain-gauge plethysmography [24]. The method uses the contralateral arm as its control, with most studies assessing percentage differences in FBF and vascular resistance between experimental and control arm after the administration of endothelium-dependent and endothelium-independent agonists. By using eNOS antagonists, such as L-NMMA, the contribution of NO to vasomotor regulation can be inferred; the technique can also be used in healthy controls and allows other vasomotor pathways to be studied in detail. Its invasive nature, however, thus limits its use to smaller studies and its clinical relevance to conduit vessel atherosclerosis is also questioned.

The noninvasive methods of measuring endothelial function are inherently more practical in that they can be more readily used in large patient groups. Flow-mediated dilatation (FMD) using ultrasound stands as the current gold-standard technique for noninvasive assessment of endothelial function. The rationale is based on the reactive blood flow in the brachial artery following a five-minute period of forearm ischemia caused by

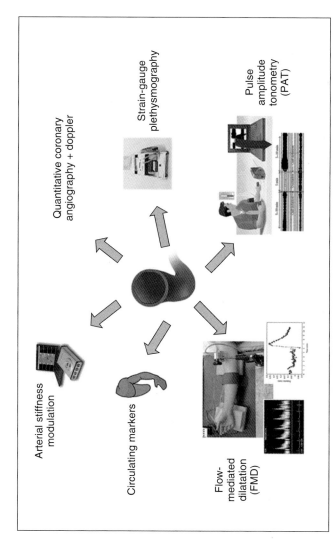

Figure 1.2 Methods for assessing human endothelial function. (Color plate 1.2).

suprasystolic inflation of a blood-pressure cuff. The increased shear stress during the resulting hyperemia stimulates NO release from the endothelium, causing smooth muscle relaxation and dilatation of the artery. By imaging the brachial artery with high-resolution 2D ultrasound and using pulsed-wave Doppler interrogation, changes in arterial diameter and blood flow can be assessed [17]. When care is paid to methodology, FMD has been demonstrated to have good reproducibility [25]. Some differences in techniques, including cuff position and duration of cuff occlusion, remain areas of controversy in using this method [26, 27, 28], although guidelines have been produced in an attempt to reduce the variability of the methodology in research [29, 30]. Despite variations in methodology, FMD stands as a reliable method of measuring endothelial function and is associated with coronary endothelial vasodilator function and circulating markers of endothelial activation, as well as being a predictor of long-term cardiovascular outcomes [21, 31].

Another useful noninvasive technique that is emerging for measuring endothelial function is pulse amplitude tonometry (PAT). The same stimulus as FMD is used and the EndoPAT system employs a probe placed on the fingertip to record changes in arterial pulsatile volume. Both fingertips are used for recordings in order to have an internal control. Measurements are made at baseline and following reactive hyperemia (RH) so as to allow an RH-PAT index (ratio) to be calculated. The RH-PAT signal is decreased with risk factor expression, has been shown to correlate well with risk factor burden, and can help to identify coronary vascular dysfunction [32, 33]. Reproducibility has been shown to be similar to that of FMD. Although the mechanism of vasodilatation is not entirely NO dependent and the autonomic nervous system may also have an influence on the fingertip pulse waveform [34], RH-PAT is widely considered to be a useful and practical tool for assessing endothelial dysfunction.

Endothelial function can also be assessed using pulse wave velocity (PWV) measurement. This method measures the speed of transit of the arterial pulse-pressure waveform through an artery, thus providing information on arterial stiffness and endothelial function. A similar protocol to that of FMD, with RH stimulus, has been devised by Naka et al. involving placing one cuff at the wrist and one on the upper arm, with RH induced following the occlusion of the wrist cuff. The subsequent NO release and reduction in arterial tone cause a slowing in PWV, reflecting the magnitude of endothelial NO release [35].

Although these newer methods, particularly RH-PAT, appear promising in their use for assessing endothelial function, FMD currently remains the technique of choice and has become widely used in clinical studies.

Circulating Markers of Endothelial Dysfunction

In addition to invasive and noninvasive methods of assessing endothelial function, such as coronary angiography or FMD, there are a number of circulating biomarkers that reflect the degree of endothelial activation and dysfunction (Table 1.1).

Given that endothelial activation and dysfunction are characterized by the change in the balance of vasomotor factors released by the endothelium, measuring circulating markers and mediators of this dysfunction have been shown to provide important pathological insights into the influence of the endothelium on atherosclerotic disease, although the systemic levels of these markers may not necessarily represent their true local effects on the vascular wall.

Endothelial activation results in vascular inflammation. Thus, an array of inflammatory cytokines, adhesion molecules, regulators of thrombosis, measures of NO biology, as well as markers of endothelial damage and repair can be evaluated to inform on these processes. These measures can be helpful markers of the severity of endothelial activation and dysfunction in a population and can complement other physiological tests of measuring endothelial function [36].

No precise circulating marker reflecting local and systemic generation of NO is available, although levels of nitrite and nitrate have been suggested as indirect measures. Asymmetric dimethylarginine (ADMA), an endogenously derived competitive antagonist of eNOS, is quantifiable; higher levels are typically present in those patients with cardiovascular risk factors, such as dyslipidemia and diabetes, and may contribute to the endothelial dysfunction. Higher levels of ADMA have been associated with reduced NO bioavailability in animal and clinical studies [37, 38]. Logistical and financial barriers currently preclude its use in routine clinical practice.

The inflammatory cytokines and adhesion molecules generated by endothelial activation, reflecting the stimuli to leucocyte migration into the subendothelium, can also be measured. Vascular cell adhesion molecule 1, intracellular adhesion molecule 1, and E- and P-selectins are examples, with E-selectin most specific for vascular endothelial activation. Circulating levels of such molecules are typically associated with adverse cardiovascular outcomes [39, 40].

In addition, MicroRNAs (miRNAs), a group of noncoding small RNAs, are emerging as important molecules in endothelial dysfunction in diabetes and may indeed shed light on these underlying disease processes. In the hyperglycemic environment, for example, miRNAs decrease endothelial cell proliferation and migration, as well as causing cell cycle inhibition,

Table 1.1 Circulating biomarkers of endothelial function.

Biomarkers
Nitric oxide
Nitrite ion
Asymmetric dimethyl arginine
Endothelin-1
Interleukins
Chemokines
Adhesion molecules (VCAM-1, ICAM-1)
Selectins (E-selectin, P-selectin)
Plasminogen activator inhibitor- 1
Tissue plasminogen activator
Von Willebrand factor
Endothelial microparticles microRNAs
Circulating endothelial cells
Endothelial progenitor cells
Endothelial microparticles

resulting in vascular endothelial dysfunction [41]. As levels of miRNA in the serum of humans have been shown to be stable, reproducible, and consistent among healthy individuals, it is thought they may become clinically useful biomarkers of vascular status in patients with diabetes [42, 43].

Similarly, markers of a prothrombotic state can be measured, which may reflect endothelial damage and activation; for example, the change in the balance of tissue plasminogen activator and its endogenous inhibitor, plasminogen activation inhibitor-1 [44].

As measures of endothelial cell injury and repair are a reflection of endothelial activation and dysfunction in the disease process, assays have been developed to examine the detachment of mature endothelial cells and microparticles derived from activated endothelial cells, reflecting damage, and the number and characteristics of circulating endothelial progenitor cells (EPC), reflecting repair. Assessment of the relationships between these populations can shed light on the balance between injury and repair (in diabetes) that may have a future role in clinical practice and in risk assessment of high-risk patients [45]. Endothelial microparticles (EMP) result from endothelial plasma membrane blebbing and carry endothelial proteins such as vascular endothelial cadherin, intercellular cell adhesion molecule (ICAM)-1, E-selectin, and eNOS [46, 47, 48]. Their shedding from activated or apoptotic endothelial cells reflects their role in coagulation, inflammation, endothelial function, and vascular homeostasis. The exact role of EMP in vascular homeostasis remains unclear. There is evidence that they can actually promote cell survival and induce endothelial regeneration [49] and, although promotion of angiogenic processes by EMP may have beneficial effects in ischemia, this could be detrimental for plaque stability and in proliferative diabetic retinopathy [50]. In diabetes it has been shown that higher levels of EMP are associated with endothelial activation and apoptosis [1, 51]. Furthermore, interventions to treat patients with type 2 diabetes with calcium channel blockers have shown decreases in EMP, suggesting the latter's potential use as biomarkers of vascular endothelial dysfunction in diabetes, although their specific clinical utility remains to be defined [52, 53].

Endothelial Cell Dysfunction

Endothelial dysfunction results from a loss of the homeostatic balance between endothelial-derived relaxing factors, such as NO, and contracting factors, such as ET-1. A number of cardiovascular risk factors have been implicated including dyslipidemia, diabetes mellitus, hypertension, and smoking. In these circumstances, the endothelium is activated, with an increased expression of leucocyte adhesion molecules, release of cytokines, and inflammatory molecules. The resulting inflammation and arterial damage continue in a self-promoting fashion, contributing to the initiation and development of atherosclerotic plaque formation and its clinical consequences such as myocardial ischemia or infarction [54, 55].

One of the defining characteristics of endothelial activation is reduced NO bioavailability. This largely occurs in the context of increased oxidative stress, when the enzyme, eNOS, may switch to generate superoxide (reactive oxygen species or ROS), a process known as "eNOS uncoupling." This is thought to occur when the key cofactor tetrahydrobiopterin is not present or when the substrate, L-arginine, is deficient [56]. In addition, ROS, in the presence of superoxide dismutase, leads to the production of hydrogen peroxide. These molecules can target cellular regulatory proteins, such as NFκB and phosphatases, promoting inflammatory gene transcription [1, 57]. The mitochondrion is thought to be an important source of ROS in which the production of free radicals and mitochondrial superoxide dismutase capacity is carefully regulated during physiological cellular homeostasis. During hypoxia, or in disease processes with increased substrate, such as obesity and type 2 diabetes with hyperglycemia and increased free fatty acids, this fine balance can be disturbed, resulting in increased free radical generation. Xanthine oxidase and NADPH oxidase are other important sources of oxidative stress in the endothelium, with xanthine oxidase activity having been shown to be increased by over 200% in patients with coronary artery disease compared with controls [58].

A further effect of prolonged exposure to cardiovascular risk factors is the effect on endothelial damage and repair. Normal endothelial integrity depends on its ability to repair and on any degree of localized injury. Endothelial cells are able to replicate locally to replace injured and lost cells, but also EPC recruited from the bone marrow circulate and are able to home to areas of injury and promote local repair processes in the endothelium [59, 60, 61]. It is known that eNOS is important in the regulation and function of EPC [62], that decreased levels of EPC are correlated with increased risk of coronary artery disease [63, 64], and that interventions, such as statin therapy, increase EPC in high-risk patients, including those with coronary artery disease [65]. In diabetes it has been shown that levels of EPC and circulating angiogenic cells (CAC) are reduced in relation to smooth muscle progenitor cells (SMPC), reflecting damage; this may therefore translate into reduced vascular repair capacity and promote macrovascular disease in type 2 diabetes [66]. The reduction in EPC in diabetes may also explain the pathogenesis of microangiopathy, as clinically significant correlations have been found in nephropathy and retinopathy [67, 68]. Furthermore, in diabetes EPC have functional defects such as impaired proliferation and adhesion, which are also likely to be of importance [69, 70]. Thus EPC are thought to play an important role in maintaining normal vascular endothelial function in diabetes.

Endothelial Cell Dysfunction in Diabetes

Both micro- and macrovascular complications are the major causes of morbidity and mortality in patients with diabetes, and endothelial cell dysfunction is believed to be pivotal in the development of associated vascular injury. There are a number of factors specific to diabetes that contribute to endothelial dysfunction (Figure 1.3).

Hyperglycemia
Hyperglycemia in both type I and type II diabetes has been implicated in the pathogenesis of microvascular complications in large clinical trials [71, 72, 73].

Oxidative stress in endothelial dysfunction in diabetes is chiefly driven by hyperglycemia. The high glucose levels up-regulate the polypol pathway, which usually converts excess intracellular glucose into sugar alcohols by the enzyme aldose reductase. Normally, very little glucose is utilized by this pathway. In diabetes, an overproduction of ROS by the mitochondrion leads to increased aldose reductase activation, with conversion of glucose to sorbitol and then oxidation to fructose. This results in increased ROS production, subsequent inactivation of NO, and inhibition of endothelium-dependent dilatation [74, 75, 76]. Intracellular

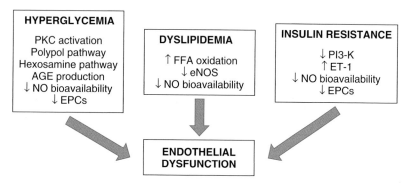

Figure 1.3 Mechanisms increasing oxidative stress and resulting in endothelial dysfunction in diabetes.

hyperglycemia also activates the hexosamine pathway, resulting in increased expression of PAI-1 [77].

Furthermore, high levels of intracellular glucose activate the enzyme protein kinase C (PKC), which can result in overexpression of the fibrinolytic inhibitor PAI-1 and activation of NFκB in endothelial cells, resulting in an increased propensity to thrombotic and atherogenic occlusion and further inflammation [78, 79]. In addition, PKC activation by hyperglycemia can cause increased vascular permeability and angiogenesis via increased expression of vascular endothelial growth factor (VEGF) in endothelial and smooth muscle cells [80].

Hyperglycemia is also causally implicated in the production of AGE, the circulating and intracellular proteins that have undergone nonenzymatic glycation. AGE have been linked to vascular inflammation, dysfunction, and injury through various mechanisms, including overproduction of ROS [81]. The main mechanism is through the binding of AGE to their receptors (RAGE), resulting in activation of NFκB and generation of ROS [76, 82, 83]. Raised plasma levels of endogenous RAGE have been noted in patients with type 2 diabetes and nephropathy [84].

It is through increased oxidative stress, as well as increased intracellular calcium, mitochondrial dysfunction, and changes in intracellular fatty acid metabolism, that hyperglycemia is thought to result in endothelial cell apoptosis [12].

In addition to its influence on oxidative stress and AGE production, hyperglycemia has also been associated with decreased NO bioavailabilty. Kawano et al. showed that hyperglycemia rapidly suppresses flow-mediated endothelium-dependent vasodilatation of the brachial artery [85]. Furthermore, in studies of human umbilical vein endothelial cells, it has been shown that elevated glucose inhibits NO production [86]. In contrast, some studies have demonstrated that NO release is increased in hyperglycemic conditions, with eNOS activity increased in the cardiac endothelium of rats with diabetes [87], leading to the suggestion that eNOS uncoupling may actually occur secondary to hyperglycemia of diabetes and explain endothelial dysfunction [88, 89]. Furthermore, endothelial dysfunction in diabetes is also related to an increase of endothelial-derived constricting factors (EDCFs), likely secondary to exposure of the endothelial cells to high glucose, causing oxidative stress and overexpression of COX-1 and COX-2, and thus involvement of COX-derived prostanoids [90]. ET-1 is also known to be present in higher levels in patients with type 2 diabetes compared with healthy subjects, and this is accompanied by increased oxidative stress and proinflammatory markers [91].

Finally, it is worth noting that the severity of hyperglycemia, as measured by HbA1c, in both type 1 and type 2 diabetes, correlates with lower levels of circulating EPC, resulting from either impaired proliferation, reduced mobilization from the bone marrow, or shorter circulating time [92, 93]. This has the potential consequence of reducing the vascular repair capacity in diabetes.

It should be noted, however, that despite evidence for hyperglycemia being responsible for these mechanisms leading to endothelial cell dysfunction, some evidence points toward endothelial dysfunction preceding marked hyperglycemia in diabetes. For example, the nonobese diabetic (NOD) mouse model for type 1 diabetes has shown that endothelial dysfunction is present, with evidence of vasoconstriction, prior to development of hyperglycemia [88]. Therefore, the cause and consequence of hyperglycemia and endothelial dysfunction may not be so obvious.

Insulin Resistance

Although hyperglycemia is common to all types of diabetes, insulin resistance is more a characteristic of type 2 diabetes and its role in endothelial cell dysfunction is important.

Endothelial cells express the cognate insulin receptor (IR) and insulin plays a vital role in normal endothelial cell homeostasis. In normal health, insulin stimulates NO release through activation of a cascade involving activation of the PI3K-Akt axis and phosphorylation of eNOS. It also has opposing actions that cause vasoconstriction through the endothelial release of ET-1. In insulin-resistant vessels there is impairment in the expression and activity of eNOS as well as impairment of the PI3K-dependent signaling, with overexpression of adhesion molecules and an increased secretion of ET-1. This results in an inflammatory endothelial microenvironment with reduced blood supply and deteriorating insulin resistance. Pharmacological blockade of ET-1 receptors improves endothelial function in obese patients with insulin resistance and those with diabetes, but not in lean, insulin-sensitive patients. It also has been suggested that endothelial dysfunction itself may be a direct causal factor in insulin resistance [88].

Insulin resistance has also been linked with reduced proliferation and differentiation of EPC as a consequence of reduced production of NO and stromal cell-derived factor (SDF)-1α, which plays a role in modulating EPC mobilization and survival [94, 95, 96].

Dyslipidemia

Both type 1 and type 2 diabetes are associated with dyslipidemia and increased levels of free fatty acids (FFA). The characteristic lipid profile associated with obesity, insulin resistance, and diabetes is reduced levels of high-density lipoprotein (HDL)-cholesterol, small dense low-density lipoprotein (LDL) particles, hypertriglyceridemia, and increased postprandial FFA flux. Both in vitro and clinical studies suggest that endothelial dysfunction in noninsulin-dependent diabetes is in part due to diabetic dyslipidemia, most specifically postprandial lipemia with associated inflammation and oxidative stress [97, 98].

Clinical Relevance of Endothelial Dysfunction in Diabetes

Endothelial dysfunction has been shown to be an earlier manifestation of vascular disease in type 2 diabetes, but is later in the course of type 1 diabetes [99]. Various studies have emerged linking endothelial dysfunction with adverse clinical outcomes of microvascular and macrovascular complications in diabetes.

In patients with type 1 diabetes, endothelial dysfunction precedes and may predict the development of microalbuminuria [100]. It has been suggested that endothelial dysfunction in patients with diabetes and normoalbuminuria could precede microalbuminuria as a risk marker for cardiovascular disease [101]. Importantly, endothelial dysfunction predicts the rate of decline in GFR in patients with nephropathy; and biomarkers of inflammation and endothelial dysfunction are associated with an increased risk of all-cause mortality and cardiovascular morbidity in patients with nephropathy [102]. Furthermore, in a cohort of patients with type 2 diabetes and microalbuminuria, endothelial dysfunction was a predictor of progression to diabetic nephropathy independent of traditional risk factors [103]. A correlation between endothelial dysfunction and diabetic retinopathy has also been made [104].

More recently, endothelial dysfunction has been shown to predict cardiovascular and renal outcome in patients with type 1 diabetes, both independently and synergistically with arterial stiffness [105]; it has also been

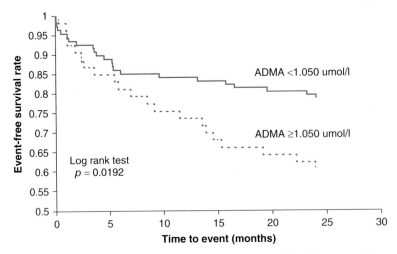

Figure 1.4 Kaplan-Meier curves for the composite outcome of death, myocardial infarction, or stroke comparing the upper tertile of baseline ADMA to the lower two tertiles combined. At 24 months, the number of patients who had experienced an event in the upper tertile was 21 (39.6%) compared with 23 (21.5%) in the lower two tertiles combined ($p = 0.0192$). (Source: Cavusoglu et al. 2010 [107]. Reproduced with permission of Elsevier.)

demonstrated that endothelial dysfunction is a determinant of aortic stiffness in hypertensive diabetic patients but not in hypertensive patients without diabetes [106].

The elevated levels of ADMA observed in patients with diabetes mellitus are implicated in the pathogenesis of endothelial dysfunction and atherosclerosis, independently predict diabetes complications, and are a strong and independent predictor of cardiovascular outcomes (including all-cause mortality) in men [107] (Figure 1.4).

Therapeutic Interventions for Endothelial Dysfunction in Diabetes

Given the importance of endothelial dysfunction in the pathogenesis of diabetes and its vascular complications, the endothelium has emerged as a compelling therapeutic target. Numerous interventions have been shown to have an effect on the endothelium. When designing and evaluating such interventional studies, aspects of the methodology used for measuring endothelial function should be carefully considered. For example, when employing FMD, external factors should be minimized (although the contribution of environmental factors to its variability is relatively small), and image acquisition quality should be considered, as well as probe position and cuff location and occlusion time, in order to standardize the methodology and analysis [108]. Such measures reduce inter- and intraobserver variability, and have a beneficial impact on sample size in the clinical trial setting [109]. The study should be large enough with adequate power to demonstrate a meaningful effect. Several treatments that have been shown to reduce cardiovascular risk also improve endothelial function both in the general population and in diabetes.

Lifestyle Interventions

Both diet and exercise exert beneficial effects on the vascular endothelium in diabetes. In those with type 2 diabetes mellitus, intervention of exercise training and a hypocaloric diet for six months improves coronary endothelial function, as assessed by acetylcholine-induced changes in coronary artery blood flow [110]. Furthermore, in patients with type 2 diabetes, eight weeks of exercise training resulted in an improvement in brachial artery FMD and forearm blood flow responses to acetylcholine [111]. Circulating markers of endothelial dysfunction have also shown an improvement following a twice-weekly, six-month, progressive aerobic training program, with decreased levels of P-selectin and ICAM-1 [112]. In those with impaired glucose tolerance (IGT), a combination of exercise and a low-calorie diet has been shown to reduce the plasma concentrations of ET-1 and NO, potentially improving the endothelial dysfunction in this "pre-diabetes" cohort [113].

Statins

The Hydroxymethylglutaryl-CoA (HMG-CoA) reductase inhibitors have been the subject of much research regarding their actions apart from their LDL-lowering effects; that is, their so-called pleiotropic effects. Particularly with regard to endothelial function, improvement has been noted following administration of statin therapy in both adults with coronary artery disease and asymptomatic adults with cardiovascular risk factors. The effect on endothelial function was independent of the type, dose, or duration of therapy and was not associated directly with lowering of cholesterol [114]. It is suggested that eNOS levels and activity are enhanced in statin therapy, resulting in increased NO bioavailability and improved FMD. Furthermore, it has been demonstrated that statins reduce inflammatory and pro-inflammatory cytokines and adhesion molecules, reduce the production of endothelin and angiotensin 1, and inhibit macrophage migration and smooth muscle cell proliferation [115, 116]. An improvement in FMD has been demonstrated in patients with diabetes receiving statin therapy, although it is suggested that the reduction in LDL cholesterol per se rather than therapeutic pleiotropy is likely to be a more important determinant of the improvement in endothelial function

[117, 118]. A recent meta-analysis showed that statins significantly improved the FMD in patients with diabetes who had better endothelial functions [119].

Insulin Sensitizers

Metformin is the principle insulin sensitizer used in the treatment of type 2 diabetes and has long been shown to have a beneficial impact on cardiovascular outcomes in patients with diabetes. Patients receiving metformin therapy undergoing coronary intervention have decreased adverse cardiovascular events, specifically death and myocardial infarction, compared with those patients not treated with insulin sensitizers [120]. Metformin is thought to improve endothelial function by reducing leukocyte interactions with human endothelial cells, and has also been shown to increase endothelium-dependent vasodilatation in subjects, independent of glycemic control [121, 122].

Thiazolidinediones, another class of insulin sensitizers, are also recognized to have beneficial effects on the endothelium via activating peroxisome proliferator receptor-gamma (PPARγ). This can result in decreased activation of transcription factors such as NFκB, which can reduce free radical generation and prevent arterial inflammation [123]. Troglitazone inhibited the expression of vascular cell adhesion molecule-1 and ICAM-1 in endothelial cells in vitro, and also reduced the migration of inflammatory cells to atherosclerotic plaques [124]. Newer thiazolidnediones, such as rosiglitazone and pioglitazone, have also been shown to improve the number and migration of EPC and the re-endothelization capacity of EPC in patients with type 2 diabetes [125]. Although the addition of rosiglitazone in patients with advanced type 2 diabetes treated with insulin appears to have a beneficial effect on endothelial function [126], it has also been associated with an increased incidence of myocardial infarction in patients with type 2 diabetes. Thus, the beneficial effects of treatments on the endothelium cannot be considered in isolation, and further research is needed to investigate why a beneficial effect on endothelial function with this class of drug does not translate into better cardiovascular prognosis.

Renin-Angiotensin-Aldosterone System Antagonists, Calcium Channel Blockers, and Beta Blockers

In patients with both type 1 and type 2 diabetes, studies have shown that angiotensin-converting enzyme (ACE) inhibitors and angiotensin II receptor antagonists improve endothelial function [127, 128, 129, 130, 131] (Figure 1.5). Initially the results of TREND (Trial on Reversing ENdothelial Dysfunction) showed that in patients with coronary artery disease,

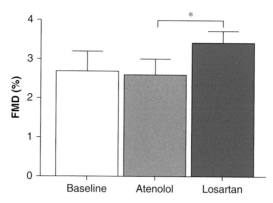

Figure 1.5 Flow-mediated dilatation (FMD) of the brachial artery was increased after 4 weeks' treatment with losartan compared to atenolol (*$p = 0.01$). (Source: Flammer et al. 2007 [130]. Reproduced with permission of Lippincott, Williams & Wilkins.)

including those with type 2 diabetes, quinapril improved endothelial dysfunction, as demonstrated by a significant net improvement in response to acetylcholine using quantitative coronary angiography after six months of treatment [132]. Other studies have since strengthened these findings. It is thought that inhibition of angiotensin II-mediated vasoconstricton, ET-1 release, ROS production, and stimulation of cytokine and growth factor expression all contribute to the benefits of these drugs [133, 134, 135]. Furthermore, a combination of angiotensin II receptor antagonist valsartan and the calcium channel blocker amlodipine improves FMD, as well as normalizing proteinuria and other markers of endothelial function in diabetic patients with stage I chronic kidney disease (CKD) and hypertension [136].

The use of beta blockers in diabetes has been cautioned against, as they can impair glycemic control. However, carvedilol possesses antioxidant properties that might provide vascular protection. In a head-to-head trial with metoprolol, carvedilol significantly improved endothelial function in patients with type 2 diabetes. Changes in glycemic control and oxidative stress did not appear fully to explain the relative improvement in FMD, suggesting other mechanisms of action [137]. A further study showed that metoprolol compared to carvedilol impairs insulin-stimulated endothelial vasomotion in patients with type 2 diabetes [138]. Therefore, the role, effects, and mechanisms of beta blockade on endothelial function in type 2 diabetes warrant further clinical evaluation.

Insulin

It has been demonstrated that insulin therapy partly restores insulin-stimulated endothelial function in patients with type 2 diabetes and ischemic heart disease [139], and that intensive insulin therapy improves endothelial function in young people with type 1 diabetes, with significantly greater improvements in E-selectin and vascular responses to acetylcholine compared with a conventional insulin therapy group [140]. Moreover, a three-and-a-half-year-study of insulin therapy with insulin glargine improved in-vivo endothelial function in patients with type 2 diabetes, improving endothelial-dependent and endothelial-independent dilatation [141]. However, the large, recently completed ORIGIN trial did not demonstrate improved clinical outcomes with early initiation of insulin glargine in patients with insulin resistance or early type 2 diabetes, despite better glycemic control and reduced progression to diabetes [142].

Other Novel Agents

The use of antioxidants as interventions in patients with diabetes have yielded conflicting results regarding their effect on endothelial function and clinical outcomes, despite early promise [143, 144]. For example, in patients with uncomplicated type 2 diabetes, endothelial dysfunction was not shown to be improved by treatment with vitamin E [145], and in those receiving vitamin C therapy, there was a lack of effect on oxidative stress and endothelial function [146].

However, other more novel agents, acting as antioxidants, are in development. Inhibition of ROS production may well be a valid mechanism targeting endothelial dysfunction in diabetes. New drugs, such as Nox inhibitors, superoxide dismutase mimetics, and glutathione peroxidise (GPx1; antioxidant enzyme) are all potential therapeutic approaches to reduce oxidative stress. Therapies that modulate and regulate eNOS are also under development [147].

The mitogen-activated protein kinase (MAPK) pathway that reduces NO production, EPC proliferation, and differentiation, as well as inducing the pro-inflammatory effects of endothelial cells, may be a further novel target for intervention [148]. Blockade of the pro-inflammatory vasoconstrictor endothelin is a further potential therapeutic approach. Indeed, it has been shown that treatment with an endothelin receptor antagonist results in improved peripheral endothelial function in patients with type 2 diabetes and microalbuminuria [149].

Although many of these drugs, including statin therapy and ACE inhibitors, have clearly demonstrated clinical benefits, questions remain regarding at what stage to intervene and with what agents in those with diabetes and subclinical endothelial dysfunction. Further studies are needed that can translate an improvement in endothelial function into a direct improvement in clinical outcomes.

Conclusions

The vascular endothelium in diabetes is the key regulator of blood vessel health and normal functioning. A loss of NO bioavailability and increased oxidative stress in diabetes, caused by factors including hyperglycemia, insulin resistance, and dyslipidemia, can cause activation of the endothelium. The resulting cascade of inflammation leads to the development of atherosclerosis and subsequent micro- and macrovascular complications. Various therapies have been associated with an improvement in endothelial function in diabetes, and a number of therapies appear promising in preventing the progression of endothelial dysfunction.

It is important to remember that endothelial dysfunction, although important, is only a component of the pathophysiological process of atherogenesis. Inflammatory, proliferative, and thrombotic pathways also act independently of the endothelium and have important influences on plaque development, destabilization, and resultant clinical sequelae. Given the physiological sensitivity of the endothelium coupled with the complexity of some of the techniques for assessing its function, it is unlikely that assessment of endothelium-dependent vasomotion will ever become a routine tool used to guide clinical decision-making outside of specialist centers. However, it will remain a core component of the clinical vascular research assessment portfolio.

Case Study 1

A 25-year-old male smoker with poorly controlled type 1 diabetes for the past five years is found to have evidence of persistent microalbuminuria at his clinic review. His blood pressure is 140/90 mmHg on no antihypertensive treatment and his cholesterol is 3.7 mmol/L (normal).

Multiple-Choice Questions

1 The most significant cause of his microalbuminuria is:
   A Hypertension
   B Hyperglycemia
   C Insulin resistance
   D Dyslipidemia
   E Smoking

2 The most appropriate option for measuring his vascular endothelial function would be:
   A Invasive coronary angiography
   B Venous occlusion strain-gauge plethysmography

    C Circulating markers

    D Flow-mediated dilatation

3 The most suitable first-line drug to improve endothelial function and microalbuminuria is:

    A Statin

    B Metformin

    C ACE inhibitor

    D Thiazolidnedione

    E Antioxidant

Answers provided after the References

Case Study 2

A 57-year-old woman with a 15-year history of type 2 diabetes, with HbA1c 7.5% (58 mmol/mol) and no evidence of nephropathy or retinopathy, has excellent blood pressure control (135/65 mmHg) on an ACE inhibitor alone. Her cholesterol is 3.6 mmol/L (normal). She has a BMI of 34 kg/m^2 (obese).

Multiple-Choice Questions

1 A conventional drug that is likely to have the most beneficial effect on endothelial function and in reducing cardiovascular events in this patient is:

    A Insulin

    B Doxazosin

    C Vitamin E

    D Metformin

    E Gliclazide

2 A novel drug to improve her endothelial dysfunction to assess in an RCT would:

    A Block the action of eNOS

    B Block ET-1 receptors

    C Stimulate ROS production

    D Reduce EPC proliferation

    E Stimulate the MAPK pathway

Answers provided after the References

Guidelines and Web Links

http://journals.lww.com/jhypertension/pages/articleviewer.aspx?year=2005&issue=01000&article=00004&type=abstract

http://www.sciencedirect.com/science/article/pii/S0735109701017466

Endothelial function and dysfunction. Part I: Methodological issues for assessment in the different vascular beds: A statement by the Working Group on Endothelin and Endothelial Factors of the European Society of Hypertension.

Guidelines for the ultrasound assessment of endothelial-dependent flow-mediated dilatation of the brachial artery: A report of the International Brachial Artery Reactivity Task Force.

References

1 Deanfield JE, Halcox JP, Rabelink TJ. Endothelial function and dysfunction: Testing and clinical relevance. *Circulation* 2007; 115: 1285–95.

2 Sita S, Tomasoni L, Atzeni F et al. From endothelial dysfunction to atherosclerosis. *Autoimmun. Rev* 2010; 9: 830–34.

3 Furchgott R and Zawadzki J. The obligatory role of endothelial cells in the relaxation of arterial smooth muscle by acetylcholine. *Nature* 1980; 288(5789): 373–6.

4 Ignarro LJ, Buga GM, Wood KS et al. Endothelium-derived relaxing factor produced and released from artery and vein is nitric oxide. *Proc Nat Acad Sci USA* 1987; 84(24): 9265–9.

5 Forstermann U, Munzel T. Endothelial nitric oxide synthase in vascular disease: From marvel to menace. *Circulation* 2006; 113: 1708–14.

6 Corson MA, James NL, Latta SE et al. Phosphorylation of endothelial nitric oxide synthase in response to fluid shear stress. *Circ Res* 1996; 79: 984–91.

7 Govers R, Rabelink TJ. Cellular regulation of endothelial nitric oxide synthase. *Am J Physiol Renal Physiol* 2001; 280: F193–F206.

8 Herrmann J, Lerman L, Lerman A. Simply say yes to NO? Nitric oxide (NO) sensor-based assessment of coronary endothelial function. *Eur Heart J* 2010; 31: 2834–6.

9 Kawashima S. The two faces of endothelial nitric oxide synthase in the pathophysiology of atherosclerosis. *Endothelium* 2004; 11(2): 99–107.

10 Halcox JP, Narayanan S, Cramer-Joyce L et al. Characterization of endothelium-derived hyperpolarizing factor in the human forearm microcirculation. *Am J Physiol Heart Circ Physiol* 2001; 280: H2470–77.

11 Moncada S, Higgs EA, Vane JR. Human arterial and venous tissues generate prostacyclin (prostaglandin x), a potent inhibitor of platelet aggregation. *Lancet* 1977; 1: 18–20.

12 van den Oever IA, Raterman HG, Nurmohamed MT et al. Endothelial dysfunction, inflammation, and apoptosis in diabetes mellitus. *Mediators Inflamm* 2010; 2010: 792393 [Epub Jun 15].

13 Tracy RP, Lemaitre RN, Psaty BM et al. Relationship of C-reactive protein to risk of cardiovascular disease in the elderly. Results from the Cardiovascular Health Study and the Rural Health Promotion Project. *Arterioscler Thromb Vasc Biol* 1997; 17(6): 1121–7.

14 Biegelsen ES, Loscalzo J. Endothelial function and atherosclerosis. *Coron Artery Dis* 1999; 10(4): 241–56.

15 Cowan DB, Langille BL. Cellular and molecular biology of vascular remodeling. *Curr Opin Lipidol* 1996; 7(2): 94–100.

16 Ludmer PL, Selwyn AP, Shook TL, et al. Paradoxical vasoconstriction induced by acetylcholine in atherosclerotic coronary arteries. *N Engl J Med* 1986; 315(17): 1046–51.

17 Celermajer DS, Sorensen KE, Gooch VM et al. Noninvasive detection of endothelial dysfunction in children and adults at risk of atherosclerosis. *Lancet* 1992; 340(8828): 1111–15.

18 Sorensen K, Celermajer DS, Georgakopoulos D et al. Impairment of endothelium-dependent dilation is an early event in children with familial hypercholesterolemia and is related to the lipoprotein (a) level. *J Clin Investig* 1994; 93(1): 50–55.

19 Celermajer D, Sorensen KE, Georgakopoulos D et al. Cigarette smoking is associated with dose-related and potentially reversible impairment of endothelium-dependent dilation in healthy young adults. *Circulation* 1993; 88(5I): 2149–55.

20 Williams SB, Cusco JA, Roddy MA et al. Impaired nitric oxide-mediated vasodilation in patients with non-insulin-dependent diabetes mellitus. *J Am Coll Cardiol* 1996; 27(3): 567–74.

21 Yeboah J, Crouse JR, Hsu FC et al. Brachial flow-mediated dilation predicts incident cardiovascular events in older adults: The cardiovascular health study. *Circulation* 2007; 115(18): 2390–97.

22 Quyyumi AA, Dakak N, Mulcahy D et al. Nitric oxide activity in the atherosclerotic human coronary circulation. *J Am Coll Cardiol* 1997; 29(2): 308–17.

23 Anderson TJ, Meredith IT, Yeung AC et al. The effect of cholesterol-lowering and antioxidant therapy on endothelium-dependent coronary vasomotion. *N Engl J Med* 1995; 332(8): 488–93.

24 Benjamin N, Calver A, Collier J et al. Measuring forearm blood flow and interpreting the responses to drugs and mediators. *Hypertension* 1995; 25: 918–23.

25 Donald AE, Charakida M, Cole TJ et al. Non-invasive techniques for assessment of endothelial function. *J Am Coll Cardiol* 2006; 48(9): 1846–50.

26 Betik AC, Luckham VB, and Hughson RL. Flow-mediated dilation in human brachial artery after different circulatory occlusion conditions. *Am J Physiol* 2004; 286(1): H442–H448.

27 Leeson P, Thorne S, Donald A et al. Non-invasive measurement of endothelial function: Effect on brachial artery dilatation of graded endothelial dependent and independent stimuli. *Heart* 1997; 78: 22–7.

28 Mullen MJ, Kharbanda RK, Cross J et al. Heterogenous nature of flow-mediated dilatation in human conduit arteries in vivo: Relevance to endothelial dysfunction in hypercholesterolemia. *Circ Res* 2001; 88(2): 145–51.

29 Corretti MC, Anderson TJ, Benjamin EJ et al. Guidelines for the ultrasound assessment of endothelial-dependent flow-mediated vasodilation of the brachial artery: A report of the international brachial artery reactivity task force. *J Am Coll Cardiol* 2002; 39(2): 257–65.

30 Deanfield J, Donald A, Ferri C et al; Working Group on Endothelin and Endothelial Factors of the European Society of Hypertension. Endothelial function and dysfunction. Part I: Methodological issues for assessment in the different vascular beds: A statement by the Working Group on Endothelin and Endothelial Factors of the European Society of Hypertension. J Hypertens 2005; 23(1): 7–17.

31 Boulanger CM, Amabile N, Tedgui A. Circulating microparticles: A potential prognostic marker for atherosclerotic vascular disease. *Hypertension* 2006; 48: 180–86.

32 Hamburg NM, Keyes MJ, Larson MG et al. Cross-sectional relations of digital vascular function to cardiovascular risk factors in the Framingham Heart Study. *Circulation* 2008; 117: 2467–74.

33 Bonetti PO, Pumper GM, Higano ST et al. Noninvasive identification of patients with early coronary atherosclerosis by assessment of digital reactive hyperemia. *J Am Coll Cardiol* 2004; 44: 2137–41.

34 Nohria A, Gerhard-Herman M, Creager MA et al. Role of nitric oxide in the regulation of digital pulse volume amplitude in humans. *J Appl Physiol* 2006; 101: 545–8.

35 Naka KK, Tweddel AC, Doshi SN et al. Flow-mediated changes in pulse wave velocity: A new clinical measure of endothelial function. *Eur Heart J* 2006; 27: 302–9.

36 Smith SC Jr., Anderson JL, Cannon RO III, et al. CDC; AHA. CDC/AHA workshop on markers of inflammation and cardiovascular disease: Application to clinical and public health practice: Report from the clinical practice discussion group. *Circulation* 2004; 110: e550–e553.

37 Rassaf T, Feelisch M, Kelm M. Circulating NO pool: Assessment of nitrite and nitroso species in blood and tissues. *Free Radic Biol Med* 2004; 36: 413–22.

38 Vallance P, Leiper J. Cardiovascular biology of the asymmetric dimethylarginine: Dimethylarginine dimethylaminohydrolase pathway. *Arterioscler Thromb Vasc Biol* 2004; 24: 1023–30.

39 Hwang SJ, Ballantyne CM, Sharrett AR et al. Circulating adhesion molecules VCAM-1, ICAM-1, and E-selectin in carotid atherosclerosis and incident coronary heart disease cases: The Atherosclerosis Risk In Communities (ARIC) study. *Circulation* 1997; 96: 4219–25.

40 Ridker PM, Hennekens CH, Roitman-Johnson B et al. Plasma concentration of soluble intercellular adhesion molecule 1 and risks of future myocardial infarction in apparently healthy men. *Lancet* 1998; 351: 88–92.

41 Shantikumar S, Caporali A, Emanueli C. Role of microRNAs in diabetes and its cardiovascular complications. *Cardiovasc Res* 2012; 93: 583–93.

42 Gilad S, Meiri E, Yogev Y et al. Serum microRNAs are promising novel biomarkers. *PloS ONE* 2008; 3: e3148.

43 Zampetaki A, Kiechl S, Drozdov I et al. Plasma microRNA profiling reveals loss of endothelial mir-126 and other microRNAs in type 2 diabetes. *Circ Res* 2010; 107: 810–17.

44 Vaughan DE. PAI-1 and atherothrombosis. *J Thromb Haemost* 2005; 3: 1879–83.

45 Sabatier F, Camoin-Jau L, Anfosso F et al. Circulating endothelial cells, microparticles and progenitors: Key players towards the definition of vascular competence. *J Cell Mol Med* 2009; 13: 454–71.

46 Dignat-George F and Boulanger CM. The many faces of endothelial microparticles. *Arterioscler Thromb Vasc Biol* 2011; 31: 27–33.

47 Chironi GN, Boulanger CM, Simon A et al. Endothelial microparticles in diseases. *Cell Tissue Res* 2009; 335: 143–51.

48 Leroyer AS, Ebrahimian TG, Cochain C et al. Microparticles from ischemic muscle promotes postnatal vasogenesis. *Circulation* 2009; 119: 2808–17.

49 Hoyer FF, Nickenig G, Werner N. Microparticles: Messenger of biological information. *J Cell Mol Med* 2010; 14(9): 2250–56.

50 Chahed S, Leroyer AS, Benzerroug M et al. Increased vitreous shedding of microparticles in proliferative diabetic retinopathy stimulates endothelial proliferation. *Diabetes* 2010; 59: 694–701.

51 Tramontano AF, Lyubarova R, Tsiakos J et al. Circulating endothelial microparticles in diabetes mellitus. *Mediators Inflamm.* 2010; 2010: 250476 [Epub Jun 16].

52 Nomura S, Inami N, Kimura Y et al. Effect of nifedipine on adiponectin in hypertensive patients with type 2 diabetes mellitus. *J Hum Hypertens* 2007; 21: 38–44.

53 Nomura S, Shouzu A, Omoto S et al. Benidipine improves oxidised LDL-dependent monocyte and endothelial dysfunction in hypertensive patients with type 2 diabetes mellitus. *J Hum Hypertens* 2005; 19: 551–7.

54 Hansson GK. Inflammation, atherosclerosis, and coronary artery disease. *N Engl J Med* 2005; 352: 1685–95.

55 Jansson P-A. Endothelial dysfunction in insulin resistance and type 2 diabetes. *J Int Medicine* 2007; 262(2): 173–83.

56 Fostermann U, Munzel T. Endothelial nitric oxide synthase in vascular disease: From marvel to menace. *Circulation* 2006; 113: 1708–14.

57 Rhee SG. Cell signalling: H$_2$O$_2$, a necessary evil for cell signalling. *Science* 2006; 312: 1882–3.

58 Spiekermann S, Landmesser U, Dikalov S et al. Electron spin resonance characterization of vascular xanthine and NAD(P)H oxidase activity in patients with coronary artery disease: Relation to endothelium-dependent vasodilation. *Circulation* 2003; 107: 1383–9.

59 Op den Buijs J, Musters M, Verrips T et al. Mathematical modeling of vascular endothelial layer maintenance: The role of endothelial cell division, progenitor cell homing and telomere shortening. *Am J Physiol Heart Circ Physiol* 2004; 287: H2651–H2658.

60 Asahara T, Murohara T, Sullivan A et al. Isolation of putative progenitor endothelial cells for angiogenesis. *Science* 1997; 275: 964–7.

61 Shi Q, Rafii S, Wu MH-D et al. Evidence for circulating bone marrow–derived endothelial cells. *Blood* 1998; 92: 362–7.

62 Aicher A, Heeschen C, Mildner-Rihm C et al. Essential role of endothelial nitric oxide synthase for mobilization of stem and progenitor cells. *Nat Med* 2003; 9: 1370–76.

63 Hill JM, Zalos G, Halcox JP et al. Circulating endothelial progenitor cells, vascular function, and cardiovascular risk. *N Engl J Med* 2003; 348: 593–600.

64 Cheng S, Cohen KS, Shaw SY et al. Association of colony-forming units with coronary artery and abdominal aortic calcification. *Circulation* 2010; 122: 1176–82.

65 Vasa M, Fichtlscherer S, Adler K et al. Increase in circulating endothelial progenitor cells by statin therapy in patients with stable coronary artery disease. *Circulation* 2001; 103: 2885–90.

66 van Ark J, Moser J, Lexis CP et al. Type 2 diabetes mellitus is associated with an imbalance in circulating endothelial and smooth muscle progenitor cell numbers. *Diabetologia* 2012; Jun 1 [Epub ahead of print].

67 Fadini GP, Sartore S, Baesso I et al. Endothelial progenitor cells and the diabetic paradox. *Diabetes Care* 2006; 29(3): 714–16.

68 Makino H, Okada S, Nagumo A et al. Decreased circulating CD34+ cells are associated with progression of diabetic nephropathy: Short report. *Diabetic Medicine.* 2009; 26(2): 171–3.

69 Fadini GP, Sartore S, Albiero M et al. Number and function of endothelial progenitor cells as a marker of severity for diabetic vasculopathy. *Arterioscler, Thromb Vasc Biol* 2006; 26(9): 2140–46.

70 Tepper OM, Galiano RD, Capla JM et al. Human endothelial progenitor cells from type II diabetics exhibit impaired proliferation, adhesion, and incorporation into vascular structures. *Circulation* 2002; 106(22): 2781–6.

71 Shamoon H, Duffy H, Fleischer N et al. The effect of intensive treatment of diabetes on the development and progression of long-term complications in insulin-dependent diabetes mellitus. *N Engl J Med* 1993; 329(14): 977–86.

72 Holman RR, Cull CA, Fox C et al. United Kingdom prospective diabetes study (UKPDS) 13: Relative efficacy of randomly allocated diet, sulphonylurea, insulin, or metformin in patients with newly diagnosed non-insulin dependent diabetes followed for three years. *Br Med J* 1995; 310(6972): 83–8.

73 Stratton IM, Adler AI, Neil HA et al. Association of glycaemia with macrovascular and microvascular complications of type 2 diabetes (UKPDS 35): Prospective observational study. *Br Med J* 2000; 321: 405–12.

74 Brownlee M. Biochemistry and molecular cell biology of diabetic complications. *Nature* 2001; 414: 813–20.

75 Wong WT, Wong SL, Tian XY et al. Endothelial dysfunction: The common consequence in diabetes and hypertension. *J Cardiovasc Pharmacol* 2010; 55: 300–7.

76 Madonna R, De Caterina R. Cellular and molecular mechanisms of vascular injury in diabetes – Part I: Pathways of vascular disease in diabetes. *Vasc Pharm* 2011; 54: 68–74.

77 Buse MG. Hexosamines, insulin resistance, and the complications of diabetes: Current status. *Am J Physiol Endocrinol Metab* 2006; 290: E1–8.

78 Feener EP, Xia P, Inoguchi T et al. Role of protein kinase C in glucose- and angiotensin II-induced plasminogen activator inhibitor expression. *Contrib. Nephrol* 1996; 118: 180–87.

79 Rikitake Y, Liao JK. Rho-kinase mediates hyperglycemia-induced plasminogen activator inhibitor-1 expression in vascular endothelial cells. *Circulation* 2005; 111: 3261–8.

80 Chakrabarti S, Cukiernik M, Hileeto D et al. Role of vasoactive factors in the pathogenesis of early changes in diabetic retinopathy. *Diabetes Metab. Res. Rev.* 2000; 16: 393–407.

81 Goldin A, Beckman JA, Schmidt AM et al. Advanced glycation end products: Sparking the development of diabetic vascular injury. *Circulation* 2006; 114: 597–605.

82 Basta G, Lazzerini G, Massaro, M et al. Advanced glycation end products activate endothelium through signal-transduction receptor RAGE: A mechanism for amplification of inflammatory responses. *Circulation* 2002; 105: 816–22.

83 Yan SF, Ramasamy R, Schmidt AM. The RAGE axis: A fundamental mechanism signaling danger to the vulnerable vasculature. *Circ. Res* 2010; 106: 842–53.

84 Gohda T, Tanimoto M, Moon JY et al. Increased serum endogenous secretory receptor for advanced glycation end-product (esRAGE) levels in type 2 diabetic patients with decreased renal function. *Diabetes Res Clin Pract* 2008; 81: 196–201.

85 Kawano H, Motoyama T, Hirashima O et al. Hyperglycaemia rapidly suppresses flow-mediated endothelium-dependent vasodilatation of brachial artery. *J Am Coll Cardiol* 1999; 34: 146–54.

86 Graier WF, Simecek S, Kukovetz WR et al. High D-glucose-induced changes in endothelial Ca2+/EDRF signaling are due to generation of superoxide anions. *Diabetes* 1996; 45: 1386–95.

87 Raij L. Nitric oxide in the pathogenesis of cardiac disease. *J Clin Hypertens* 2006; 8: 30–39.

88 Xu J, Zou M-H. Molecular insights and therapeutic targets for diabetic endothelial dysfunction. *Circulation* 2009; 120: 1266–86.

89 Triggle CR, Ding H. A review of endothelial dysfunction in diabetes: A focus on the contribution of a dysfunctional eNOS. *J Am Soc Hypertens* 2010; 4(3): 102–15.

90 Tesfamariam B, Brown ML, Deykin D et al. Elevated glucose promotes generation of endothelium-derived vasoconstrictor prostanoids in rabbit aorta. *J Clin Invest* 1990; 85: 929–32.

91 el-Mesallamy H, Suwailem S, Hamdy N. Evaluation of C-reactive protein, endothelin-1, adhesion molecule(s), and lipids as inflammatory markers in type 2 diabetes mellitus patients. *Mediators Inflamm* 2007; 2007: 73635.

92 Tepper OM, Galiano RD, Capla JM et al. Human endothelial progenitor cells from type II diabetics exhibit impaired proliferation, adhesion, and incorporation into vascular structures. *Circulation* 2002; 106: 2781–6.

93 Loomans CJ, de Koning, EJ, Staal FJ et al. Endothelial progenitor cell dysfunction: A novel concept in the pathogenesis of vascular complications of type 1 diabetes. *Diabetes* 2004; 53: 195–9.

 94 Gallagher KA, Liu ZJ, Xiao M et al. Diabetic impairments in NO-mediated endothelial progenitor cell mobilization and homing are reversed by hyperoxia and SDF-1 alpha. *J. Clin. Invest* 2007; 117: 1249–59.

 95 Zheng H, Dai T, Zhou B et al. SDF-1α/CXCR4 decreases endothelial progenitor cells apoptosis under serum deprivation by PI3K/Akt/eNOS pathway. *Atherosclerosis* 2008; 201: 36–42.

 96 Zheng H, Shen CJ, Qiu FY et al. Stromal cell-derived factor 1alpha reduces senescence of endothelial progenitor subpopulation in lectinbinding and DiLDL-uptaking cell through telomerase activation and telomere elongation. *J. Cell. Physiol* 2010; 23(3): 757–63.

 97 Evans M, Khan N, Rees A, Diabetic dyslipidaemia and coronary heart disease: New perspectives. *Curr Opin Lipidol* 1999; 10(5): 387–91.

 98 Woodman RJ, Chew GT, Watts GF. Mechanisms, significance and treatment of vascular dysfunction in type 2 diabetes mellitus: Focus on lipid-regulating therapy. *Drugs* 2005; 65(1): 31–74.

 99 Clarkson P, Celermajer DS, Donald AE et al. Impaired vascular reactivity in insulin-dependent diabetes mellitus is related to disease duration and low density lipoprotein cholesterol levels. *J Am Coll Cardiol* 1996; 28: 573–9.

100 Stehouwer CD, Fischer HR, van Kuijk AW et al. Endothelial dysfunction precedes development of microalbuminuria in IDDM. *Diabetes* 1995; 44: 561–4.

101 Dogra G, Rich L, Stanton K et al. Endothelium-dependent and independent vasodilation studies at normoglycaemia in type I diabetes mellitus with and without microalbuminuria. *Diabetologia* 2001; 44: 593–601.

102 Astrup AS, Tarnow L, Pietraszek L et al. Markers of endothelial dysfunction and inflammation in type 1 diabetic patients with or without diabetic nephropathy followed for 10 years: Association with mortality and decline of glomerular filtration rate. *Diabetes Care* 2008; 31(6): 1170–76.

103 Persson F, Rossing P, Hovind P et al. Endothelial dysfunction and inflammation predict development of diabetic nephropathy in the Irbesartan in Patients with Type 2 Diabetes and Microalbuminuria (IRMA 2) study. *Scand J Clin Lab Invest.* 2008; 68(8): 731–8.

104 Klein BE, Knudtson MD, Tsai MY et al. The relation of markers of inflammation and endothelial dysfunction to the prevalence and progression of diabetic retinopathy: Wisconsin epidemiologic study of diabetic retinopathy. *Arch Ophthalmol* 2009; 127(9): 1175–82.

105 Theilade S, Lajer M, Jorsal A et al. Arterial stiffness and endothelial dysfunction independently and synergistically predict cardiovascular and renal outcome in patients with type 1 diabetes. *Diabet Med* 2012; Mar 13. doi: 10.1111/j.1464-5491.2012.03633.x [Epub ahead of print].

106 Bruno RM, Penno G, Daniele G et al. Type 2 diabetes mellitus worsens arterial stiffness in hypertensive patients through endothelial dysfunction. *Diabetologia* 2012; Mar 13 [Epub ahead of print].

107 Cavusoglu E, Ruwende C, Chopra V et al. Relation of baseline plasma ADMA levels to cardiovascular morbidity and mortality at two years in men with diabetes mellitus referred for coronary angiography. *Atherosclerosis* 2010; 210(1): 226–31.

108 Charakida M, Masi S, Lüscher TF et al. Assessment of atherosclerosis: The role of flow-mediated dilatation. *Eur Heart J.* 2010; 31(23): 2854–61.

109 Donald AE, Halcox JP, Charakida M et al. Methodological approaches to optimise reproducibility and power in clinical studies of flow-mediated dilatation. *J Am Coll Cardiol* 2008; 51: 1959–64.

110 Sixt S, Beer S, Blüher M et al. Long- but not short-term multifactorial intervention with focus on exercise training improves coronary endothelial dysfunction in diabetes mellitus type 2 and coronary artery disease. *Eur Heart J* 2010; 31(1): 112–19.

111 Maiorana A, O'Driscoll G, Cheetham C et al. The effect of combined aerobic and resistance exercise training on vascular function in type 2 diabetes. *J Am Coll Cardiol* 2001; 38: 860–66.

112 Zoppini G, Targher G, Zamboni C et al. Effects of moderate-intensity exercise training on plasma biomarkers of inflammation and endothelial dysfunction in older patients with type 2 diabetes. *Nutr Metab Cardiovasc Dis* 2006; 16(8): 543–9.

113 Kasımay O, Ergen N, Bilsel S et al. Diet-supported aerobic exercise reduces blood endothelin-1 and nitric oxide levels in individuals with impaired glucose tolerance. *J Clin Lipidol* 2010; 4(5): 427–34.

114 Ray KK, Cannon CP. Intensive statin therapy in acute coronary syndromes: Clinical benefits and vascular biology. *Curr Opin Lipidol* 2004; 15: 637–43.

115 Tsiara S, Elisaf M, Mikhailidis DP. Early vascular benefits of statin therapy. *Curr Med Res Opin* 2003; 19: 540–56.

116 Charakida M, Masi S, Loukogeorgakis SP et al. The role of flow-mediated dilatation in the evaluation and development of antiatherosclerotic drugs. *Curr Opin Lipidol* 2009; 20: 460–66.

117 Settergren M, Bohm F, Ryden L et al. Cholesterol lowering is more important than pleiotropic effects of statins for endothelial function in patients with dysglycaemia and coronary artery disease. *Eur Heart J* 2008; 29: 1753–60.

118 Tomizawa A,, Hattori Y, Suzuki K et al. Effects of statins on vascular function in hypercholesterolaemic patients with type 2 diabetes mellitus: Fluvastatin vs. *Rosuvastatin. Int J Cardiol* 2010; 144(1): 108–9.

119 Zhang L, Gong D, Li S et al. Meta-analysis of the effects of statin therapy on endothelial function in patients with diabetes mellitus. *Atherosclerosis* 2012; Jan 23 [Epub ahead of print].

120 Kao J, Tobis J, McClelland RL et al. Relation of metformin treatment to clinical events in diabetic patients undergoing percutaneous intervention. *Am J Cardiol* 2004; 93: 1347–50, A1345.

121 Mamputu JC, Wiernsperger NF, and Renier G. Antiatherogenic properties of metformin: The experimental evidence. *Diabetes Metab* 2003; 29(2): 6S71–6.

122 Vitale C, Mercuro G, Cornoldi A et al. Metformin improves endothelial function in patients with metabolic syndrome. *J Intern Med* 2005; 258: 250–56.

123 Jiang C, Ting AT, Seed B. PPAR-gamma agonists inhibit production of monocyte inflammatory cytokines. *Nature* 1998; 391: 82–6.

124 Pasceri V, Wu HD, Willerson JT et al. Modulation of vascular inflammation in vitro and in vivo by peroxisome proliferator-activated receptor-gamma activators. *Circulation* 2000; 101: 235–8.

125 Sorrentino SA, Bahlmann FH, Besler C et al. Oxidant stress impairs in vivo reendothelialization capacity of endothelial progenitor cells from patients with type 2 diabetes mellitus: Restoration by the peroxisome proliferator-activated receptor-γ agonist rosiglitazone. *Circulation* 2007; 116: 163–73.

126 Naka KK, Papathanassiou K, Bechlioulis A et al. Rosiglitazone improves endothelial function in patients with type 2 diabetes treated with insulin. *Diab Vasc Dis Res* 2011; 8(3): 195-201.

127 Arcaro G, Zenere BM, Saggiani F et al. ACE inhibitors improve endothelial function in type 1 diabetic patients with normal arterial pressure and microalbuminuria. *Diabetes Care* 1999; 22: 1536–42.

128 O'Driscoll G, Green D, Maiorana A et al. Improvement in endothelial function by angiotensin-converting enzyme inhibition in noninsulin-dependent diabetes mellitus. *J Am Coll Cardiol* 1999; 33: 1506–11.

129 Cheetham C, Collis J, O'Driscoll G et al. Losartan, an angiotensin type 1 receptor antagonist, improves endothelial function in non-insulin dependent diabetes. *J Am Coll Cardiol* 2000; 36: 1461–6.

130 Flammer AJ, Hermann F, Wiesli P et al. Effect of losartan, compared with atenolol, on endothelial function and oxidative stress in patients with type 2 diabetes and hypertension. *J Hypertens* 2007; 25: 785–91.

131 Yilmaz MI, Axelsson J, Sonmez A et al. Effect of renin angiotensin system blockade on pentraxin 3 levels in type-2 diabetic patients with proteinuria. *Clin J Am Soc Nephrol* 2009; 4: 535–41.

132 Mancini JGB, Henry GC, Macaya C et al. Angiotensin-converting enzyme inhibition with quinapril improves endothelial vasomotor dysfunction in patients with coronary artery disease. The TREND (Trial on Reversing ENdothelial Dysfunction) Study. *Circulation* 1996; 94: 258–65.

133 Braga MF, Leiter LA. Role of renin-angiotensin system blockade in patients with diabetes mellitus. *Am J Cardiol* 2009; 104: 835–9.

134 Klahr S, Morrissey JJ. The role of vasoactive compounds, growth factors and cytokines in the progression of renal disease. *Kidney Int Suppl* 2000; 75: S7–S14.

135 Raij L. Workshop: Hypertension and cardiovascular risk factors: Role of the angiotensin II-nitric oxide interaction. *Hypertension* 2001; 37: 767–73.

136 Yilmaz MI, Carrero JJ, Martín-Ventura JL et al. Combined therapy with renin-angiotensin system and calcium channel blockers in type 2 diabetic hypertensive patients with proteinuria: Effects on soluble TWEAK, PTX3, and flow-mediated dilation. *Clin J Am Soc Nephrol* 2010 Jul; 5(7): 1174–81.

137 Bank AJ, Kelly AS, Thelen AM et al. Effects of carvedilol versus metoprolol on endothelial function and oxidative stress in patients with type 2 diabetes mellitus. *Am J Hypertens* 2007; 20: 777–83.

138 Kveiborg B, Hermann TS, Major-Pedersen A et al. Metoprolol compared to carvedilol deteriorates insulin-stimulated endothelial function in patients with type 2 diabetes – a randomized study. *Cardiovasc Diabetol* 2010 May 25; 9: 21.

139 Rask-Madsen N, Ihlemann T, Krarup E et al. Insulin therapy improves insulin-stimulated endothelial function in patients with type 2 diabetes and ischemic heart disease. *Diabetes* 2001; 50: 2611–18.

140 Franklin VL, Khan F, Kennedy G et al. Intensive insulin therapy improves endothelial function and microvascular reactivity in young people with type 1 diabetes. *Diabetologia* 2008; 51(2): 353–60.

141 Vehkavaara S, Yki-Järvinen H. 3.5 years of insulin therapy with insulin glargine improves in vivo endothelial function in type 2 diabetes. *Arterioscler Thromb Vasc Biol* 2004; 24(2): 325–30.

142 The ORIGIN Trial Investigators. Basal insulin and cardiovascular and other outcomes in dysglycemia. *N Engl J Med* 2012; Jun 11 [Epub ahead of print]

143 Ting HH, Timimi FK, Boles KS et al. Vitamin C improves endothelium-dependent vasodilation in patients with non-insulin-dependent diabetes mellitus. *J Clin Invest* 1996; 97: 22–8.

144 Timimi FK, Ting HH, Haley EA et al. Vitamin C improves endothelium-dependent vasodilation in patients with insulin-dependent diabetes mellitus. *J Am Coll Cardiol* 1998; 31(3): 552–7.

145 Gazis A, White DJ, Page SR et al. Effect of oral vitamin E (alphatocopherol) supplementation on vascular endothelial function in Type 2 diabetes mellitus. *Diabet Med* 1999; 16: 304–11.

146 Darko D, Dornhorst A, Kelly FJ et al. Lack of effect of oral vitamin C on blood pressure, oxidative stress and endothelial function in type II diabetes. *Clin Sci* 2002; 103: 339–44.

147 Sharma A, Bernatchez PN, de Haan JB. Targeting endothelial dysfunction in vascular complications associated with diabetes. *Int J Vasc Med* 2012; 2012: 750126.

148 Madonna R, De Caterina R. Cellular and molecular mechanisms of vascular injury in diabetes – Part II: Cellular mechanisms and therapeutic targets. *Vasc Pharm* 2011; 54: 75–9.

149 Rafnsson A, Böhm F, Settergren M et al. The endothelin receptor antagonist bosentan improves peripheral endothelial function in patients with type 2 diabetes mellitus and microalbuminuria: A randomised trial. *Diabetologia* 2012 Mar; 55(3): 600–7.

Answers to Multiple-Choice Questions for Case Study 1

1 B

2 D

3 C

Answers to Multiple-Choice Questions for Case Study 2

1 D

2 B

CHAPTER 2

New Biomarkers of Cardiovascular Disease in Diabetes

Hitesh Patel[1], Sujay Chandran[1] and Kausik K. Ray[2]

[1] *St Georges Hospital, London, UK*
[2] *St George's University of London, London, UK*

Key Points

- Biomarkers can be useful to guide clinical decision-making for individual patients, but do not replace the need for clinical judgment.

- When evaluating a biomarker, its robustness must be evaluated by independent association (hazards ratio), AUC (c-statistic), calibration, and reclassification.

- Only a few trials have used the biomarker in question to guide clinical judgment in a randomized and controlled fashion, which is gold standard.

- The Reynolds risk score incorporates CRP measurement and family history in its scoring for CVD, components that are not used in the Framingham risk score.

- The National Lipid Association panel recommends that in patients with intermediate risk, hs-CRP should be measured routinely in men > 50 years of age and women > 60 years of age given its capacity to enhance risk prediction, especially when used with the Reynolds risk score.

- The American Diabetes Association and American College of Cardiology have recommended that apoB be added to risk assessment in patients at elevated cardiometabolic risk.

- Lp (a), which has a regression dilution ratio of 0.87 suggesting that levels are remarkably stable over time, is recommended by the EAS for further refining risk in those with intermediate CVD risk, a FH of premature CHD, or those with progressive disease despite good risk-factor control.

- The EAS Consensus Panel recommends niacin (nicotinic acid, 1–3 g day) as the primary treatment for lowering elevated Lp (a) levels, based on its efficacy in reducing levels by 30–40% and in reducing cardiovascular disease in individuals at risk.

- Coronary artery calcium scoring and carotid intimal thickness may be demonstrating premature atherosclerosis and hence have a role in guiding treatment decisions in asymptomatic diabetics who do not fulfill criteria for initiation of primary prevention medications.

- There is no clear role of genetic biomarkers for guiding treatments for CVD prevention among diabetic patients.

Managing Cardiovascular Complications in Diabetes, First Edition.
Edited by D. John Betteridge and Stephen Nicholls.
© 2014 John Wiley & Sons, Ltd. Published 2014 by John Wiley & Sons, Ltd.

Introduction

Diabetes mellitus (DM) is associated with a twofold increase in myocardial infarction (MI) and a twofold increase in stroke [1]. A study by Wannamethee et al. [2] demonstrated that the risk of cardiovascular disease (CVD) and all-cause mortality was proportional to the duration of diabetes. In particular, a mean duration of diabetes of about a decade appears to confer an equivalent risk of CVD to a prior history of MI. In addition, recent work has shown that a history of DM results in six years of life years lost, mostly from CVD [3]. These data highlight the importance of preventing diabetes and identifying patients early to modify the atherosclerotic disease process that is accelerated with duration of diabetes in this population.

To prevent the clinical manifestation of CVD among those with DM, clinical care focuses on optimizing the control of "traditional" risk factors, which include lipids, glycemia, blood pressure, smoking, weight, alcohol consumption, and uptake of exercise. There remains unmodifiable risk from family history, gender, and age. However, 20% of all vascular events occur in patients without any traditional risk factors, necessitating the need for more precise clinical tools that aid clinicians in identifying those at highest risk [4]. To help achieve this goal, there is growing interest in the development and exploitation of new biomarkers.

What Is a Biomarker?

A biomarker was defined by a National Institutes of Health (NIH) working group as "a characteristic that is objectively measured and evaluated as an indicator of normal biological processes, pathogenic processes, or pharmacologic responses to a therapeutic intervention" [5]. Biomarkers are used in a variety of ways, including screening, diagnosis, staging, prognostication, and monitoring of disease.

An example of an established biomarker is the use of an elevated troponin I or T in distinguishing between an acute myocardial infarction and unstable angina in a patient who presents with chest pain. It is important to stress that a biomarker is useful as an addition to a thorough clinical assessment rather than an alternative. All patients with a positive troponin have not necessarily had an acute myocardial infarction and similarly, a negative troponin does not mean that the patient does not have significant coronary artery disease.

A biomarker should meet several criteria to be deemed clinically useful. This is structured around three fundamental questions [6]:

1 Is the biomarker measurable?
2 Does the biomarker add new information?
3 Will the biomarker help the clinician to manage patients?

Additional criteria include cost-effectiveness, safety, and replication of the biomarker in clinical scenarios.

Biomarker discovery is currently undertaken by two complementary processes: knowledge based, in which markers for different stages in a known biological process (e.g., atherosclerosis) are investigated; and an inductive strategy, which is more labor intensive, involving analysis of thousands of often unrelated molecules with respect to a disease stage [6].

How Are Biomarkers Evaluated?

An ideal biomarker should enable the clinician to change patient management and improve outcomes above that of current standard care. To achieve this goal, ideally, it has to hold true against four criteria: risk association, discrimination, calibration, and reclassification [6].

Risk Association

There has to be a statistically significant association between the biomarker and the outcome. When defining the outcome, it is probably more desirable to use "hard" endpoints such as death or myocardial infarction rather than "softer" ones such as coronary artery stenosis. Risk association is described using hazards ratios or odds ratios; however, these do not provide meaningful information for predicting whether or not an individual who is "positive" or has elevated levels will develop the outcome of interest over and above other factors. This is partly because the methods used in defining an abnormal biomarker threshold aim to minimize false-positive rates and as a consequence sensitivity declines.

There are three main methods for defining abnormal biomarker levels [6]: reference limits (usually arbitrarily chosen between the 95th and 99th percentiles) of the distribution of the biomarker values in a healthy population; discrimination limits, which are derived from the biomarker-level distribution curves in populations with and without disease; and identifying a threshold above which the risk of disease escalates significantly. It is clinically attractive to dichotomize biomarkers into either a "positive" or "negative" result, but it is important to bear in mind that certain biomarkers have a continuous relationship with risk, such that the higher the level of biomarker, the higher the risk.

Discrimination

Discrimination is the ability of a test to separate two outcome classes. It is performed by measuring the area under the receiver-operating-characteristic curve (AUC), which plots sensitivity (proportion of patients with the disease with a positive result) on the y-axis against 1-specificity (proportion of patients without the disease with a negative result) on the x-axis. The AUC is normally used in case-control studies and is similar to the c-statistic employed in prospective studies. A value of 0.5 suggests that the biomarker does not help to discriminate between individuals who will and will not develop the disease, whereas a value of 1.0 indicates perfect discrimination.

To put a novel biomarker into perspective, the Framingham risk scores for coronary heart disease give a c-statistic of approximately 0.75. The AUC method is dependent on sensitivity and specificity, so factors that affect these values will influence discrimination; for example, whether the sample population includes a predominantly high- or low-risk cohort.

Calibration

A biomarker should give an indication of predicted future risk that should agree with the actual observed outcome. A good model will have a goodness-of-fit statistic (e.g., Hosmer-Lemeshow) p value of >0.05. Clinically, this is useful as the model can be used to give an estimated 10-year risk for an event and hence identify higher-risk patients who would benefit from interventions in a cost-effective manner.

Reclassification

This is a relatively new concept, but potentially the most clinically relevant as it assesses the ability of a test to reclassify individuals correctly into a different risk category; for example, an intermediate-risk subject into a high-risk subject, or a low-risk subject into an intermediate-risk subject. If this results in a change in clinical decision-making as somebody moves into a category requiring treatment or one that does not, then this is referred to as net clinical reclassification. The ability of the new test to achieve reclassification can be statistically examined by net reclassification improvement (NRI) or integrated discrimination improvement (IDI). The NRI method, which is determined by the proportion of individuals whose risk is correctly escalated or de-escalated, is more useful in primary prevention, where well-accepted categories of risk exist. The IDI estimates the change in predicted probability of an outcome between those with and without the outcome after the biomarker is added to the prediction model. The larger the value of the NRI or the IDI, the better the biomarker.

Categories of Biomarkers of Cardiovascular Disease

The three main subtypes of biomarkers can be summarized as circulating, imaging, or genetic biomarkers, as in Figure 2.1, by linking them to different stages in the disease processes [7].

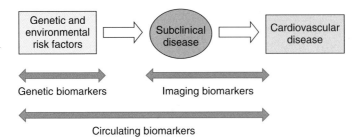

Figure 2.1 Progression from risk factors to cardiovascular disease. (Source: Wang 2011 [7]. Reproduced with permission of Wolters Kluwer Health.)

This chapter does not intend to be a comprehensive overview of all biomarkers in cardiovascular disease, but instead to provide a summary of the key ones that have the support of a large body of evidence and are hence more likely to have a clinical utility. We will discuss in turn each biomarker subtype briefly described above and present the evidence base for use of these novel biomarkers in cardiovascular disease, relating this as much as possible to the diabetic population.

Circulating Biomarkers

The National Lipid Association evaluated the use of selected biomarkers in clinical practice as either tools to improve risk assessment or markers to adjust therapy once a decision to treat had been made [8]. During the course of this chapter we will discuss some of the key biomarkers from Table 2.1 as well as other novel and emerging biomarkers that may be used in clinical practice.

CRP
Pathophysiology
Considerable in vitro and clinical data link inflammation to cardiovascular disease. Hence, there has been considerable interest in a blood-based test that provides information on subclinical inflammation. CRP is a nonspecific acute phase protein produced by hepatocytes and is the most studied biomarker of inflammation and CVD risk. It is a downstream marker of inflammation with levels largely derived from Interleukin-6 mediated hepatic production, and recent genetic studies [9] do not suggest a causal role for CRP. In most cases, CRP indicates high-sensitivity CRP (hs-CRP), which detects levels of low-grade inflammation below the level of standard assays and is the assay that is recommended for use in clinical practice. Hs-CRP can be elevated in other inflammatory states, so its clinical utility is debatable in the setting of an active infection, malignancy, or chronic inflammatory disease for CVD risk prediction. In addition, although it is widely accepted

Table 2.1 Summary and recommendations for measurement of inflammatory markers and advanced lipoprotein/subfraction testing in initial clinical assessment and on-treatment management decisions. (Source: Davidson et al. 2011 [8]. Reproduced with permission of Elsevier.)

	Initial Clinical Assessment					
	CRP	Lp-PLA$_2$	Apo B	LDL-P	Lp(a)	HDL or LDL Subfractions
Low risk (<5% 10-year CHD event risk)	Not recommended	Not recommended	Not recommended	Not recommended	Not recommended	Not recommended
Intermediate risk (5-20% 10-year CHD event risk)	Recommended for routine measurement	Consider for selected patients	Reasonable for many patients	Reasonable for many patients	Consider for selected patients	Not recommended
CHD or CHD Equivalent	Consider for selected patients	Consider for selected patients	Consider for selected patients	Consider for selected patients	Consider for selected patients	Not recommended
Family History	Reasonable for many patients	Consider for selected patients	Reasonable for many patients	Reasonable for many patients	Reasonable for many patients	Not recommended
Recurrent Events	Reasonable for many patients	Consider for selected patients	Reasonable for many patients	Reasonable for many patients	Reasonable for many patients	Not recommended

	On-Treatment Management Decisions					
	CRP	Lp-PLA$_2$	Apo B	LDL-P	Lp(a)	HDL or LDL Subfractions
Low risk (<5% 10-year CHD event risk)	Not recommended	Not recommended	Not recommended	Not recommended	Not recommended	Not recommended
Intermediate risk (5-20% 10-year CHD event risk)	Reasonable for many patients	Not recommended	Reasonable for many patients	Reasonable for many patients	Not recommended	Not recommended
CHD or CHD Equivalent	Reasonable for many patients	Not recommended	Reasonable for many patients	Reasonable for many patients	Consider for selected patients	Not recommended
Family History	Consider for selected patients	Not recommended	Consider for selected patients	Consider for selected patients	Consider for selected patients	Not recommended
Recurrent Events	Reasonable for many patients	Not recommended	Reasonable for many patients	Reasonable for many patients	Consider for selected patients	Not recommended

Apo, apolipoprotein; CHD, coronary heart disease; CRP, C-reactive protein; HDL, high-density lipoprotein; Lp-PLA$_2$, lipoprotein-associated phospholipase A$_2$; LDL, low-density lipoprotein; LDL-P, LDL particle number/concentration; Lp(a), lipoprotein (a). (Color plate 2.1).

that inflammation plays a role in atherosclerosis, there is little evidence from randomized clinical trials to suggest that CRP itself is directly a contributor to the atherogenic process. This being said, CRP via activation of complement may increase infarct size during ischemia. Studies suggest that CRP inhibitors used in animal models of ischemia may reduce infarct size, which is the only direct evidence to date for a direct causal role of CRP [10].

Technique and Measurement

Hs-CRP assays detect concentrations of CRP below 3 mg/L [11]. They are the assays used to assess cardiovascular risk because they are able to quantitate CRP within the range normally seen in asymptomatic patients (<3 mg/L). A statement from the Centers for Disease Control and Prevention and the American Heart Association (CDC/AHA) provides some guidance on the use of serum hs-CRP to estimate CVD risk [12]:

- Low-, average-, and high-risk values can be defined as <1, 1 to 3, and >3 mg/L, which also correspond to approximate tertile risk values.
- A value above 10 mg/L should initiate a search for a source of infection or inflammation.
- Due to the variability of measurements in an individual, the average of two assays, fasting or nonfasting, and optimally obtained two weeks apart provides a more stable estimate than a single value.

Population Studies

One of the earliest studies to demonstrate an association between hs-CRP and cardiovascular disease was the Women's Health Study (WHS) [13], which had 28,263 apparently healthy postmenopausal women enrolled in it. The cohort was monitored prospectively for future risk of incident vascular events. In this study, several putative markers of risk were assessed and hs-CRP was found to be more predictive of CVD events, outperforming homocysteine, lipoprotein(a), and LDL-C. However, establishing an independent association does not necessarily improve clinical decision-making or target people more appropriately as likely to benefit from therapeutic interventions. The value of hs-CRP with regard to reclassification is uncertain. Addition of hs-CRP to standard risk models in the WHS reclassified 20% of intermediate-risk individuals. Approximately three-quarters of these individuals were reclassified down to low risk. Only 4% of the intermediate risk group were reclassified from intermediate to high risk. The NRI in this study was of modest magnitude (5.7%). This has been incorporated into the Reynolds risk score.

   In the largest study to date, the Emerging Risk Factors Collaboration (ERFC) meta-analysed individual records of 160,309 people without a history of vascular disease from 54 long-term worldwide prospective studies, comprising 1.31 million person-years at risk and nearly 28,000 fatal or nonfatal coronary heart disease (CHD) outcomes [14]. Log-transformed hs-CRP concentrations were linearly associated with most established risk factors and several inflammatory markers, including interleukin-6. Log hs-CRP concentrations once adjusted for age and sex were also strongly associated with the risk of coronary heart disease (risk ratio [RR] 1.37, 95% CI 1.27–1.48), ischemic stroke (RR 1.44, 95% CI 1.32–1.57), vascular mortality (RR 1.71, 95% CI 1.53–1.91), and even nonvascular mortality (RR 1.55, 95% CI 1.41–1.69). However, adjustment for several conventional risk factors and plasma fibrinogen resulted in considerable weakening of associations of hs-CRP concentration with risk of coronary heart disease (RR 1.23, 95% CI 1.07–1.42). Such adjustment also attenuated associations of hs-CRP concentration with ischemic stroke (RR 1.32, 95% CI 1.18–1.49) and deaths from nonvascular diseases (RR 1.34, 95% CI 1.20–1.50). It can therefore be concluded from this study that hs-CRP associations with ischemic vascular disease depend considerably on conventional risk factors and other markers of inflammation (Figure 2.2). Furthermore, the nonspecific associations between CRP and a range of vascular and nonvascular endpoints make it unlikely that CRP is a causal factor for CHD.

Hs-CRP may also be a useful measure of residual risk among those who are aggressively treated with contemporary therapy. In the Pravastatin or Atorvastatin Evaluation and Infection Therapy-Thrombolysis in Myocardial Infarction (PROVE-IT-TIMI) trial, 4,162 ACS patients randomly assigned to intensive (Atorvastatin 80 mg) therapy had a lower risk of CVD compared to standard (Pravastatin 40 mg) statin therapy by virtue of having achieved a lower LDL-C level [15]. However, observational data from that study suggested that even among those subjects achieving a very low LDL-C level of <70 mg/dl, risk varied considerably in part based on hs-CRP levels, with those <2 mg/L having a lower risk of CVD than those >2 mg/L, and with the lowest rates observed among those with hs-CRP levels <1 mg/L. Based on this study, monitoring of CRP might offer a way to identify high-risk individuals for more intensive risk-factor control. A study by Ray et al. [16] in the same population showed that in both statin groups "on treatment CRP levels" correlated with the number of uncontrolled risk factors present, therefore among those with elevations in CRP, more intensive control of weight, blood pressure, triglycerides, glucose, raising HDL, and stopping smoking would be expected to lower CRP and potentially used as a motivational tool for patients.

Clinical Use

The Reynolds risk score (http://www.reynoldsriskscore.org) incorporates CRP measurement and family history in its scoring for CVD, components that are not used in the Framingham risk score. In studies by Ridker et al., the Reynolds risk score reclassified 40% to 50% of women [17] at intermediate risk into higher- or lower-risk categories and similarly, for men [18], reclassified approximately 20% of men into higher- or lower-risk categories when compared with the traditional Framingham risk score. Therefore, both of these studies show that a prediction model that incorporates hs-CRP and family history modestly improves global cardiovascular risk prediction. However, among high-risk individuals such as those with diabetes who are already candidates for treatment, it is unclear what these additional measurements would offer.

Currently, the ESC and the AHA offer no official recommendation with regard to the routine measurement of hs-CRP. However, the National Lipid Association panel recommends that in patients with intermediate risk

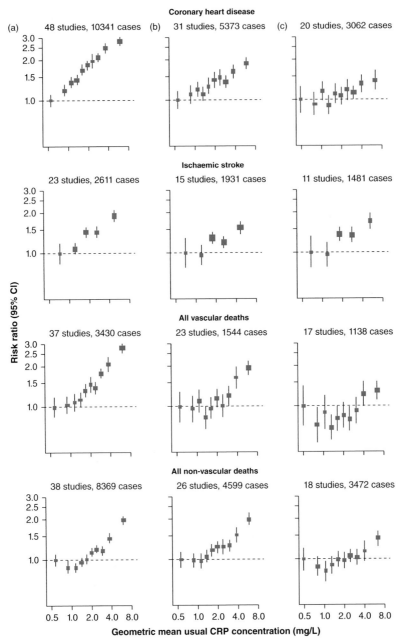

Figure 2.2 Risk ratios for coronary artery disease, stroke, and nonvascular outcomes by quantiles of C-reactive protein (CRP) concentration, with different degree of adjustment for potential confounders. Adjusted study-specific $\log_e$ risk ratios were combined by use of multivariate random-effects meta-analysis. The adjustments were age, sex, and study only (a); age, sex, study, systolic blood pressure, smoking, history of diabetes, body-mass index, concentrations of $\log_e$ triglycerides, non-HDL cholesterol, and HDL cholesterol, and alcohol consumption (b); and (a) plus (b) plus fibrinogen (c). Studies with fewer than 10 cases of any outcome were excluded from the analysis of that outcome. Error bars represent the 95% CIs, calculated using floating absolute risk technique. The sizes of the boxes are proportional to the inverse of the variance of the risk ratios. (Source: ERFC 2010 [14]. Reproduced with permission of Elsevier.)

(520% 10-year risk), hs-CRP should be measured routinely in men >50 years of age and women >60 years of age, given its capacity to enhance risk prediction, especially when used with the Reynolds risk score [8].

Apolipoproteins
Pathophysiology
Apolipoproteins are multifunctional proteins that serve as templates for the assembly of lipoprotein particles. They also maintain the structure and direct metabolism of lipoproteins by binding to membrane receptors and the regulation of enzyme activity. The most important clinical application of apolipoprotein measurements is in the assessment of those individuals where atherogenic risk may not be accurately captured by LDL-C alone; for example, in genetic dyslipidemia and for cardiovascular risk assessment among those with insulin resistance. Most of the data relating to cardiovascular risk revolves around ApoB and ApoAI.

The plasma concentration of ApoB is positively associated and that of ApoAI inversely associated with cardiovascular risk [19]. The ApoB/ApoAI ratio has been interpreted similarly to that for TC/HDL-C as a reflection of the pro-atherogenic potential of the fractions in total cholesterol versus the anti-atherogenic properties of HDL, although more accurately this ratio reflects the non-HDL-C/HDL-C ratio. There is evidence that ApoB is a better marker of cardiovascular risk than TC or LDL-C. This is in part intuitive, as TC includes HDL-C, which has an inverse relationship with CHD risk. LDL-C incompletely captures CHD risk in particular among those with insulin resistance syndromes where VLDL-C and IDL-C levels are high with relatively normal levels of LDL-C.

Technique and Measurement
Tests for either ApoB or ApoAI do not require fasting samples. The reference range for Apo B is 60–120 mg/dL and for ApoAI, 90–200 mg/dL. The ranges for both assays are age and sex dependent.

Population studies
The Apolipoprotein-Related Mortality Risk Study (AMORIS) [20] included 175,553 individuals followed up for approximately 65 months. The relative risk of fatal myocardial infarction associated with 1 standard deviation (SD) increase in ApoB concentration was approximately 2.7, which increased to 3.6 in individuals younger than 70 years. The ApoB/AI ratio was associated with an even higher relative risk of almost 4. However, this study only adjusted for age and sex and HDL-C levels were estimated from ApoA levels.

Since then, several individual studies of subjects free from CVD at baseline have failed to show a superiority of Apo B over non-HDL-C or Apo

A over HDL-C. These include the MONICA/KORA Augsburg study of men and women followed up for 13 years, which demonstrated that the predictive power of ApoB/AI and TC/HDL-C was comparable [21]. Similar findings were observed in the Framingham cohort [22] and the WHS [23].

The largest prospective study to date included individual participant data on 302,430 subjects without initial vascular disease from 68 long-term prospective studies with 2.7 million person-years of follow-up (ERFC) [24]. This study standardized a range of lipid parameters and compared the values of non-HDL-C and HDL-C with ApoB and ApoAI in the assessment of vascular risk. After adjustment for standard CV risk factors, in fully adjusted models the associations with risk were similar for both the groups. The hazard ratios for CHD were 1.50 (95% CI, 1.38–1.62) with the ratio of non-HDL-C/HDL-C and 1.49 (95% CI, 1.39–1.60) with the ratio of Apo B/Apo AI. The group concluded that lipid assessment in vascular disease can be measured by either cholesterol levels or apolipoproteins, depending on what is cost-effective or more efficient to obtain. More recently, work from the same group showed that the addition of apolipoproteins to traditional risk parameters for CVD risk prediction only yielded modest improvement in the model's discrimination, with C-index change of 0.0006 (95% CI, 0.0002–0.0009) for the combination of ApoB and A-I. There was also a modest change in net reclassification. Additional testing with a combination of ApoB and A-I reclassified 1.1% of people to a 20% or higher predicted CVD risk category and, therefore, in need of statin treatment under Adult Treatment Panel (ATP) III guidelines [25].

In the Air Force/Texas Coronary Prevention Study, on treatment apolipoproteins were also shown to predict cardiovascular risk in patients treated with statins [26]. This showed that on treatment, ApoB rather than LDL-C was the best predictor of the first acute event. However, this study did not evaluate all lipoprotein variables, for example, non HDL-C. In the PROVE IT trial [27], non-HDL-C and ApoB provided similar risk associations with CVD. The Treat to New Target (TNT) and Incremental Decrease in End Points through Aggressive Lipid Lowering (IDEAL) studies directly compared the strength of the relationships with CVD event occurrence for LDL-C, non-HDL-C, and ApoB, as well as ratios of total/HDL cholesterol, LDL/HDL-C, and ApoB/A-I in patients receiving statin therapy [28]. The study demonstrated that in patients receiving statin therapy, on-treatment levels of non-HDL-C and ApoB were more closely associated with CVD outcome than were levels of LDL-C. More recently, a meta-analysis of 62,154 patients enrolled in 8 statin trials published between 1994 and 2008 has shown that of the lipid parameters, non HDL-C is the best parameter for assessing on-treatment risk of CVD, being slightly superior to ApoB, and both being superior to LDL-C [29].

Clinical Use

The American Diabetes Association and American College of Cardiology have recommended that ApoB be added to risk assessment in patients at elevated cardiometabolic risk [30]. In high-risk patients – i.e. patients with at least two or more major CVD risk factors – an Apo B target <90 mg/dl is recommended. In patients categorized as being at the greatest risk, including those with established CVD or diabetes, and at least one other cardiometabolic risk factor, an ApoB concentration of <80 mg/dl is recommended. The Canadian guidelines recommend an ApoB level of <80 mg/dl in moderate to-high risk patients as a secondary optional treatment target once LDL-C is at goal. Based on the lack of clinical data for specific targets, it therefore remains uncertain on what basis these recommendations have been made. Further iterations in ATP IV should help clarify this further.

Lp (a)
Pathophysiology
Lipoprotein (a) is a plasma lipoprotein consisting of a cholesterol-rich LDL particle with one molecule of apoB100 and apo (a) attached via a disulfide bond. The apo (a) chain is comprised of cysteine-rich domains called kringles. The fourth kringle is homologous with the fibrin-binding domain of plasminogen. In vitro Lp (a) may act as a carrier for cholesterol esters, which by virtue of its size are deposited in the subendothelial space. Elevated Lp (a) levels can potentially increase the risk of CVD through the homology of Lp (a) with plasminogen increasing the thrombotic tendency of those individuals with elevated levels, and through accelerated atherogenesis as a result of intimal deposition of Lp (a) cholesterol.

Plasma levels of Lp (a) are similar in men and women and are skewed in the population with a tail toward the highest levels [31]. The distribution of Lp (a) also varies between racial groups. Levels are lowest in Caucasians, Eastern Asian, and Asian Indian populations, slightly higher in Hispanics, and even higher in the black population [32].

Serum Lp (a) levels are primarily genetically determined. In families without familial hypercholesterolemia, greater than 90% of the variability in Lp (a) levels can be explained by polymorphisms at the apo (a) gene locus (isoforms), also referred to as the LPA gene [27]. Genetic data from mendelian randomization studies [33] have suggested that those individuals with genetically higher levels of Lp (a) have a higher risk of CHD, in keeping with the expected risk from plasma levels.

Technique and Measurement
Several types of Lp (a) assays are currently available, the most prominent among them enzyme-linked immunosorbent assays (ELISAs),

noncompetitive ELISAs, latex immunoassays, immunoturbidometric and fluorescence assays [34].

Population Studies

In one of the earliest studies, Danesh et al. [35] reported a meta-analysis of 18 prospective studies of the association between the plasma concentration of Lp (a) and 4000 CHD cases before the year 2000. Overall, in the 18 population-based cohorts, the combined risk ratio for the comparison of CHD rates in the top third of baseline Lp (a) measurement versus those in the bottom third was 1.7 (95% CI 1.4–1.9, $2P<0.00001$).

The largest epidemiological study to date on Lp (a) and CVD assessed individual records of 126,634 participants in 36 prospective studies [36], comprising 1.3 million years of follow-up. Associations of Lp (a) with CHD risk were broadly continuous in shape. In 24 cohort studies, the rate of CHD in the top and bottom thirds of baseline Lp (a) distributions, respectively, were 5.6 (95% CI, 5.4–5.9) per 1,000 person-years and 4.4 (4.2–4.6) per 1,000 person-years. The risk ratio (RR) for CHD, adjusted for age and sex only, was 1.16 (1.09–1.18) per 3.5-fold higher usual Lp (a) concentration and 1.13 (1.09–1.18) following further adjustments for lipids and other conventional risk factors. The adjusted RR were 1.10 (1.02–1.18) for ischemic stroke, 1.01 (0.98–1.05) for the aggregate of nonvascular mortality, 1.00 (0.97–1.04) for all cancer deaths, 1.03 (0.97–1.09) for smoking-related cancer deaths, and 1.00 (0.95–1.06) for nonvascular deaths other than cancer. This study provided large-scale evidence of a continuous, independent, and modest association of Lp (a) concentration with risk of CHD and stroke that appeared exclusive to vascular outcomes independent of levels of LDL or non-HDL cholesterol.

These data are supported by studies that investigated genetic variation in Lp (a) and risk for heart disease [31, 37]. Two variants of Lp (a), present in one in six people, together explained about 36% of the variation in plasma Lp (a) levels. Individuals with two or more of these variants had more than 2.5-fold increase in heart disease risk [38].

Clinical Use

The European Atherosclerosis Society (EAS) suggests that Lp (a) should be measured once in the following groups as knowledge of Lp (a) levels may alter clinical risk management [37]:

- Premature CVD.
- Familial hypercholesterolaemia.
- A family history of premature CVD and/or elevated Lp (a).
- Recurrent CVD despite statin treatment.

- ≥3% 10-year risk of fatal CVD according to the risk-prediction tools that use SCORE.
- ≥10% 10-year risk of fatal and/or nonfatal CHD according to risk-prediction tools that use Framingham, but below the conventional risk for statin therapy.

The EAS suggests that repeat measurement is only necessary if treatment for high Lp (a) levels is initiated in order to evaluate therapeutic response, as levels have a correlation of 0.87 over time, known as the regression dilution ratio. This is considerably higher than that for total cholesterol (0.65), suggesting that Lp (a) levels are remarkably stable over time.

The EAS Consensus Panel recommends niacin (nicotinic acid, 1–3 g daily) as the primary treatment for lowering elevated Lp (a) levels, based on its efficacy in reducing levels by 30–40% and in reducing cardiovascular disease in individuals at risk (see Table 2.2) [39]. However, there is a need for further studies in both primary and secondary prevention settings to better define who to treat and to what targets.

Although many observational studies have found a significant association between Lp (a) and cardiovascular events, there is little data to demonstrate whether measurement of Lp (a) improves discrimination, calibration, or classification. Recently, work from ERFC showed that the addition of Lp (a) to traditional risk parameters for CVD risk yielded a modest improvement in the model's discrimination, with a C-index change of 0.0016 (95% CI, 0.00090.0023) for Lp (a). Lp (a) also reclassified 4.1% of people to a 20% or higher predicted CVD risk category and, therefore, in need of statin treatment under Adult Treatment Panel III guidelines.

Table 2.2 Desirable levels for low-density lipoprotein cholesterol and lipoprotein (a) levels in the fasting or nonfasting state. (Source: Nordestgaard et al. 2010 [37]. Reproduced with permission of Oxford University Press.)

	Patients with CVD and/or diabetes	Other patients and individuals	Highest level of evidence for treatment
LDL cholesterol	<2 mmol/L (<77 mg/dL)	<3 mmol/L (116 mg/dL)	I[a]: meta-analysis of randomized, controlled trials of statin treatment
Lp (a)	<80th percentile (<~50 mg/dL[b])	<80th percentile (<~50 mg/dL[b])	I[a]: meta-analysis of randomized, controlled trials of niacin treatment

Notes:
[a] According to the 2007 European guidelines.
[b] The 80th percentile roughly corresponds to 50 mg/dL in Caucasians.

Imaging Biomarkers

Imaging tests offer an advantage in that they provide a measure of the presence or absence of the atherosclerotic disease process itself, in contrast to some circulating and all genetic biomarkers. This has an advantage in the short to medium term, as individuals with subclinical atherosclerosis may be more likely to have an acute cardiovascular event compared with those who do not have evidence of subclinical atherosclerotic disease, merely a predisposition by virtue of risk factors. Examples of imaging modalities include coronary calcium scoring and carotid ultrasound.

Coronary Artery Calcium Score (CACS)
Pathophysiology
Vascular calcification in part reflects an age-related phenomenon secondary to precipitation of calcium and phosphate within the vascular intima, and has been indentified in up to 93% of men and 75% of women above the age of 70 [40]. However, there is growing evidence that vascular calcification is an active process that in part reflects inflammatory processes and that shares pathways that are similar to bone calcification [41].

Coronary artery calcification is an index of the burden of atherosclerosis and does not occur in the absence of atherosclerosis in otherwise normal arteries [42, 43]. Individuals with CAC are also more likely to have noncalcified or "soft" plaque (which cannot be identified on X-ray-based imaging), which is more likely to rupture and cause an acute coronary syndrome [44].

CAC occurs via two distinct mechanisms: atherosclerotic and medial artery calcification [45]. The former pathway takes place in plaque with initial cartilage formation followed by lamellar bone formation. Medial artery calcification (Monckeberg's sclerosis) progresses to intramembranous bone formation without the need for the intermediate step of cartilage formation. It is common in the diabetic and renal failure population and can cause a distinct "railroad" outline of the relevant artery on a standard radiograph.

Technique
Electron-beam computed tomography (EBCT) and the newer multidetector-computed tomography (MDCT) are the currently available modalities of quantifying CACS. They both employ fast imaging protocols that take thin cuts through the heart. A typical scan takes less than 15 minutes to complete with no need for contrast agents. No clinically meaningful difference between EBCT and MDCT has been shown. However, MDCT is likely to be more available and can also be used to perform a CT coronary angiogram. The average cost of the scan is between US $300 and $400.

The detected calcium can be summarized either into the Agatston score [46] (based on plaque size and density at a fixed slice thickness of 3 mm) or the volume method [47] (less dependent on slice thickness). The results can be generated for a specific coronary artery or for the entire coronary tree. The Agastson score, which has been used in a large number of databases and outcomes-based research, is still widely quoted by most interpreting physicians. A score <0 suggests minimal risk of plaque, whereas a score >400 suggests significant risk [48].

With respect to radiation exposure, EBCT (up to 1.3 millisievert [mSv]) is associated with less exposure than prospective MDCT (up to 1.8 mSv). This compares well to the average annual background radiation exposure in the United States, which is 3.-3.6 mSv [49].

Clinical Use

The two main indications being proposed for CACS are in CHD risk assessment of asymptomatic patients at intermediate or low 10-year CVD risk, and in patients who are otherwise at low risk for CHD but who present with atypical stable chest pain symptoms that may or may not represent myocardial ischemia. For the latter group, CACS is unlikely to offer a change in clinical decision-making, as diabetic patients are often classified as a CHD risk equivalent. The utility of CACS to predict risk of CVD events in the diabetic population has been relatively well researched and four key studies are discussed below.

The PREDICT study [50] examined the utility of CACS in predicting the risk of cardiovascular death, angina, or stroke in 589 patients with type 2 diabetes but without CVD, compared to traditional risk factors. During the 4-year (median) follow-up, 66 (11.2%) of patients experienced primary events. The study showed that CACS was an independent predictor of CVD endpoints above and beyond the more traditional risk factors. When added to either the UKPDS CVD or Framingham CHD risk prediction model, CACS significantly increased the ROC area under the curve from 0.63 to 0.73. For every doubling in CACS, CVD risk increased by 29%. Of the 23% of patients who had a low calcium score (Agatston units <10), only two experienced a significant event over the follow-up period.

Anand et al. [51] similarly had shown a few years earlier an improved ROC AUC curve for cardiovascular event prediction with CACS over Framingham and UKPDS models (Figure 2.3). These authors undertook a study in 510 asymptomatic patients with T2DM to see whether CACS could predict silent myocardial ischemia by nuclear myocardial perfusion scanning. All patients with a CACS>100 ($n = 136$) underwent perfusion scanning as well as a random selection of 53 from those with a score <100 ($n = 374$). In total, 57 patients had perfusion abnormalities suggestive of silent ischemia. In their short 2.2-year follow-up, 20 patients had CVD events,

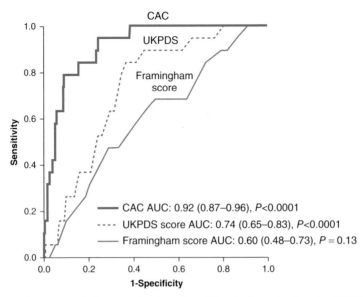

Figure 2.3 ROC analysis comparing the value of Framingham risk function, UKPDS risk engine, and the CAC score for predicting cardiovascular events. AUC, area under the curve. (Source: Anand et al. 2006 [51]. Reproduced with permission of Oxford University Press.)

82% of whom had a calcium score of >400 AU. None of the patients (n = 15) with a CACS of <10 had a perfusion abnormality. On multivariable logistic regression analysis, only CACS was a predictor of myocardial perfusion abnormality.

The Diabetes Heart Study [52] was a longitudinal cohort study of 1,051 patients with type 2 DM that assessed the relationship between CACS and all-cause mortality. During 7.4 years of follow-up, 178 (17%) of participants died. Subjects with a CACS of 0 had an estimated annual mortality of only 0.9% compared to 2.7% per annum in patients where the score was 1,000. Individuals with a score of >1,000 were also 58 times more likely to suffer a CVD event. These findings were further supported in a cohort of low-risk patients in the Multi-Ethnic Study of Atherosclerosis (MESA) [53]. Here, 6,814 patients (883 with diabetes) were followed up for a median of 6.4 years. The annual CHD rate in the diabetic population was 1.5% and in the nondiabetic cohort was 0.5%. When CACS was added to traditional risk factors, the AUC for CVD and CHD events increased significantly from 0.72 to 0.78. Patients with diabetes and a low CACS (<100) had similar hazard ratios for a CVD event compared to patients without diabetes and a similar calcium score (2.9 vs 2.6).

In summary, CACS improves risk prediction for cardiovascular mortality and events in patients (including those with DM) above and beyond traditional risk models. The data that exist so far show good discrimination, but there is little statistical interpretation for the more day-to-day clinically meaningful reclassification. There is also little evidence that widespread implementation of therapies in these high-risk diabetics would further improve outcomes based on a given CACS, nor is there any evidence from randomized controlled trials that reducing the intensity of therapy in low CACS individuals would not worsen outcomes. In part reflecting the lack of adequate randomized controlled trials using this modality, the American Heart Association (AHA) has given CACS a Class IIa recommendation (level of evidence B) in the risk assessment of asymptomatic diabetic patients above the age of 40 [54]. However, in an editorial, Budoff has identified three possible roles of the usage of CACS [55]:

1 In patients with type 1 diabetes, as at least 50% of them could be identified as low risk after a negative scan (score=0).
2 Noncompliant patients who can get visual incentives to take the medicines if they have an elevated score.
3 Screening younger type 2 diabetics in particular to identify those who would benefit from earlier statin and ACE inhibitor treatment.

Carotid Intimal Thickness (CIMT) and Carotid Plaque (CP)
Pathophysiology
Symptomatic CVD occurs when atherosclerotic plaque progresses to a flow-limiting stenosis or becomes unstable and causes an acute occlusion. Hence, there is considerable interest in techniques that visualize the process of arterial injury or atherosclerosis, such as CIMT and CP imaging. While it may be difficult to visualize the coronary atheroma noninvasively, thickening of the intima-medial portion of the carotid arteries is easily visualized and appears to predate plaque formation as a general measure of atherosclerotic tendency. Hence, CIMT is likely to be an earlier biomarker of atherosclerosis than coronary artery calcium, which tends to reflect healed plaque [56].

Technique
Thickness of the far wall of the intima and media of the common carotid artery, as well as visualization of plaque in the common and internal carotid artery, can be assessed by *B*-mode ultrasound. Standardized techniques have been reported by the American Society of Echocardiography that include imaging at least a 1 cm length of artery at at least three different angles [57]. As the testing is noninvasive and leads to no radiation exposure, it can be repeated easily to assess the progression of subclinical disease. Ultrasound machines to undertake this investigation are widely available and this test can be performed with minimal expense, making it attractive as the noninvasive technique of choice.

Clinical Use

In the largest study to date [58], Nambi et al investigated 13,145 patients in a prospective study (ARIC) assessing the clinical utility of CIMT and CP in predicting risk for CVD. Patients with a prior history of CVD were excluded and approximately 10% of the population had diabetes. The AUC, NRI, and calibration were calculated for a 10-year follow-up. Using traditional risk factors the AUC was 0.742 and this was significantly increased to 0.755 by the addition of CIMT and CP. There was good calibration between expected outcomes and observed outcomes when the CIMT and CP were used on top of the classical Framingham risk score. Using the carotid ultrasound data, 21.7% of subjects at intermediate risk were reclassified either into the high-risk or low-risk group; 62% of these intermediate-risk patients were reclassified into the low-risk group, with the remainder into the high-risk group. This analysis from ARIC suggested that the addition of CIMT and CP estimation to the traditional risk model improved risk estimation for future CVD events as assessed by discrimination, calibration, and reclassification.

While there are data in cohort studies that CIMT or CP predict risk, it remains unclear based on these observational data whether changes in CIMT or CP are useful measures of risk or of response to therapy on a large scale. Several studies have used CIMT as a measure of efficacy of different therapeutic regimens such as statins or niacin. Surrogate markers of atherosclerosis have been used to obtain a licensed indication for atherosclerosis regression. For instance, the METEOR (Measuring Effects on Intima-Media Thickness: An Evaluation of Rosuvastatin) study randomly assigned statin therapy to individuals with <10% 10-year Framingham risk scores whose only risk factor was either age or hypercholesterolemia (i.e., a group that would not normally qualify for treatment) [59]. They showed that those patients who were randomized to statin therapy had a lower rate of CIMT progression. Even though METEOR did not show that lowering CIMT progression reduced CV events (it was not powered to do so), other trials have shown that a reduction in CIMT progression is congruent with a reduction in CV events [60].

As individuals with diabetes are more prone to diffuse atherosclerosis and are at high risk of CVD, ultrasound techniques may offer an initial and useful screening tool in this population. In an asymptomatic population of individuals with diabetes consisting of 98 consecutive patients, CIMT was significantly related to myocardial perfusion abnormalities (SPECT) on multivariable analysis. Only 3% of patients with a normal CIMT were found to have severely abnormal perfusion, compared to 28% of those with increased CIMT. While no correlation with outcome data are available, this study correlated CIMT with myocardial perfusion abnormalities, which have been shown to be prognostically relevant in the diabetic population [61].

The American Society of Echocardiography published a consensus statement in 2008 [57]. It suggested that a CIMT thickness above the 75th centile was associated with a high CVD risk, as was the presence of CP. It recommended CIMT measurement in the following scenarios:

- Patients with an intermediate CVD risk without established disease or diabetes.
- Patients with a family history of premature CVD.
- Patients less than 60 years in age with a severe abnormality in just one risk factor (e.g., hypercholesterolemia) who otherwise do not qualify for treatment.

The 2010 ACC/AHA has given CIMT measurement a Class IIa recommendation with a level of evidence of B for cardiovascular risk assessment in intermediate risk cohorts.

Genetic Markers

Pathophysiology

Cardiovascular disease is a complex process involving multiple genes and multiple environmental factors. The strongest evidence of a role for genetic factors in CVD arises from twin studies. In a cohort study of 21,004 twins born in Sweden and followed for 26 years, where one twin died from CAD (male <55 years, female <65 years), the hazard ratio of the remaining twin dying from CAD was approximately 8 for monozygotes and 3 for dizygotes [62]. Having at least one parent (father <55 years, mother <65 years) with premature coronary artery disease is associated with a doubling of the multivariate odds ratio of CV events in the offspring [63].

Family history (a surrogate for inherited genes) of premature cardiovascular disease has an independent association with cardiovascular events. However, the clinical utility of family history was questioned in the EPIC-Norfolk study, a prospective cohort study of at least 25,000 individuals aged 40–79 [64]. This showed that in the intermediate-risk group, the addition of family history to the model resulted in a modest increase in the NRI by 2%. This study included a large cohort of patients greater than 60 years of age, which is relevant as the effect of genes on CVD risk prediction declines with age.

Searching for genetic biomarkers as opposed to merely relying on family history to predict CVD is clinically appealing, as it can be tested for from birth, allowing for theoretically better risk prediction, diagnosis, and disease management, particularly with respect to lifetime risk.

Technique

In cardiac disease there are two approaches that can be used to investigate genetic markers: candidate gene studies, in which individual genes that are responsible for monogenic diseases (e.g., Brugada syndrome) are identified; and genomic studies, which are ideal for polygenic conditions as the whole genome is studied. The complex genetics of CVD and diabetes lend themselves to genomic studies. Markers such as single nucleotide polymorphisms (SNP) are investigated by either linkage or association studies. SNP are variants at a single DNA base pair and can be easily exploited as a genetic biomarker due to their high frequency in the genome and the relative technological ease of identifying them [65].

In linkage studies, family data is required to identify nonrandomly inherited segments of the genome in relation to the studied disease process. With association studies, the whole genome is studied in a cohort of cases and controls to find an association between certain genetic loci and the cases (this usually requires a large number of individuals) [65]. A big concern with association studies is the lack of reproducibility of results, with a large amount of type-1 errors (false positives) [66]. However, with the more recently developed, large-scale, genome-wide association studies (GWAS) some of these concerns have been addressed.

Genetic biomarkers are tested only in specialist laboratories. The investigation can be undertaken on both blood and tissue samples.

Clinical Use

One of the first identified genetic biomarkers for CVD was the 9p21 loci. In a meta-analysis of 4,645 patients with CAD and 5,177 controls, a SNP at chromosome 9p21 was associated with an odd ratio for CAD of 1.3 per copy of risk allele [67]. However, in observational studies the clinical utility of 9p21 loci SNP has been questioned. In two large studies, one involving only men [68] and the other women as well [69], 9p21 SNP did not discriminate well (nonsignificant change in the c-statistic). However, the c-statistic, which has been broadly used to evaluate diagnostic tests, may not be the best tool for risk-prediction models. Talmud et al. [68] did find that the 9p21 loci SNP improved calibration (predicted risk corresponds better to observed risk) and that genetic marker moved 13.5% of patients into a more accurate risk category; in particular, 3.3% of intermediate-risk patients were moved to a high-risk category. At present there is no reliable large-scale evidence that genetic testing will improve risk prediction. Currently, genetic testing for this loci is not routinely undertaken.

The most recent summary suggests there are now 27 loci that confer risk for CAD [70]. Herder et al. [70] have summarized the key studies related to genetic risk models for the prediction of coronary artery disease. The studies reviewed showed only minimal improvement in the AUC of less than <0.04 for each chromosomal loci and only a few of these allowed clinically usefully reclassification [70]. There is a great theoretical hope for genetic biomarkers, but much more research needs to be undertaken.

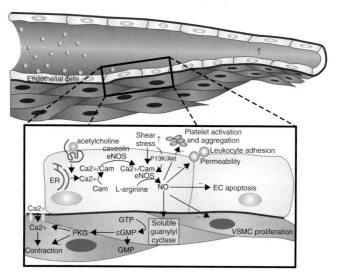

Color plate 1.1 Illustration of the stimulation of endothelial NO synthase by acetylcholine and shear stress leading to increased nitric oxide (NO) production in endothelial cells by receptor and nonreceptor and calcium-dependent and noncalcium-dependent pathways. (Source: Herrmann J et al. 2010 [8]. Reproduced with permission of Oxford University Press.)

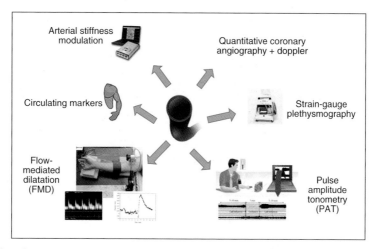

Color plate 1.2 Methods for assessing human endothelial function.

Color plate 2.1 Summary and recommendations for measurement of inflammatory markers and advanced lipoprotein/subfraction testing in initial clinical assessment and on-treatment management decisions. (Source: Davidson et al. 2011 [8]. Reproduced with permission of Elsevier.)

	Initial Clinical Assessment					
	CRP	Lp-PLA$_2$	Apo B	LDL-P	Lp(a)	HDL or LDL Subfractions
Low risk (<5% 10-year CHD event risk)	Not recommended	Not recommended	Not recommended	Not recommended	Not recommended	Not recommended
Intermediate risk (5-20% 10-year CHD event risk)	Recommended for routine measurement	Consider for selected patients	Reasonable for many patients	Reasonable for many patients	Consider for selected patients	Not recommended
CHD or CHD Equivalent	Consider for selected patients	Consider for selected patients	Consider for selected patients	Consider for selected patients	Consider for selected patients	Not recommended
Family History	Reasonable for many patients	Consider for selected patients	Reasonable for many patients	Reasonable for many patients	Reasonable for many patients	Not recommended
Recurrent Events	Reasonable for many patients	Consider for selected patients	Reasonable for many patients	Reasonable for many patients	Reasonable for many patients	Not recommended

	On-Treatment Management Decisions					
	CRP	Lp-PLA$_2$	Apo B	LDL-P	Lp(a)	HDL or LDL Subfractions
Low risk (<5% 10-year CHD event risk)	Not recommended	Not recommended	Not recommended	Not recommended	Not recommended	Not recommended
Intermediate risk (5-20% 10-year CHD event risk)	Reasonable for many patients	Not recommended	Reasonable for many patients	Reasonable for many patients	Not recommended	Not recommended
CHD or CHD Equivalent	Reasonable for many patients	Not recommended	Reasonable for many patients	Reasonable for many patients	Consider for selected patients	Not recommended
Family History	Consider for selected patients	Not recommended	Consider for selected patients	Consider for selected patients	Consider for selected patients	Not recommended
Recurrent Events	Reasonable for many patients	Not recommended	Reasonable for many patients	Reasonable for many patients	Consider for selected patients	Not recommended

Apo, apolipoprotein; CHD, coronary heart disease; CRP, C-reactive protein; HDL, high-density lipoprotein; Lp-PLA$_2$, lipoprotein-associated phospholipase A$_2$; LDL, low-density lipoprotein; LDL-P, LDL particle number/concentration; Lp(a), lipoprotein (a).

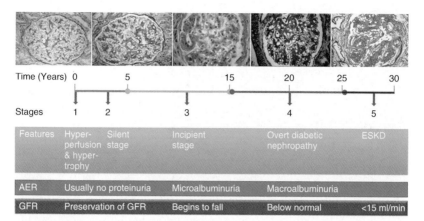

Time (Years)	0	5		15	20	25	30
Stages	1	2		3	4	5	
Features	Hyper-perfusion & hyper-trophy	Silent stage		Incipient stage	Overt diabetic nephropathy	ESKD	
AER	Usually no proteinuria			Microalbuminuria	Macroalbuminuria		
GFR	Preservation of GFR			Begins to fall	Below normal	<15 ml/min	

Color plate 3.1 The course of diabetic nephropathy. (Source: Kidney Check Australia Taskforce, Chronic Kidney Disease and Diabetes, Workshop Module, 2013. Reproduced with permission of Kidney Health Australia.)

Composite ranking for relative risks by GFR and albuminuria (KDIGO 2009)				Albuminuria stages, description and range (mg/g)				
				A1		A2	A3	
				Optimal and high-normal		High	Very high and nephrotic	
				<10	10–29	30–299	300–1999	≥2000
GFR stages, description and range (ml/min per 1.73 m²)	G1	High and optimal	>105					
			90–104					
	G2	Mild	75–89					
			60–74					
	G3a	Mild-moderate	45–59					
	G3b	Moderate-severe	30–44					
	G4	Severe	15–29					
	G5	Kidney failure	<15					

Color plate 3.2 New classification of chronic kidney disease. (Source: Levey et al. 2011 [42]. Reproduced with permission of Nature Publishing Group.)

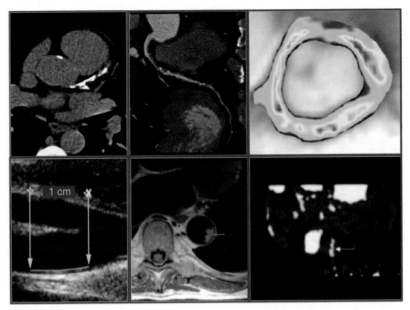

Color plate 4.1 Noninvasive arterial wall imaging modalities. Clockwise from upper left: computed tomography calcium scoring, computed tomography coronary angiography, molecular imaging of vascular cell adhesion molecule-1 (VCAM-1) in plaque, fluorodeoxyglucose (FDG) positron emission tomography (PET) imaging of plaque inflammation, magnetic resonance imaging, and carotid intima-medial thickness evaluation on B-mode ultrasound.

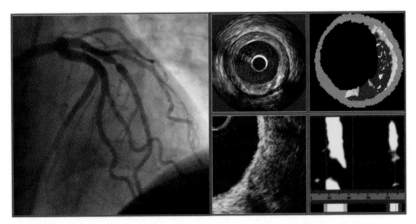

Color plate 4.2 Invasive arterial wall imaging modalities. Clockwise from left: coronary angiography, intravascular ultrasound, ultrasound radiofrequency plaque composition analysis, near-infrared spectroscopy, and optical coherence tomography.

Genetic biomarkers reflect disease susceptibility, but only provide static information. They do not provide any information as to whether or not the individual has actually developed risk factors or indeed cardiovascular disease.

The AHA has given genomic testing in risk assessment in asymptomatic adults a Class III recommendation (no benefit) with a level of evidence of B, highlighting the current lack of clear clinical role [71].

Conclusions

In patients with diabetes, biomarkers may be useful for screening asymptomatic patients for indolent atherosclerosis (e.g., CIMT), or for prognosis (e.g., CACS, BNP, hSCRP). Perhaps the greatest potential clinical utility for both clinicians and patients is for biomarkers in primary prevention. The burden of cardiovascular disease is high in patients with diabetes; while biomarkers may offer clinical utility in this field, there is scant data on cost-effectiveness or differential benefit from specific treatments. Nonetheless, there has been progress in this field over the last few years such that a few biomarkers have been included in national guidelines.

It is logical to assume that if one biomarker measure gives a small incremental gain in risk prediction, multiple biomarkers would result in a larger one. However, trials of multiple biomarkers have disappointingly only shown at best a moderate improvement in usefulness when compared to standard risk factors [72]. It has been suggested that the multimarker model could be improved if it included biomarkers that were unrelated; for example, in a model that included hs-CRP (which is a marker of inflammation), one would expect little incremental value in adding other markers of inflammation, but the value might be higher if NTproBNP were added. Currently, genomic studies are being undertaken to identify biomarkers involved in differing pathways, and these raise the possibility that biomarkers may play a more central role in primary prevention.

Ultimately, all emerging biomarkers should have a valid, reproducible assay with a small coefficient of variation and be standardized. Beyond independent association, they should perform well under biostatistical analysis, which may include discrimination, calibration, and reclassification. However, before it is fully adopted into clinical practice, the biomarker should be incorporated into a randomized controlled trial that demonstrates that a treatment reduces clinical events in cohorts identified using a high-risk biomarker phenotype. These data are largely lacking for most of the novel biomarkers.

> **Case Study 1**
>
> A 62-year-old asymptomatic female smoker with a background of treated hypertension and a family history of coronary artery disease presents to her family practitioner for a routine check-up. She has some blood tests that show her to have a total cholesterol level of 5.3 mmol/L, LDL cholesterol of 3.5 mmol/L, and a HDL cholesterol of 0.9 mmol/L. Her Framingham 10-year risk score for future coronary events is 10%. She does not currently meet the criteria for lipid-lowering therapy.

Multiple-Choice Question

1 Which biomarker would help further risk stratify her as well as guiding the need for lipid-lowering therapy?

   A BNP

   B Echocardiography

   C HbA1C

   D HsCRP

   E Troponin

   Answer provided after the References

> **Case Study 2**
>
> A 42-year-old man is reviewed in clinic. He has type 2 diabetes. His blood pressure is 125/75. His total cholesterol is 5.1 mmol/L and LDL-cholesterol is 2.2 mmol/L. He smokes and at this stage is not willing to give up. His HBA1C is 6.8%. His drug history consists only of metformin 500 mg three times a day. His father recently had a heart attack at the age of 67; the man is concerned about his risk and wants to know if any other tablets would help. His UKPDS 10-year risk for coronary heart disease puts him at intermediate risk.

Multiple-Choice Question

1 Which one of the following in the most appropriate next step in his management?

   A ACE inhibitor

   B Carotid intimal thickness measurement

   C Coronary calcium score

   D Genetic profiling

   E Statin therapy

   Answer provided after the References

Guidelines and Web Links

http://content.onlinejacc.org/article.aspx?articleid=1143998
http://content.onlinejacc.org/article.aspx?articleid=1188641
http://www.escardio.org/guidelines-surveys/esc-guidelines/guidelinesdocuments
  /guidelines-dyslipidemias-ft.pdf

2010 ACCF/AHA Guideline for Assessment of Cardiovascular Risk in Asymptomatic Adults: Executive Summary.

ACCF/AHA 2007 Clinical Expert Consensus Document on Coronary Artery Calcium Scoring By Computed Tomography in Global Cardiovascular Risk Assessment and in Evaluation of Patients With Chest Pain.

ESC/EAS guidelines for the management of dyslipidemias.

References

1 The Emerging Risk Factors Collaboration. Diabetes mellitus, fasting blood glucose concentration, and risk of vascular disease: A collaborative meta-analysis of 102 prospective studies. *Lancet* 2010 June 26; 375: 2215–22.

2 Wannamethee S, Shaper A, Whincup P, Lennon L, Sattar N. Impact of diabetes on cardiovascular disease risk and all-cause mortality in older men influence of age at onset, diabetes duration, and established and novel risk factors. *Arch Intern Med* 2011; 171(5): 404–10.

3 The Emerging Risk Factors Collaboration. Diabetes mellitus, fasting glucose and risk of cause-specific death. *N Engl J Med* 2011; 364: 829–41.

4 Khot UN, Khot MB, Bajzer CT et al. Prevalence of conventional risk factors in patients with coronary heart disease. *JAMA* 2003; 290: 898–904.

5 Biomarkers Definitions Working Group. Biomarkers and surrogate endpoints: Preferred definitions and conceptual framework. *Clin Pharmacol Ther* 2001; 69: 89–95.

6 Vasan R. Biomarkers of cardiovascular disease: Molecular basis and practical considerations. *Circulation* 2006; 113: 2335–62.

7 Wang T. Assessing the role of circulating, genetic, and imaging biomarkers in cardiovascular risk prediction. *Circulation* 2011; 123: 551–65.

8 Davidson MH, Ballantyne CM, Jacobson TA et al. Clinical utility of inflammatory markers and advanced lipoprotein testing: Advice from an expert panel of lipid specialists. *J Clin Lipidol* 2011; 5: 338–67.

9 C Reactive Protein Coronary Heart Disease Genetics Collaboration (CCGC). Association between C reactive protein and coronary heart disease: Mendelian randomization analysis based on individual participant data. *Br Med J* 2011; 342: d548.

10 Pepys MB, Hirschfield GM. C reactive protein and atherothrombosis. *Ital Heart J* 2001 Mar; 2(3): 196–9.

11 Ridker PM. Clinical application of C-reactive protein for cardiovascular disease detection and prevention. *Circulation* 2003; 107: 36.

12 Pearson TA, Mensah GA, Alexander RW et al. Markers of inflammation and cardiovascular disease: Application to clinical and public health practice: A statement for healthcare professionals from the Centers for Disease Control and Prevention and the American Heart Association. *Circulation* 2003; 107: 499.

13 Ridker PM, Hennekens CH, Buring JE, Rifai N. C-reactive protein and other markers of inflammation in the prediction of cardiovascular disease in women. *N Engl J Med* 2000; 342: 836–43.

14 Emerging Risk Factors Collaboration, Kaptoge S, Di Angelantonio E, Lowe G et al. C-reactive protein concentration and risk of coronary heart disease, stroke, and mortality: An individual participant meta-analysis. *Lancet* 2010; 375: 132–40.

15 Ahmed S, Cannon CP, Murphy SA, Braunwald E. Acute coronary syndromes and diabetes: Is intensive lipid lowering beneficial? Results of the PROVE IT-TIMI 22 trial. *Eur Heart J* 2006; 27: 2323–9.

16 Ray KK, Cannon CP, Cairns R et al.; PROVE IT-TIMI 22 Investigators. Relationship between uncontrolled risk factors and C-reactive protein levels in patients receiving standard or intensive statin therapy for acute coronary syndromes in the PROVE IT-TIMI 22 trial. *J Am Coll Cardiol* 2005; 46: 1417–24.

17 Ridker PM, Buring JE, Rifai N, Cook NR. Development and validation of improved algorithms for the assessment of global cardiovascular risk in women: The Reynolds Risk Score. *JAMA* 2007; 297: 611–19.

18 Ridker PM, Paynter NP, Rifai N, Gaziano JM, Cook NR. C-reactive protein and parental history improve global cardiovascular risk prediction: The Reynolds Risk Score for men. *Circulation* 2008; 118: 2243–51.

19 Andrikoula M, McDowell IFW. The contribution of apoB and apoA1 measurements to cardiovascular risk assessment. *Diabetes Obes Metab* 2008; 10: 271–8.

20 Walldius G, Jungner I, Holme I et al. High apolipoprotein B, low apolipoprotein A-1, and improvement in the prediction of fatal myocardial infarction (AMORIS study): A prospective study. *Lancet* 2001; 358: 2026–33.

21 Meisinger C, Loewel H, Mraz W, Koenig W. Prognostic value of apolipoprotein B and A-1 in the prediction of myocardial infarction in middle-aged men and women: Results from the MONICA/KORA. *Eur Heart J* 2005; 26: 271–8.

22 Ingelsson E, Schaefer EJ, Contois JH et al. Clinical utility of different lipid measures for prediction of coronary heart disease in men and women. *JAMA* 2007; 298: 776–85.

23 Ridker PM, Rifai N, Cook NR, Bradwin G, Buring JE. Non-HDL cholesterol, apolipoproteins A-I and B100, standard lipid measures, lipid ratios, and CRP as risk factors for cardiovascular disease in women. *JAMA* 2005; 294(3): 326–33.

24 The Emerging Risk Factor Collaboration. Major lipids, apolipoproteins, and risk of vascular disease. *JAMA* 2009; 302: 1993–2000.

25 The Emerging Risk Factor Collaboration. Lipid-related markers and cardiovascular disease prediction. *JAMA* 2012; 307(23): 2499–506.

26 Gotto AM, Whitney E, Stein EA et al. Relation between baseline and on-treatment lipid parameters and first acute major coronary events in the Air Force/Texas Coronary Atherosclerosis Prevention Study (AF-CAPS/TexCAPS). *Circulation* 2000; 101: 477–84.

27 Miller M, Cannon CP, Murphy SA, Qin J, Ray KK, Braunwald E; PROVE IT-TIMI 22 Investigators. Impact of triglyceride levels beyond low-density lipoprotein cholesterol after acute coronary syndrome in the PROVE IT-TIMI 22 trial. *J Am Coll Cardiol* 2008; 51: 724–30.

28 Kastelein JJ, van der Steeg WA, Holme I et al.; TNT Study Group; IDEAL Study Group. Lipids, apolipoproteins, and their ratios in relation to cardiovascular events with statin treatment. *Circulation* 2008 Jun 10; 117: 3002–9.

29 Boekholdt SM, Arsenault BJ, Mora S et al. Association of LDL cholesterol, non-HDL cholesterol, and apolipoprotein B levels with risk of cardiovascular events among patients treated with statins: A meta-analysis. *JAMA* 2012 Mar 28; 307(12): 1302–9.

30 Brunzell JD, Davidson M, Furberg CD et al. Lipoprotein management in patients in cardiometabolic risk: Conference report from the American Diabetes Association and the American College of Cardiology Foundation. *JACC* 2008; 51: 1512–24.

31 Kamstrup PR, Tybjaerg-Hansen A, Steffensen R, Nordestgaard BG. Genetically elevated lipoprotein(a) and increased risk of myocardial infarction. *JAMA* 2009; 301: 2331.

32 Matthews KA, Sowers MF, Derby CA, Stein E, Miracle-McMahill H, Crawford SL,Pasternak RC. Ethnic differences in cardiovascular risk factor burden among middle-aged women: Study of Women's Health Across the Nation (SWAN). *Am Heart J* 2005; 149: 1066–73.

33 Boerwinkle E, Leffert CC, Lin J et al. Apolipoprotein(a) gene accounts for greater than 90% of the variation in plasma lipoprotein(a) concentrations. *J Clin Invest* 1992; 90: 52.

34 Marcovina SM, Koschinsky ML, Albers JJ, Skarlatos S. Report of the National Heart, Lung, and Blood Institute Workshop on Lipoprotein(a) and Cardiovascular Disease: Recent advances and future directions. *Clin Chem* 2003; 49: 1785–96.

35 Danesh J, Collins R, Peto R. Lipoprotein(a) and coronary heart disease: Meta-analysis of prospective studies. *Circulation* 2000; 102: 1082–5.

36 The Emerging Risk Factors Collaboration. Lipoprotein (a) concentration and the risk of coronary heart disease, stroke, and nonvascular mortality. *JAMA* 2009; 302: 412–23.

37 Nordestgaard BG, Chapman MJ, Ray K et al; European Atherosclerosis Society Consensus Panel. Lipoprotein (a) as a cardiovascular risk factor. *Eur Heart J* 2010; 31: 2844–53.

38 Clarke R, Peden JF, Hopewell JC et al. Genetic variants associated with Lp(a) lipoprotein level and coronary disease. *N Engl J Med* 2009; 361: 2518–28.

39 Chapman MJ, Redfern JS, McGovern ME, Giral P. Niacin and fibrates in atherogenic dyslipidemia: Pharmacotherapy to reduce cardiovascular risk. *Pharmacol Ther* 2010; 126: 314–45.

40 Wong ND, Kouwabunpat D, Vo AN, Detrano RC, Eisenberg H, Goel M, Tobis JM. Coronary calcium and atherosclerosis by ultrafast computed tomography in asymptomatic men and women: Relation to age and risk factors. *Am Heart J* 1994; 127: 422–30.

41 Bostrom K, Watson KE, Horn S, Wortham C, Herman IM, Demer LL. Bone morphogenetic protein expression in human atherosclerotic lesions. *J Clin Invest* 1993; 91: 1800–9.

42 Mintz GS, Pichard AD, Popma JJ et al. Determinants and correlates of target lesion calcium in coronary artery disease: A clinical, angiographic and intravascular ultrasound study. *J Am Coll Cardiol* 1997; 29: 268–74.

43 Blankenhorn DH. Coronary arterial calcification: A review. *Am J Med Sci* 1961; 242: 41–9.

44 Rumberger JA, Simons DB, Fitzpatrick LA, Sheedy PF, Schwartz RS. Coronary artery calcium area by electron-beam computed tomography and coronary atherosclerotic plaque area: A histopathologic correlative study. *Circulation* 1995; 92: 2157–62.

45 Johnson RC, Leopold JA, Loscalzo J. Vascular calcification: Pathobiological mechanisms and clinical implications. *Circ Res* 2006; 99: 1044–59.

46 Agatston AS, Janowitz WR, Hildner FJ, Zusmer NR, Viamonte M Jr,, Detrano R. Quantification of coronary artery calcium using ultrafast computed tomography. *J Am Coll Cardiol* 1990; 15: 827–32.

47 Callister TQ, Cooil B, Raya SP, Lippolis NJ, Russo DJ, Raggi P. Coronary artery disease: Improved reproducibility of calcium scoring with electron-beam CT volumetric method. *Radiology* 1998; 208: 807–14.

48 Pletcher MJ, Tice JA, Pignone M, Browner WS. Using the coronary artery calcium score to predict coronary heart disease events: A systematic review and meta-analysis. *Arch Intern Med* 2004; 164: 1285–92.

49 Hunold P, Vogt FM, Schmermund A et al. Radiation exposure during cardiac CT: Effective doses at multi-detector row CT and electron-beam CT. *Radiology* 2003; 226: 145–52.

50 Elkeles R, Godsland I, Feher M et al. Coronary calcium measurement improved prediction of cardiovascular events in asymptomatic patients with patients with type 2 diabetes: The Predict study. *Eur Heart J* 2008; 29: 2244–51.

51 Anand D, Lim E, Hopkins D et al. Risk stratification in uncomplicated type 2 diabetes: Prospective evaluation of the combined use of coronary artery calcium imaging and selective myocardial perfusion scintigraphy. *Eur Heart J* 2006; 27: 713–21.

52 Agarwal S, Morgan T, Herrington D et al. Coronary calcium score and prediction of all-cause mortality in diabetes: The Diabetes Heart Study. *Diabetes Care* 2011; 34: 1219–24.

53 Malik S, Budoff M, Katz R et al. Impact of subclinical atherosclerosis on cardiovascular disease events in individuals with metabolic syndrome and diabetes: The multi-ethnic study of atherosclerosis. *Diabetes Care* 2011; 34: 2285–90.

54 Budoff MJ, Achenbach S, Blumenthal RS et al. Assessment of coronary artery disease by cardiac computed tomography: A scientific statement from the American Heart Association Committee on Cardiovascular Imaging and Intervention, Council on Cardiovascular Radiology and Intervention, and Committee on Cardiac Imaging, Council on Clinical Cardiology. *Circulation* 2006; 114: 1761–91.

55 Budoff M. Not all diabetics are created equal (in cardiovascular risk). *Eur Heart J* 2008; 29: 2193–4.

56 Sharma K, Blaha MJ, Blumenthal RS, Musunuru K. Clinical and research applications of carotid intima-media thickness. *Am J Cardiol.* 2009; 103: 1316–20.

57 Stein J, Korcarz C, Hurst T et al. ASE Consensus Statement: Use of carotid ultrasound to identify subclinical vascular disease and evaluate cardiovascular disease risk: A consensus statement from the American Society of Echocardiography Carotid Intima-Media Thickness Task Force. *JASE* 2008; 21: 93–111.

58 Nambi V, Chambless L, Folsom A et al. Carotid intima-media thickness and presence or absence of plaque improves prediction of coronary heart disease risk: The ARIC (Atherosclerosis Risk In Communities) Study. *J Am Coll Cardiol* 2010; 55(15): 1600–7.

59 Crouse JR III, Raichlen JS, Riley WA et al. Effect of rosuvastatin on progression of carotid intima-media thickness in low-risk individuals with subclinical atherosclerosis: The METEOR trial. *JAMA* 2007; 297: 1344–53.

60 Espeland MA, O'Leary DH, Terry JG, Morgan T, Evans G, Mudra H. Carotid intimal-media thickness as a surrogate for cardiovascular disease events in trials of HMG-CoA reductase inhibitors. *Curr Control Trials Cardiovasc Med.* 2005; 6: 3.

61 Kang X, Berman DS, Lewin HC et al. Incremental prognostic value of myocardial perfusion single photon emission computed tomography in patients with diabetes mellitus. *Am Heart J* 1999; 138: 1025–32.

62 Marenberg ME, Risch N, Berkman LF, Floderus B, de Faire U. Genetic susceptibility to death from coronary heart disease in a study of twins. *N Engl J Med* 1994; 330: 1041–6.

63 Lloyd-Jones DM, Nam BH, D'Agostino RB Sr, et al. Parental cardiovascular disease as a risk factor for cardiovascular disease in middle-aged adults: A prospective study of parents and offspring. *JAMA* 2004; 291: 2204–11.

64 Sivapalaratnam S, Boekholdt S, Trip M, Sandhu M, Luben R, Kastelein J, Wareham N, Khaw K. Family history of premature coronary heart disease and risk prediction in the EPIC-Norfolk prospective population study Heart 2010; 96: 1985–9.

65 Gibbons G, Liew C, Goodarzi M et al. Genetic markers: Progress and potential for cardiovascular disease. *Circulation* 2004; 109: IV-47–IV-58.

66 Sturm A. Cardiovascular genetics: Are we there yet? *J Med Genet* 2004; 41: 321–32.

67 Schunkert H, Gotz A, Braund P, McGinnis R et al. Repeated replication and a prospective meta-analysis of the association between chromosome 9p21.3 and coronary artery disease. *Circulation* 2008; 117: 1675–84.

68 Talmud PJ, Cooper JA, Palmen J et al. Chromosome 9p21.3 coronary heart disease locus genotype and prospective risk of CHD in healthy middle-aged men. *Clin Chem* 2008; 54: 467–74.

69 Paynter NP, Chasman DI, Buring JE et al. Cardiovascular disease risk prediction with and without knowledge of genetic variation at chromosome 9p21.3. *Ann Intern Med* 2009; 150: 65–72.

70 Herder C, Karakas M, Koenig W. Biomarkers for the prediction of type 2 diabetes and cardiovascular disease. *Nature* 2011; 90: 52–66.

71 Arnett DK, Baird AE, Barkley RA et al. Relevance of genetics and genomics for prevention and treatment of cardiovascular disease: A scientific statement from the American Heart Association Council on Epidemiology and Prevention, the Stroke Council, and the Functional Genomics and Translational Biology Interdisciplinary Working Group. *Circulation* 2007; 115: 2878–901.

72 Wang T. Multiple biomarkers for predicting cardiovascular events: Lessons learned. *J Am Coll Cardiol* 2010; 55: 2092–5.

Answer to Multiple-Choice Question for Case Study 1

1 D

HsCRP would be recommended in this situation since this patient has intermediate risk for CHD and is above 60 years of age (National Lipid Association recommendation). Consistent with the JUPITER trial, a hsCRP level >2.0 mg/L might warrant intensive risk-factor control in the form of statin therapy.

Answer to Multiple-Choice Question for Case Study 2

1 E

According to the ADA guidelines, this patient fulfills the criteria for statin therapy as he is above 40 years of age and has other risk factors. No further investigation is required for risk stratification.

CHAPTER 3
Kidney Disease in Diabetes

Amanda Y. Wang, Meg Jardine and Vlado Perkovic
The George Institute for Global Health, Sydney, NSW, Australia

---

Key Points

- Diabetic kidney disease is a complication of diabetes and affects 20–40% of people with diabetes.

- Diabetic kidney disease is characterized by increased urine albumin excretion (micro- or macroalbuminuria) and/or reduced kidney function in the absence of other causes for kidney disease.

- Hyperglycemia, hypertension, a genetic predisposition, smoking, and dyslipidemia are major risk factors for diabetic kidney disease.

- Early detection of diabetic kidney disease is crucial. Annual screening tests for urine albumin excretion and kidney function are recommended. Micro- and macro-albuminuria are risk factors for cardiovascular events, kidney failure, and death in people with diabetes.

- Reduced kidney function (glomerular filtration rate) is also a separate and independent risk factor for cardiovascular events, kidney failure, and death, and the additional risk is additive to that associated with increased urine albumin excretion.

- Coexisting hypertension accelerates the development of renal failure.

- Multifactorial approaches including optimization of blood glucose and blood pressure control, management of risk factors, and lifestyle modification can slow the progression of the kidney disease.

- Reno-protective agents targeting the renin-angiotensin-aldosterone system are the first-line therapy for reduction of microalbuminuria and blood pressure control.

- Glucose-lowering therapy should be tailored for individuals with diabetic kidney disease. Dose adjustment is required for most agents.

- Timely referral of CKD patients to a nephrologist is important for those with advanced or deteriorating diabetic kidney disease.

Definition

Kidney disease in diabetic patients can be caused by diabetes itself or other coexisting conditions such as hypertension or vascular disease. Diabetic kidney disease (or diabetes-associated chronic kidney disease)

Managing Cardiovascular Complications in Diabetes, First Edition.
Edited by D. John Betteridge and Stephen Nicholls.
© 2014 John Wiley & Sons, Ltd. Published 2014 by John Wiley & Sons, Ltd.

is a clinical diagnosis and is defined by the presence of albuminuria, often with associated abnormal kidney function (an increase in creatinine or a decrease in creatinine clearance or estimated glomerular filtration rate [eGFR]), in an appropriate clinical setting. A classic case would be a person with longstanding diabetes and coexistent diabetic retinopathy and/or neuropathy. Diabetic nephropathy is a histological diagnosis, characterized by typical histopathological features including mesangial expansion, glomerular basement membrane thickening, and glomerulosclerosis with Kimmelstiel–Wilson lesions. Diabetic kidney disease is most commonly caused by diabetic nephropathy, but other kidney pathologies may be present such as nephroangiosclerosis, atheromatous embolism, atherosclerotic renal artery disease, or glomerulonephritis.

As people with diabetic kidney disease are uncommonly biopsied unless there are clinical features suggesting a different diagnosis, most patients will not have a diagnosis of diabetic nephropathy confirmed. In this chapter, we will therefore focus on diabetic kidney disease.

Natural History and Courses of Diabetic Kidney Disease

Diabetic kidney disease is a chronic complication of diabetes and affects approximately one third of all diabetic patients [1, 2]. It is the most common cause of kidney failure requiring renal replacement therapy in Western countries [3] and can occur in both type 1 and type 2 diabetes with equivalent risks [4]. The natural history and prognosis of diabetic kidney disease differ somewhat based on the type of diabetes and whether microalbuminuria is present (Figure 3.1) [5]. In people with type 1 diabetes who have microalbuminuria, if left untreated, approximately 80% will develop macroalbuminuria (also called overt nephropathy) within 6–14 years [6, 7]. Subsequently, half of these will develop end-stage kidney disease (ESKD) over 10 years if there is still a lack of specific intervention. In contrast, approximately 20–40% of people with type 2 diabetes and microalbuminuria develop macroalbuminuria without intervention, and ESKD has been reported to develop in 20% of patients with overt nephropathy within 20 years [8]. Some of these differences may relate to the older age and greater burden of comorbidity experienced by people with type 2 diabetes for a given duration of diabetes, meaning that more of them will die of cardiovascular and other complications before developing kidney disease.

There are five stages of diabetic kidney disease: stage one has only functional changes and maintains normal glomerular structures, while stage

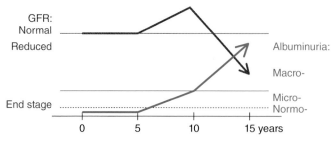

Figure 3.1 Natural history of nephropathy in diabetes. Microalbuminuria generally develops after between 5 and 15 years' duration of diabetes. There is a high chance of progression to macro albuminuria over the next 10 years. Sometime after the onset of clinical albuminuria, the GFR begins to fall, and a large proportion of patients reach ESKD by 20 years after the onset of clinical albuminuria.

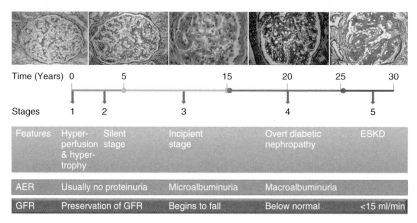

Figure 3.2 The course of diabetic nephropathy. (Source: Kidney Check Australia Taskforce, Chronic Kidney Disease and Diabetes, Workshop Module, 2013. Reproduced with permission of Kidney Health Australia.) (Color plate 3.1).

five is ESKD (Figure 3.2). Patients with diabetic kidney disease have a markedly increased risk of cardiovascular events and mortality [9].

Pathophysiology of Diabetic Nephropathy

Both hemodynamic and metabolic factors play important roles in the development of diabetic nephropathy. The early signs of diabetic nephropathy are glomerular hyperperfusion due to decreased resistance of afferent and efferent arterioles of the glomerulus. This functional change further leads to an activation of the renin-angiotensin-aldosterone system and endothelin, causing structural abnormalities in the kidneys.

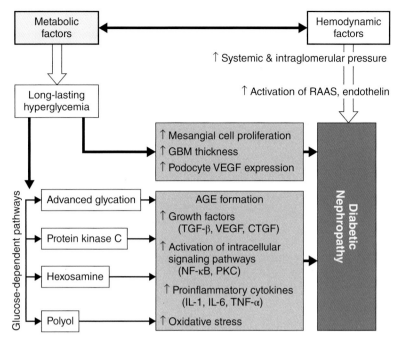

Figure 3.3 Metabolic factors in the pathogenesis of diabetic nephropathy. AGE: advanced glycation end product; CTGF: connective tissue growth factor; GBM: glomerular basement membrane; IL: interleukin; NF: nuclear factor; PKC: protein kinase C; RAAS: renin-angiotensin-aldosterone system; TGF: transforming growth factor; TNF: tumor necrosis factor; VEGF: vascular endothelial growth factor. (Source: Turgut 2010 [10]. Reproduced with permission of Elsevier.)

In addition, long-standing hyperglycemia directly induces mesangial expansion, thickening of the glomerular basement membrane (GBM), and an increase in podocyte vascular endothelial growth factor (VEGF) expression. Meanwhile, an activation of advanced glycation, protein kinase C, hexosamine, and polyol also contributes to the development of diabetic nephropathy. Damage to the glomerular filtration barrier (GFB) subsequently occurs, leading to increasing urinary protein levels, inflammation, fibrosis, and eventually glomerular filtration rate (GFR) reduction and kidney failure (Figure 3.3) [10].

Risk Factors for Diabetic Kidney Disease

The main risk factors for the development of diabetic kidney disease include hyperglycemia, arterial hypertension, smoking, dyslipidemia, race, and genetic predisposition.

Glycemic Control

Hyperglycemia is a significant risk factor for the development of microalbuminuria in both type 1 and type 2 diabetes [11, 12]. Patients with worse glycemic control are more likely to develop diabetic kidney disease, while a reduction of HbA1c by 1% is associated with a 37% decrease in microvascular endpoints [13, 14]. More recently, data from the ADVANCE trial [2] have suggested that intensive glucose control based on a sulfonylurea reduces the risk of kidney failure by two-thirds [15].

Hypertension

Prospective studies have noted an association between the development of diabetic kidney disease and higher blood pressures [16, 17]. UKPDS analysis demonstrated that every 10 mmHg reduction in systolic blood pressure (BP) is associated with a 13% decrease in the risk of microvascular complications, with the smallest risk among those patients with systolic BP <120 mmHg [18].

Smoking

Smoking increases albuminuria and might contribute to the progression of diabetic kidney disease [19]. It is also associated with an increased risk for cardiovascular events, including a decreased survival for people with kidney failure requiring dialysis.

Dyslipidemia

Dyslipidemia, as a well-established risk factor for cardiovascular disease, is strikingly common in patients with type 2 DM, affecting almost 50% of this population [20]. Dyslipidemia is associated with the development of diabetic kidney disease in both type 1 and type 2 diabetes. In type 1 DM, increased serum triglycerides, total and LDL-cholesterol were associated with micro- and macroalbuminuria [21, 22], and high serum cholesterol also appears to contribute to GFR loss [23]. In type 2 DM, dyslipidemia is mainly attributed to insulin resistance [24] and its presence increases the risk of renal impairment [12, 16].

Genetic Predisposition

Genetic factors also play a role in diabetic kidney disease. A number of studies have shown that the angiotensin-converting enzyme (ACE) gene genotype is a potential genetic risk factor. However, definitive genetic markers have yet to be identified.

Race

The incidence of diabetic kidney disease is three- to sixfold higher in black people compared to Caucasians. Mexican Americans and Pima Indians with type 2 diabetes are also more likely to develop diabetic kidney disease.

Clinical Manifestation

Diabetic kidney disease has a heterogeneous presentation. Early stages are often asymptomatic and only detected by abnormal laboratory tests (albuminuria and changes in GFR). Albuminuria is one of the earliest detectable features of diabetic kidney disease, with a prevalence of 25% after 10 years of diabetes [25], although reduced GFR in the absence of albuminuria/proteinuria is also recognized in an increasing proportion of type 2 diabetic patients [26]. Patients with diabetic kidney disease become symptomatic once the kidney disease is severe enough, causing uremic symptoms and hypertension [26].

As diabetes manifests as a systemic disease, patients with type 1 DM almost always have other signs of diabetic microvascular complications, such as retinopathy and neuropathy. Diabetic retinopathy usually precedes the onset of overt nephropathy, while the relationship between diabetic kidney disease and retinopathy is less predictable in type 2 diabetes. Type 2 diabetics with marked proteinuria and retinopathy most likely have diabetic nephropathy, while those without retinopathy have a high frequency of nondiabetic glomerular disease. Therefore, the K/DOQI guidelines suggest that chronic kidney disease should be attributed to diabetic nephropathies in most patients with diabetes if albuminuria and diabetic retinopathy are both present [27].

Screening and Diagnosis of Diabetic Kidney Disease (Algorithm 3.1)

As diabetic kidney disease is associated with poor outcomes, early diagnosis and subsequent intervention are essential to improve prognosis. Current guidelines recommended that diabetic patients should be screened for albuminuria and GFR at least annually. Both are used as independent but additive risk factors for CKD [28, 29, 30].

Urinary Albumin Excretion (UAE)

Microalbuminuria is the earliest marker of diabetic kidney disease [31, 32] detectable with widely available laboratory tests, and the presence of microalbuminuria is associated with increased risk of cardiovascular morbidity and mortality, as well as kidney failure, in both type 1 and type 2 diabetes. Patients with proteinuria have a 2.5-fold higher mortality rate than those without proteinuria [33], and hence current guidelines suggest that albuminuria changes are an important marker of CKD progression [34, 35].

There are three ways to screen for increased urine albumin excretion (UAE): measurement of the albumin to creatinine ratio (ACR) in a random

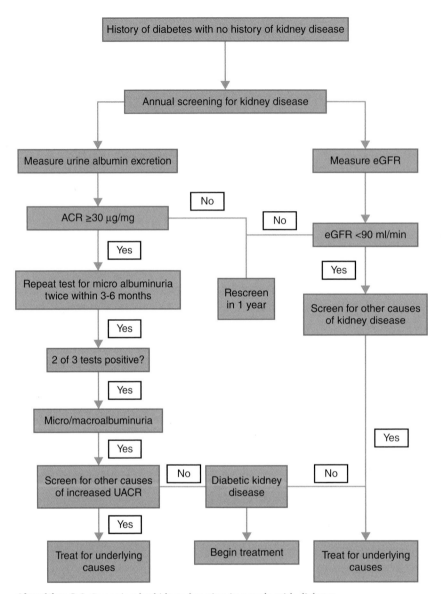

Algorithm 3.1 Screening for kidney function in people with diabetes.

spot urine collection, 24-hour urine collection, and timed (e.g., 4-hour or overnight) urine collection [36]. UAE is most easily assessed using a spot urine ACR, preferably a first morning void spot specimen, which has been shown to correlate well with more complicated urine collections. For people with type 1 diabetes, approximately 20–30% will have microalbuminuria after a mean duration of diabetes of 15 years [37, 38]. Similarly, 25% of individuals with type 2 diabetes have microalbuminuria after

Table 3.1 Classification of abnormal urinary albumin excretion. [31, 41, 42]

	24-hr urine albumin (mg/24 hr)	Overnight urine albumin (µg/24 hr)	Spot urine Albumin:creatinine ratio			Recommended follow-up
			Gender	mg/mmol	mg/g	
Normal	< 15	< 10	M	< 1.25	< 10	Every 1–2 years and annually for people with diabetes or hypertension
			F	< 1.75	< 15	
High normal	15 to < 30	10 to < 20	M	1.25 to < 2.5	10 to < 20	
			F	1.75 to < 3.5	15 to < 30	
Microalbuminuria	30 to < 300	20 to < 200	M	2.5 to < 25	20 to < 200	Repeat 2 times over 3–6 months Confirm microalbuminuria if 2 out of 3 tests are positive
			F	3.5 to < 35	30 to < 300	
Macroalbuminuria	> 300	> 200	M	> 25	> 200	Quantify urine protein excretion by 24 hours urine protein

10 years, according to UKPDS [25]. Transient elevation of UAE can be seen in hyperglycemia, vigorous physical exercise, urinary tract infections, marked hypertension, heart failure, acute febrile illnesses or systemic diseases, and hematuria [39]. Therefore, abnormal albuminuria tests should be confirmed in two of three samples collected at a three- to six-month interval [40] (Table 3.1).

Kidney function

The first manifestation of diabetic kidney disease is an increase in GFR due to hyperfiltration; however, this is difficult to detect using eGFR estimated from serum creatinine levels. People with diabetic kidney disease often develop reduced kidney function and, in fact, it can occur in the absence of albuminuria. Therefore, routine measurement of kidney function assessed by eGFR is also recommended as part of screening for diabetic kidney disease. The eGFR is derived from an estimating equation, taking serum creatinine, age, gender, body weight, and race into consideration. Normal GFR values for young individuals are 90 to 130 ml/min/l.73 m^2, with a steady fall with increasing age, in the order of 10 ml/min/decade after the age of 50 years [43]. Current guidelines classify chronic kidney

Table 3.2 Stages of chronic kidney disease. (Source: Levey et al. 2011 [42]. Reproduced with permission of Nature Publishing Group.)

Stage	Description	eGFR (mL/min/1.73 m^2)
1	Kidney damage with normal or ↑ eGFR plus persistent albuminuria	≥ 90
2	Kidney damage with mild ↓ eGFR plus persistent albuminuria	60–89
3	Moderate ↓ eGFR	30–59
4	Severe ↓ eGFR	15–29
5	Kidney failure	< 15 (or dialysis)

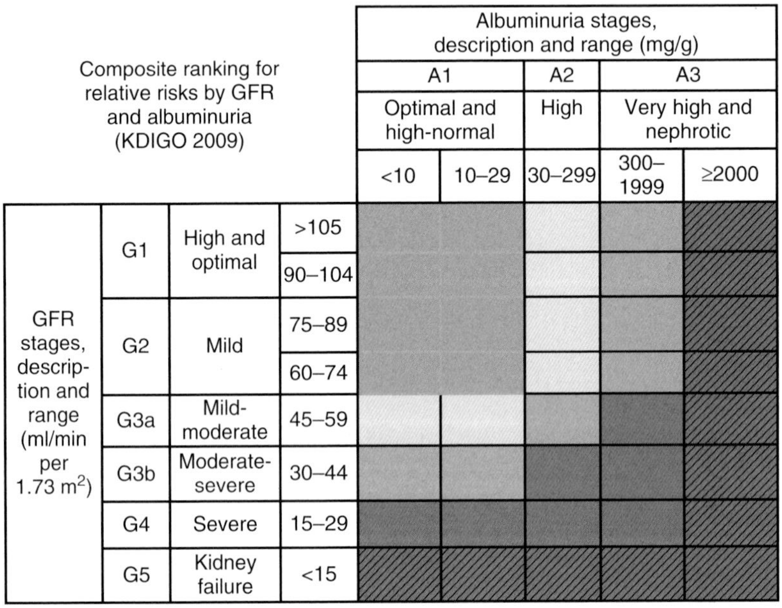

Figure 3.4 New classification of chronic kidney disease. Colors reflect the ranking of adjusted relative risk. The ranks were averaged across all five outcomes for the 28 GFR and albuminuria categories. The categories with mean rank numbers 1–8 are green, mean rank numbers 9–14 are yellow, mean rank numbers 15–21 are orange, and mean rank numbers 22–28 are red. Color for twelve additional cells with diagonal hash marks is extrapolated based on results from the meta-analysis of chronic kidney disease cohorts. The highest level of albuminuria is termed 'nephrotic' to correspond with nephrotic range albuminuria and is expressed here as > 2000 mg/g. column and row labels are combined to be consistent with the numbers of estimated GFR (eGFR) and albuminuria stages agreed on at the conference. (Source: Levey et al. 2011 [42]. Reproduced with permission of Nature Publishing Group.) (Color plate 3.2).

disease into five stages according to eGFR level and other markers of kidney disease, specifically albuminuria (Table 3.2 and Figure 3.4).

Decline of eGFR usually occurs in people with macroalbuminuria, but is less common in those with microalbuminuria. The eGFR may remain stable for years [44], but often declines with more advanced diabetic kidney disease [45].

Diabetic kidney disease is diagnosed by the presence of micro- or macro-albuminuria and/or reduced kidney function in the absence of other causes for kidney disease. Renal biopsy is usually not necessary, but may be considered in some situations to rule out important nondiabetic kidney diseases. Nondiabetic kidney disease was reported to occur in 12–38% of people with type 2 diabetes [46, 47] and should be considered in people with recent onset diabetes, acute onset of kidney disease, or clinical features suggesting another renal or systemic diagnosis.

Prognosis of Diabetic Kidney Disease

Proteinuria and abnormal kidney function are independent risk factors for renal outcomes in diabetes [28]. Diabetic kidney disease is the leading cause of ESKD requiring renal replacement therapy.

There is also an increasing recognition that diabetic kidney disease is a potent risk factor for cardiovascular disease, and is associated with an increased risk of cardiovascular morbidity and mortality [9]. Kidney disease also predicts a worse prognosis after a cardiovascular event. The US Renal Data System reported that the two-year mortality rate after a myocardial infarction (MI) was 44% among patients without CKD, compared with 58% in patients with stage 3 CKD and 68% in those with stage 4–5 CKD. Survival of patients with diabetic kidney disease is to a large extent determined by cardiovascular comorbidities.

Management of Diabetic Kidney Disease

The goal of managing diabetic kidney disease is not only to slow the progression of albuminuria and the decline of kidney function, but also to reduce the risk of cardiovascular complications. The treatment principle is a holistic approach, involving multiple and intensive strategies (Algorithm 3.2).

Lifestyle Modification

Weight reduction, dietary salt restriction, DASH diet (fruits, vegetables, low-fat and low-calorie diet) [48], physical activity, and moderate alcohol consumption all have been shown to reduce systolic blood pressure by 5–20 mmHg. Weight loss has also been associated with a significant reduction in microalbuminuria in obese diabetic patients [49]. These lifestyle changes should therefore be recommended to all people with diabetic kidney disease.

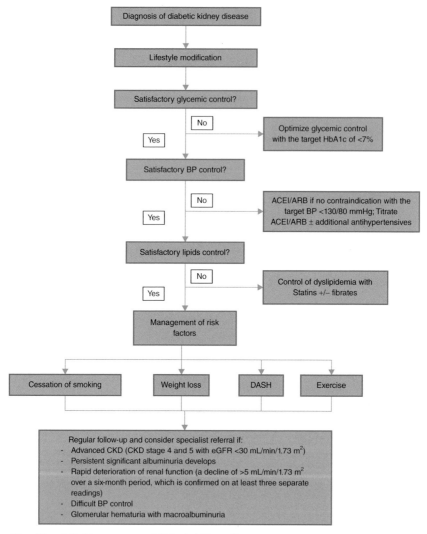

Algorithm 3.2 Management of diabetic kidney disease.

Glycemic Control

An accumulative body of literature has shown that intensive glycemic control reduces the risk of microalbuminuria, and slows the progression of diabetic retinopathy and neuropathy in both type 1 and type 2 DM (Table 3.3) [13, 50, 51, 52]. For example, the DCCT and UKPDS illustrated that lower HbA1c values were associated with a lower risk of developing microvascular complications, including CKD [13, 52]. Furthermore, the UKPDS follow-up study found that the risk reduction for microvascular and macrovascular complications associated with tight glycemic control

Table 3.3 Clinical trials for effect of glycemic control on diabetic nephropathy.

Name	Abbreviation	Conclusion
Type 1 DM		
The Diabetes Control and Complications Trial	DCCT [53]	Intensive diabetes therapy can significantly reduce the risk of the development of microalbuminuria and overt nephropathy in people with diabetes.
The Stockholm Diabetes Intervention Study	SDIS [54]	Compared with regular treatment, intensified conventional treatment significantly reduced HbA1c level. Less retinopathy and progression of microalbuminuria was observed in ICT group, but at the expense of an increased frequency of serious hypoglycemia.
Type 2 DM		
The United Kingdom Prospective Diabetes Study	UKPDS [51]	Intensive glucose control can significantly reduce the risk of the development of microalbuminuria and overt nephropathy in people with diabetes.
The Kumatomo Study	Ohkubo [55]	Intensive glycemic control by administering multiple insulin injection delayed the onset of diabetic retinopathy, nephropathy, and neuropathy in Japanese patients with type 2 diabetes.
Action in Diabetes and Vascular Disease: Preterax and Diamicron Modified-Release Controlled Evaluation	ADVANCE [14]	There were clinical benefits (reduced microvascular outcomes and ESKD) with no harm (with respect to CVD or mortality) of intensive control (HbA1c target of ≤6.5%) versus conventional control (HbA1c target defined by local guidelines).
The Veterans Affairs Diabetes Trial	VADT [56]	The incidence of CVD events was not significantly lower in the intensive arm. Post hoc subgroup analyses suggested that duration of diabetes interacted with randomization such that participants with duration of diabetes less than about 12 years appeared to have a CVD benefit of intensive glycemic control, while those with longer duration of disease before study entry had a neutral or even adverse effect of intensive glycemic control.
Action to Control Cardiovascular Risk in Diabetes	ACCORD [57]	The primary outcome (MI, stroke, or cardiovascular death) was reduced in the intensive glycemic control group due to a reduction in nonfatal MI, although this finding was not statistically significant. However, the study was terminated early due to increased mortality in the intensive arm caused by severe hypoglycemia.

in T2DM patients extended beyond the period of intensive therapy. Most recently, the Action in Diabetes and Vascular Disease: Preterax and Diamicron Modified-Release Controlled Evaluation (ADVANCE) trial [2] compared the effect of an intensive glucose-lowering strategy based on gliclazide MR (HbA1c target ≤6.5%) versus standard glucose control on renal outcome. After a median of five years, intensive glucose control reduced the risk of ESRD by 65%, microalbuminuria by 9%, macroalbuminuria by 30%, and progression of albuminuria. These results suggest that improved glucose control will prevent major kidney outcomes in people with type 2 diabetes.

In addition, patients with diabetic kidney disease are at increased risk of hypoglycemia. Hypoglycemia can lead to serious outcomes including coronary ischemia, cardiac arrhythmia, and sudden death [58]. The causes for the increased risk of Hypoglycemia in people with diabetic kidney disease are likely to be multifactorial, including decreased clearance of medications, prolonged half-life of insulin, and impaired kidney gluco-neogenesis. New classes of antihyperglycemic agents, such as dipeptidyl peptidase 4 (DPP-4) inhibitors, are likely to require dose reduction in patients with renal impairment due to accumulation and possibly an increased risk of hypoglycemia, although linagliptin is hepatically excreted and does not require dose adjustment. Therefore, greater care with monitoring and selection of glucose-lowering agents is necessary in this group of patients [59].

Selection of Glucose-Lowering Agents in Patients with Diabetic Kidney Disease

Some of the most widely used oral glucose-lowering agents, including metformin (due to an increased risk of lactic acidosis) and some sulfony-lureas, are not suitable in patients with moderate to severe chronic kidney disease. A proposed recommendation for use of metformin based on eGFR [60] stated that metformin can be used if eGFR is between 45 and 60 mL/min per $1.73\,m^2$, but renal function should be monitored closely (every three to six months). Dose reduction for metformin is considered if eGFR is 30–45 mL/min per $1.73\,m^2$, and renal function should be monitored closely (every three months). Metformin should be stopped once eGFR is below 30 mL/min per $1.73\,m^2$.

An individualized approach to treatment should be adopted, taking into account the degree of renal impairment and the need for dose adjustment [61, 61, 63]. Insulin is the mainstay of treatment in type 2 DM patients with advanced CKD. Several of the meglitinides can be used in mild to moderate CKD, and mitiglinide does not need dose adjustment for moderate to severe CKD [64]. Newer agents, dipeptidyl peptidase 4 (DPP-4) inhibitors, most notably linagliptin, may have a role to play in the management of type 2

Table 3.4 Recommendations for noninsulin hyperglycemic drug therapy for patients with moderate to severe CKD. [66, 67, 68, 69, 70]

Class	Drug	Dosing recommendation in moderate to severe CKD	Complication
Second generation of sulfonylurea	Glipizide Gliclazide	Contraindicated when GFR <30 ml/min	Hypoglycemia
Biguanide	Metformin	Contraindicated when GFR <30 ml/min	Lactic acidosis
α-glucosidase inhibitors	Acarbose	Not recommended when serum Creatinine >2 mg/dl	Hepatic toxicity
Thiazolidinediones	Rosiglitazone Pioglitazone	No dose adjustment	Volume retention, CHF
Meglitinides	Mitiglinides	No dose adjustment	Hypoglycemia
Incretin mimetics (GLP1 analogue)	Exenatide	Contraindicated when GFR <30 ml/min	Gastrointestinal discomfort, hypoglycemia
DPP4 inhibitors	Sitagliptin	Reduce dose by 50% when GFR <50 mL/min; by 75% (25 mg/day) when GFR <30 mL/min	? Nil

DM in patients with renal impairment (Table 3.4). A recent randomized clinical trial showed that linagliptin has antiproteinuric efficacy in people with type 2 diabetes and proteinuria [65]. Linagliptin significantly lowered adjusted UACR by 33% with no significant short-term effect on kidney function and blood pressure. Detailed information on the management of glycemia in diabetes is covered in Chapter 7.

Blood Pressure Control in Diabetic Kidney Disease [71, 72]

Blood pressure control in patients with diabetes and CKD may reduce the risk of progressive loss of kidney function, CVD, and progression of diabetic retinopathy. In the United Kingdom Prospective Diabetes Study (UKPDS) [51] comparing intensive with less intensive blood pressure control, intensive control led to a 32% reduction in mortality, predominantly from cardiovascular disease but also from a decrease in microalbuminuria. The effect of lowering blood pressure on delaying the progression of renal failure was investigated in the ADVANCE study [73]. Compared with placebo, the combination of perindopril and indapamide reduced the risk for renal events by 21% in type 2 diabetic patients, which was attributed to a reduction in risks for developing microalbuminuria and macroalbuminuria.

A recent systematic review [71] showed that intensive blood pressure control reduced the risk of albuminuria progression by approximately 10% and kidney failure by 27%, and there is also a trend toward benefit for retinopathy (Figure 3.5). Therefore, current Kidney Disease-Improving Global Outcomes (KDIGO) guidelines recommended that blood pressure-lowering therapy should be commenced if BP>140/90 mmHg in people with diabetes and coexisting CKD who have a urine albumin excretion <30 mg per 24 hours, with a target blood pressure of <140 mmHg systolic and <90 mmHg diastolic (1B) [27]. More intensive blood pressure control is required for patients with micro- or macro-albuminuria of >30 mg per 24 hours; blood pressure-lowering therapy should be commenced at a blood pressure above 130/80 mmHg with a target blood pressure of <130 mmHg systolic and <80 mmHg diastolic (2D). BP should be monitored at least six-monthly in all people with diabetes, and more frequent follow-up is recommended if micro- or macro-albuminuria develops [74].

Blood pressure control in diabetes often requires multiple blood pressure-lowering agents. The KDIGO guidelines recommend an ARB or ACEI be used as first-line therapy in adults with CKD and diabetes with high blood pressure [27]. RAAS blockade has reno-protective effects and provides additional benefits in diabetes with micro- or macro-albuminuria. Captopril [75], when used in microalbuminuric type 1 diabetic patients, can slow the progression of CKD. More pronounced beneficial effects were observed in overt nephropathy, especially with baseline creatinine levels above 132 umol/L. The effect of ACEI in type 2 diabetic patients has been less well studied. A recent systematic review found that ACEI prevented new-onset diabetic kidney disease and death in normoalbuminuric people with diabetes [72]. Compared with placebo, ACEI reduced the risk of new onset of microalbuminuria, macroalbuminuria, or both.

Control of Albuminuria in Diabetes

The presence of micro- or macro-albuminuria in diabetes is associated with increased risk of kidney failure and cardiovascular events. The KDIGO guidelines recommend ACEIs and ARBs as first-line therapy in patients with diabetic and CKD with urine albumin excretion of 30 to 300 mg per 24 hours (2D). A systematic review [76] assessed the effects of ACEI or ARB on mortality and renal outcomes in diabetic kidney disease, and showed survival benefits for ACEI but not ARB for patients with diabetic kidney disease (Figure 3.6). There is also strong evidence that ACEI and ARB prevent the progression of microalbuminuria to macroalbuminuria and kidney failure (Figure 3.7). Furthermore, a systematic review [77] including 85 randomized controlled trials demonstrated that ACEI and ARB both reduced the progression of microalbuminuria to macroalbuminuria and the development of end-stage kidney disease, as well as nonfatal cardiovascular mortality. However, the effects of combining ACEI and ARB with each other or with renin inhibitors remain uncertain, with the

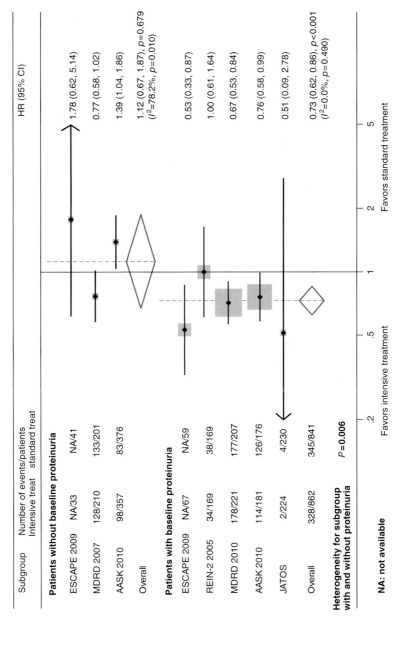

Figure 3.5 The effect of intensive blood pressure lowering on kidney failure between patients with or without proteinuria. (Source: Lv et al. 2012 [71].)

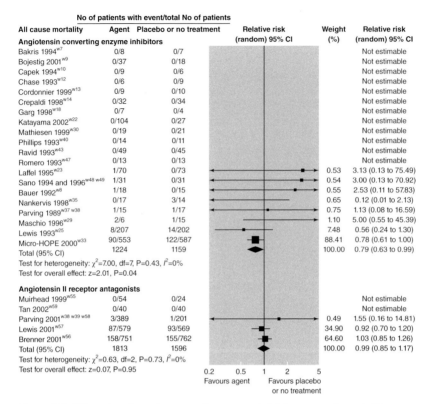

Figure 3.6 Effect of angiotensin-converting enzyme inhibitors or angiotensin II receptor antagonists compared with placebo or no treatment on overall mortality. (Source: Strippoli et al. 2004 [76]. Reproduced with permission of BMJ Publishing Group Ltd.)

balance of currently available evidence suggesting likely harm [78]. At this time, single-agent RAAS blockade is therefore recommended.

Dyslipidemia
Statins

Both statin and fibrates therapy have been investigated for potential reno-protective effects (Table 3.5). A systematic review demonstrated that statin therapy significantly reduced lipid concentrations and cardiovascular endpoints in patients with chronic kidney disease [79].

Post hoc analyses demonstrated beneficial effects of statin therapy on renal function in diabetic patients with CKD and CVD [80, 83]. In the Heart Protection Study, simvastatin improved renal function in patients with type 2 diabetes [80]. However, its mechanism of action remains unclear [80].

The SHARP trial [84] investigated the lipid-lowering effect of a combination of simvastatin and ezetimibe versus placebo in patients with chronic

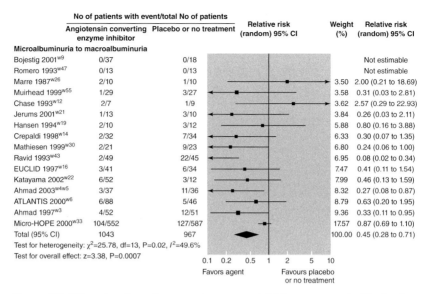

	No of patients with event/total No of patients		Relative risk (random) 95% CI	Weight (%)	Relative risk (random) 95% CI
	Angiotensin converting enzyme inhibitor	Placebo or no treatment			
Microalbuminuria to macroalbuminuria					
Bojestig 2001[w9]	0/37	0/18			Not estimable
Romero 1993[w47]	0/13	0/13			Not estimable
Marre 1987[w26]	2/10	1/10		3.50	2.00 (0.21 to 18.69)
Muirhead 1999[w55]	1/29	3/27		3.58	0.31 (0.03 to 2.81)
Chase 1993[w12]	2/7	1/9		3.62	2.57 (0.29 to 22.93)
Jerums 2001[w21]	1/13	3/10		3.84	0.26 (0.03 to 2.11)
Hansen 1994[w19]	2/10	3/12		5.88	0.80 (0.16 to 3.88)
Crepaldi 1998[w14]	2/32	7/34		6.33	0.30 (0.07 to 1.35)
Mathiesen 1999[w30]	2/21	9/23		6.80	0.24 (0.06 to 1.00)
Ravid 1993[w43]	2/49	22/45		6.95	0.08 (0.02 to 0.34)
EUCLID 1997[w16]	3/41	6/34		7.47	0.41 (0.11 to 1.54)
Katayama 2002[w22]	6/52	3/12		7.99	0.46 (0.13 to 1.59)
Ahmad 2003[w4w5]	3/37	11/36		8.32	0.27 (0.08 to 0.87)
ATLANTIS 2000[w6]	6/88	5/46		8.79	0.63 (0.20 to 1.95)
Ahmad 1997[w3]	4/52	12/51		9.36	0.33 (0.11 to 0.95)
Micro-HOPE 2000[w33]	104/552	127/587		17.57	0.87 (0.69 to 1.10)
Total (95% CI)	1043	967		100.00	0.45 (0.28 to 0.71)

Test for heterogeneity: χ^2=25.78, df=13, P=0.02, I^2=49.6%

Test for overall effect: z=3.38, P=0.0007

0.1 0.2 0.5   1   2   5 10

Favors agent   Favours placebo or no treatment

Figure 3.7 Effect of angiotensin-converting enzyme inhibitors compared with placebo or no treatment on risk of progression from microalbuminuria to macroalbuminuria. (Source: Strippoli et al. 2004 [76]. Reproduced with permission of BMJ Publishing Group Ltd.)

kidney disease, including people with diabetes. It demonstrated that combined therapy reduced average LDL cholesterol with no excess side effects, and lowered the risk of major cardiovascular events by 17%, with similar effects in people with and without diabetes, but had no effect on kidney function. As a result, lipid lowering is now routinely recommended in people with kidney disease.

Fibrates

The Diabetes Atherosclerosis Intervention Study (DAIS) [82] studied the effect of fibrates. Compared with placebo, fenofibrate significantly reduced microalbuminuria in addition to improving the lipid profile in type 2 diabetes. The effect of fenofibrate on reduction in microalbuminuria might be attributed to suppression of inflammation, decreased production of type 1 collagen in mesangial cells, and increased activity of peroxisome proliferator-activated receptor (PPAR)-alpha [85, 86]. The FIELD study [87] assessed the long-term effect of fenofibrates on cardiovascular events in patients with type 2 diabetes. Fenofibrate therapy was associated with a reduction in total cardiovascular events, less albuminuria progression, and less retinopathy needing laser treatment. A recent systematic review examined the effect of fibrates on kidney disease [88]. Overall, fibrate therapy reduced total cholesterol and triglycerides, and increased HDL level in patients with mild to moderate chronic kidney disease. In addition,

Table 3.5 Clinical trials for effect of lipid-lowering agents on diabetic nephropathy.

Name	Abbreviation	Conclusion
Study of Heart and Renal protection	SHARP	Compared with either placebo or simvastatin alone, ezetimibe in combination with simvastatin was not associated with any excess of myopathy, hepatic toxicity, or biliary complications during the first year of follow-up. Compared with placebo, combination therapy reduced average LDL cholesterol by 43 mg/dL (1.10 mmol/L) at 1 year and 33 mg/dL (0.85 mmol/L) at 2.5 years.
The Scandinavian Simvastatin Survival Study	4S	The lipid-lowering effects were similar in diabetic and nondiabetic groups. Simvastatin improves the prognosis of diabetic patients with CHD.
Fenofibrate Intervention and Event Lowering in Diabetes	FIELD	Fenofibrate therapy was associated with a reduction in total cardiovascular events, less albuminuria progression, and less retinopathy needing laser treatment.
Heart Protection Study	HPS [80]	Simvastatin 40 mg daily decreased vascular event rates and GFR decline in diabetic patients by 25%, independent of baseline cholesterol levels.
Collaborative Atorvastatin Diabetes Study	CARDS [81]	Statins reduced cardiovascular events in DM patients, and atorvastatin showed a moderate beneficial effect on eGFR, particular in those with albuminuria.
Diabetes Atherosclerosis Intervention Study	DAIS [82]	Compared with placebo, fenofibrate significantly reduced microalbuminutia in addition to lower lipid profile in type 2 diabetes.

fibrates reduced the risk of major cardiovascular events and cardiovascular death, but not all-cause mortality. Subgroup analysis showed that in people with diabetes, fibrates reduced the risk of albuminuria progression at the expense of an elevation in serum creatinine and a reduction in calculated GFR. However, no effect on the risk of end-stage kidney disease was detected.

Multifactorial Approach

The Steno-2 study showed that in type 2 DM, intensive combined therapy, including BSL and BP control as well as lipid lowering, is likely to be the optimal therapeutic approach to patients with diabetes, demonstrating a reduction in cardiovascular but not renal events (Table 3.6).

Referral to a Nephrologist

The early stage of diabetic kidney disease can be managed by a primary care physician; however, referral to a nephrologist is recommended when advanced CKD (CKD stage 4 and 5 with eGFR $<30 \, mL/min/1.73 \, m^2$) and/or persistent macro-albuminuria develops. Nephrological input is

Table 3.6 Clinical trials on multifactorial approaches for diabetic nephropathy.

Name	Conclusion
Steno type 2 trial [89, 90]	The intensive regimen consisted of behavioral therapy (including advice concerning diet, exercise, and smoking cessation) and pharmacologic intervention (consisting of the administration of an ACE inhibitor and multiple other agents to attain several aggressive therapeutic goals). Intensive therapy reduced both microvascular and macrovascular disease. Significant improvements in albumin excretion (−20 versus +30 mg/day) and in progression to overt nephropathy.
Manto A [91]	Treatment consisted of an intensive insulin regimen (which lowered the hemoglobin A1c concentration from 8.7 to 6.5%), dietary protein restriction, and antihypertensive therapy with an ACE inhibitor (which lowered the blood pressure to 120/75). At the end of three years, the glomerular filtration rate had increased to 84 mL/min and albumin excretion had fallen to 92 mg/day.

also recommended for patients with rapid deterioration of renal function (a decline of $>5\,mL/min/1.73\,m^2$ over a six-month period, which is confirmed on at least three separate readings), difficult BP control, or glomerular hematuria.

Treatment Options for ESKD Caused by Diabetic Kidney Disease

As with treatment strategies for end-stage kidney disease secondary to other causes, dialysis and renal transplantation are both options for treatment for ESKD caused by diabetes. Lower survival rates have been observed for people with ESKD caused by diabetic kidney disease, with five years' survival of 30%, according to USRDS data. Cardiovascular disease remains the most common cause of death, accounting for 50% of cases.

Conclusion

Diabetic kidney disease is a common complication of diabetes mellitus and is associated with increased cardiovascular morbidity and mortality. Its early detection with regular surveillance of albuminuria and GFR and prompt intervention is crucial to retard the progression and reduce the risk of renal and cardiovascular complications. Multifaceted approaches including lifestyle modification, optimizing blood glucose and blood pressure levels, and lipid lowering are recommended to minimize cardiovascular risk, slow the progression of kidney disease, and reduce mortality. Renin-angiotensin-aldosterone blockade provides additional reno-protective effects and should be first-line therapy for diabetic kidney disease.

Case Study 1

A 70-year-old Caucasian male was referred by his family doctor for further investigation of proteinuria and renal impairment. His medical history includes type 2 diabetes (10 years), transient ischemic attack, gastro-oesophageal reflux disease, and osteoarthritis of the knees. The patient is currently receiving Glargine 10 units daily, Metformin 500 mg three times a day, aspirin 100 mg daily, Pantoprazole 40 mg daily, and paracetamol 1 g three times a day. His family history is significant for type 2 diabetes on his paternal side. His father died of heart attack at age of 65. He is a retired businessman who has lived with his wife for 46 years. He is an ex-smoker and stopped smoking 20 years ago. He consumes two standard drinks a day.

On examination, he was alert and orientated, and obese with a BMI of 31. His BP was 150/80 mmHg and pulse was 75 beats per minute. The respiratory and cardiovascular examination was unremarkable. The abdomen was soft and nontender. There was no peripheral edema. Neurological examination revealed glove-stoking sensory loss. Fundoscopy showed moderate nonproliferative retinopathy, consistent with diabetic retinopathy.

Laboratory parameters showed normal electrolytes. The urea was 12 mmol/L and serum creatinine was 130 mmol/L, corresponding to an eGFR of 52 ml/min. Urine analysis showed protein +++, with an inactive sediment. Urine albumin/creatinine ratio (ACR) was 35 mg/g, consistent with microalbuminuria. The renal tract ultrasound showed kidney sizes of 11 cm bilaterally and there was no urinary tract obstruction. HbA1c was 8.0%, fasting blood sugar level (BSL) was 9.5 mmol/L, and two hours postprandial BSL was 14 mmol/L.

Multiple-Choice Questions

1 The most likely diagnosis for the kidney disease in this patient is:
   A He has hypertensive glomerulosclerosis
   B He has confirmed diabetic nephropathy
   C He has diabetic kidney disease, most likely due to diabetic nephropathy
   D A kidney biopsy is essential
   E The most likely diagnosis is focal segmental glomerulonephritis

2 What is the most appropriate treatment? (There can be more than one option.)
   A Optimize glycemic control
   B Optimize blood pressure control
   C Commence corticosteroids
   D Refer to a hematologist
   E Monitor renal function and refer to a nephrologist if kidney function declines

Answers provided after the References

> ### Case Study 2
>
> A 65-year-old Chinese woman was brought into the hospital by ambulance after being found unconscious at home. Her Glasgow Coma Score (GCS) was 3 on arrival. She was afebrile, BP was 90/60 mmHg, and pulse rate was 60 per minute. She appeared dehydrated. The physical examination was unremarkable except for bronchial breath sounds and crackles at the right lower lobe.
>
> Her past medical history was significant for type 2 diabetes mellitus (15 years) and asthma (20 years). Her regular medications were Gliclazide MR 120 mg daily, Metformin 500 mg tds, Fluticasone propionate/salmeterol xinafoate inhaler 250/25 mg twice a day, and Salbutamol inhaler as prn. She is single and lives alone at home, independently managing her activities of daily living. She is a nonsmoker and a social drinker. She has not visited her general practitioner for about five years; the last blood and urine tests were performed five years ago, and were unremarkable.
>
> Her blood gas showed profound metabolic acidosis with PH 7.25, PaO_2 90 mmHg and $PaCO_2$ 40 mmHg. Her serum bicarbonate was 13 mmol/L with a base excess of -10 mmol/L. The lactate was 5 mmol/L. The blood biochemistry showed a sodium of 150 mmol/L and potassium of 6.5 mmol/L. The urea was 34 mmol/L and creatinine was 515 mmol/L. The blood glucose was 4.5 mmol/L and creatinine kinase was normal. Her hematological parameters were unremarkable except for leukocytosis with a white cell count of 18×10^9/ml. Chest X-ray demonstrated right lower lobe consolidation.
>
> She was intubated and Metformin and Perindopril were ceased on admission. She was hydrated with intravenous normal saline and treated with Ceftriaxone and Azithromycin for presumed community-acquired pneumonia. Hyperkalemia was treated with medical therapy including glucose and insulin, and calcium gluconate. However, she was anuric and therefore continuous venous-venous hemodialysis (CVVHD) was commenced at the intensive care unit. She was clinically progressing well and was extubated on day 3 ICU admission. She was successfully able to come off CVVHD on day 5 and started urinating thereafter.

Multiple-Choice Questions

1 The most likely diagnosis for the kidney disease in this patient is:

   A Acute renal injury due to metformin induced nephrotoxicity

   B Rapid progressive glomerulonephritis (RPGN)

   C Acute on chronic kidney disease secondary to underlying diabetic kidney disease

   D Acute kidney injury due to dehydration

   E Acute kidney injury due to sepsis

2 In order to confirm the diagnosis, what would you do next? (There can be more than one option.)

   A Serum and urine electrophoresis

   B 24 hours' urine protein measurement and urine albumin/creatinine ratio (ACR)

   C Bone marrow biopsy

   D Renal biopsy if renal function rapidly deteriorates

   E Light chain assay

Answers provided after the References

Guidelines and Web Links

http://www.kidney.org/professionals/kdoqi/guideline_diabetes

European guidelines for diabetes and chronic kidney disease.

Inzucchi SE, Bergenstal RM, Buse JB et al. Management of hyperglycemia in type 2 diabetes: A patient-centered approach: Position statement of the American Diabetes Association (ADA) and the European Association for the Study of Diabetes (EASD). *Diabetes Care* 2012; 35(6): 1364–79. Epub Apri 21.

KDOQI Clinical Practice Guidelines and Clinical Practice Recommendations for Diabetes and Chronic Kidney Disease.

References

1 Cameron AJ, Welborn TA, Zimmet PZ et al. Overweight and obesity in Australia: The 1999–2000 Australian Diabetes, Obesity and Lifestyle Study (AusDiab). *Med J Aust* 2003; 178(9): 427–32. Epub May 2.

2 Perkovic V, Heerspink HJL, Chalmers J et al. Intensive glucose control improves kidney outcomes: The impact of endpoint definition on the results of the ADVANCE trial. *Kidney Int* (in press). 2012.

3 Rossert J. Le patient diabetique: un insuffisant renal comme les autres? [The diabetic patient: Renal insufficiency like other kidney failures?]. *Nephrol Ther* 2006; 2(Suppl 3): S187–9. Epub March 21.

4 Held PJ, Port FK, Webb RL et al. The United States Renal Data System's 1991 annual data report: An introduction. *Am J Kidney Dis* 1991; 18(5 Suppl 2): 1–16. Epub November 1.

5 Nielsen S, Schmitz A, Rehling M, Mogensen CE. The clinical course of renal function in NIDDM patients with normo- and microalbuminuria. *J Intern Med* 1997; 241(2): 133–41. Epub February 1.

6 Mogensen CE, Christensen CK. Predicting diabetic nephropathy in insulin-dependent patients. *New Eng J Med* 1984; 311(2): 89–93. Epub July 12.

7 Parving HH, Oxenboll B, Svendsen PA, Christiansen JS, Andersen AR. Early detection of patients at risk of developing diabetic nephropathy: A longitudinal study of urinary albumin excretion. *Acta Endocrinol (Copenh)* 1982; 100(4): 550–55. Epub August 1.

8 Koro CE, Lee BH, Bowlin SJ. Antidiabetic medication use and prevalence of chronic kidney disease among patients with type 2 diabetes mellitus in the United States. *Clin Ther* 2009; 31(11): 2608–17. Epub January 30.

9 Groop PH, Thomas MC, Moran JL et al. The presence and severity of chronic kidney disease predicts all-cause mortality in type 1 diabetes. *Diabetes* 2009; 58(7): 1651–8. Epub April 30.

10 Turgut F, Bolton WK. Potential new therapeutic agents for diabetic kidney disease. *Am J Kidney Dis* 2010; 55(5): 928–40. Epub February 9.

11 Marshall SM, Collins A, Gregory W et al. Predictors of the development of microalbuminuria in patients with type 1 diabetes mellitus: A seven-year prospective study. The Microalbuminuria Collaborative Study Group. *Diabetic Med* 1999; 16: 918–25.

12 Gall MA, Hougaard P, Borch-Johnsen K, Parving HH. Risk factors for development of incipient and overt diabetic nephropathy in patients with non-insulin dependent diabetes mellitus: Prospective, observational study. *Brit Med J* 1997; 314(7083): 783–8. Epub March 15.

13 Stratton IM, Adler AI, Neil HA et al. Association of glycaemia with macrovascular and microvascular complications of type 2 diabetes (UKPDS 35): Prospective observational study. *Brit Med J* 2000; 321(7258): 405–12. Epub August 11.

14 Patel A, MacMahon S, Chalmers J et al. Intensive blood glucose control and vascular outcomes in patients with type 2 diabetes. *New Eng J Med* 2008; 358(24): 2560–72. Epub June 10.

15 Perkovic V, Heerspink HL, Chalmers J et al. Intensive glucose control improves kidney outcomes in patients with type 2 diabetes. *Kidney Int.* 2013; 83(3): 517–23. Epub November 1.

16 Ravid M, Brosh D, Ravid-Safran D, Levy Z, Rachmani R. Main risk factors for nephropathy in type 2 diabetes mellitus are plasma cholesterol levels, mean blood pressure, and hyperglycemia. *Arch Intern Med* 1998; 158(9): 998–1004. Epub May 20.

17 Park JY, Kim HK, Chung YE, Kim SW, Hong SK, Lee KU. Incidence and determinants of microalbuminuria in Koreans with type 2 diabetes. *Diabetes Care* 1998; 21(4): 530–34. Epub May 8.

18 Adler AI, Stratton IM, Neil HA et al. Association of systolic blood pressure with macrovascular and microvascular complications of type 2 diabetes (UKPDS 36): Prospective observational study. *Brit Med J* 2000; 321(7258): 412–19. Epub August 11.

19 Sawicki PT, Didjurgeit U, Muhlhauser I, Bender R, Heinemann L, Berger M. Smoking is associated with progression of diabetic nephropathy. *Diabetes Care* 1994; 17(2): 126–31. Epub February 1.

20 Saydah SH, Fradkin J, Cowie CC. Poor control of risk factors for vascular disease among adults with previously diagnosed diabetes. *JAMA* 2004; 291(3): 335–42. Epub January 22.

21 Chaturvedi N, Fuller JH, Taskinen MR. Differing associations of lipid and lipoprotein disturbances with the macrovascular and microvascular complications of type 1 diabetes. *Diabetes Care* 2001; 24(12): 2071–7. Epub November 28.

22 Jenkins AJ, Lyons TJ, Zheng D et al. Lipoproteins in the DCCT/EDIC cohort: Associations with diabetic nephropathy. *Kidney Int* 2003; 64(3): 817–28. Epub August 13.

23 Mulec H, Johnsen SA, Wiklund O, Bjorck S. Cholesterol: A renal risk factor in diabetic nephropathy? *Am J Kidney Dis* 1993; 22(1): 196–201. Epub July 1.

24 Adiels M, Olofsson SO, Taskinen MR, Boren J. Diabetic dyslipidaemia. *Curr Opin Lipidol* 2006; 17(3): 238–46. Epub May 9.

25 Adler AI, Stevens RJ, Manley SE, Bilous RW, Cull CA, Holman RR. Development and progression of nephropathy in type 2 diabetes: The United Kingdom Prospective Diabetes Study (UKPDS 64). *Kidney Int* 2003; 63(1): 225–32. Epub December 11, 2002.

26 Ritz E, Zeng XX, Rychlik I. Clinical manifestation and natural history of diabetic nephropathy. *Contrib Nephrol* 2011; 170: 19–27. Epub June 11.

27 KDIGO Clinical Practice Guideline for the Management of Blood Pressure in Chronic Kidney Disease. *Kidney Int Supp.* 2012; 2(5): 337–414.

28 Ninomiya T, Perkovic V, de Galan BE et al. Albuminuria and kidney function independently predict cardiovascular and renal outcomes in diabetes. *J Am Soc Nephrol* 2009; 20(8): 1813–21. Epub May 16.

29 Heerspink HJ, Holtkamp FA, de Zeeuw D, Ravid M. Monitoring kidney function and albuminuria in patients with diabetes. *Diabetes Care* 2011; 34(Suppl 2): S325–9. Epub May 6.

30 Go AS, Chertow GM, Fan D, McCulloch CE, Hsu CY. Chronic kidney disease and the risks of death, cardiovascular events, and hospitalization. *New Eng J Med* 2004; 351(13): 1296–305. Epub September 24.

31 de Jong PE, Curhan GC. Screening, monitoring, and treatment of albuminuria: Public health perspectives. *J Am Soc Nephrol* 2006; 17(8): 2120–26. Epub July 11.

32 Weir MR. Microalbuminuria and cardiovascular disease. *Clin J Am Soc Nephrol* 2007; 2(3): 581–90. Epub August 19.

33 Perkovic V, Verdon C, Ninomiya T et al. The relationship between proteinuria and coronary risk: A systematic review and meta-analysis. *PLoS Med* 2008; 5(10): e207. Epub October 24.

34 Levey AS, Cattran D, Friedman A. Proteinuria as a surrogate outcome in CKD: Report of a scientific workshop sponsored by the National Kidney Foundation and the US Food and Drug Administration. *Am J Kidney Dis* 2009; 54(2): 205–26.

35 Khwaja A, Throssell D. A critique of the UK NICE guidance for the detection and management of individuals with chronic kidney disease. *Nephron Clin Pract* 2009; 113(3): c207–13. Epub August 20.

36 Incerti J, Zelmanovitz T, Camargo JL, Gross JL, de Azevedo MJ. Evaluation of tests for microalbuminuria screening in patients with diabetes. *Nephrol Dial Transplant.* 2005; 20(11): 2402–7. Epub August 18.

37 Orchard TJ, Dorman JS, Maser RE et al. Prevalence of complications in IDDM by sex and duration. Pittsburgh Epidemiology of Diabetes Complications Study II. *Diabetes* 1990; 39(9): 1116–24. Epub September 1.

38 Newman DJ, Mattock MB, Dawnay AB et al. Systematic review on urine albumin testing for early detection of diabetic complications. *Health Technol Assess* 2005; 9(30): iii–vi, xiii–163. Epub August 13.

39 Mogensen CE, Vestbo E, Poulsen PL et al. Microalbuminuria and potential confounders: A review and some observations on variability of urinary albumin excretion. *Diabetes Care* 1995; 18(4): 572–81. Epub April 1.

40 Gross JL, de Azevedo MJ, Silveiro SP, Canani LH, Caramori ML, Zelmanovitz T. Diabetic nephropathy: Diagnosis, prevention, and treatment. *Diabetes Care* 2005; 28(1): 164–76. Epub December 24, 2004.

41 Chadban S, Howell M, Twigg S et al. The CARI guidelines: Assessment of kidney function in type 2 diabetes. *Nephrology (Carlton)* 2010; 15 Suppl 1: S146–61. Epub April 1.

42 Levey AS, de Jong PE, Coresh J et al. The definition, classification, and prognosis of chronic kidney disease: A KDIGO Controversies Conference report. *Kidney Int* 2011; 80(1): 17–28. Epub December 15.

43 Granerus G, Aurell M. Reference values for 51Cr-EDTA clearance as a measure of glomerular filtration rate. *Scand J Clin Lab Invest* 1981; 41(6): 611–16. Epub October 1.

44 Friedman R, Gross JL. Evolution of glomerular filtration rate in proteinuric NIDDM patients. *Diabetes Care* 1991; 14(5): 355–9. Epub May 1.

45 Nosadini R, Velussi M, Brocco E et al. Course of renal function in type 2 diabetic patients with abnormalities of albumin excretion rate. *Diabetes* 2000; 49(3): 476–84. Epub June 27.

46 Christensen PK, Larsen S, Horn T, Olsen S, Parving HH. Renal function and structure in albuminuric type 2 diabetic patients without retinopathy. *Nephrol Dial Transplant* 2001; 16(12): 2337–47. Epub December 6.

47 Huang F, Yang Q, Chen L, Tang S, Liu W, Yu X. Renal pathological change in patients with type 2 diabetes is not always diabetic nephropathy: A report of 52 cases. *Clinical Nephrol* 2007; 67(5): 293–7. Epub June 5.

48 Craddick SR, Elmer PJ, Obarzanek E, Vollmer WM, Svetkey LP, Swain MC. The DASH diet and blood pressure. *Curr Atheroscler Rep* 2003; 5(6): 484–91. Epub October 4.

49 Morales E, Valero MA, Leon M, Hernandez E, Praga M. Beneficial effects of weight loss in overweight patients with chronic proteinuric nephropathies. *Am J Kidney Dis* 2003; 41(2): 319–27. Epub Jan 29.

50 Reichard P, Pihl M, Rosenqvist U, Sule J. Complications in IDDM are caused by elevated blood glucose level: The Stockholm Diabetes Intervention Study (SDIS) at 10-year follow up. *Diabetologia* 1996; 39(12): 1483–8. Epub December 1.

51 Intensive blood-glucose control with sulphonylureas or insulin compared with conventional treatment and risk of complications in patients with type 2 diabetes (UKPDS 33). UK Prospective Diabetes Study (UKPDS) Group. *Lancet* 1998; 352(9131): 837–53. Epub September 22.

52 Diabetes Control and Complications Trial Research Group. The effect of intensive treatment of diabetes on the development and progression of long-term complications in insulin-dependent diabetes mellitus. *N Eng J Med* 1993; 329: 977–86.

53 The effect of intensive treatment of diabetes on the development and progression of long-term complications in insulin-dependent diabetes mellitus. The Diabetes Control and Complications Trial Research Group. *New Eng J Med* 1993; 329(14): 977–86. Epub September 30.

54 Reichard P, Britz A, Cars I, Nilsson BY, Sobocinsky-Olsson B, Rosenqvist U. The Stockholm Diabetes Intervention Study (SDIS): 18 months' results. *Acta Med Scand* 1988; 224(2): 115–22. Epub January 1.

55 Ohkubo Y, Kishikawa H, Araki E et al. Intensive insulin therapy prevents the progression of diabetic microvascular complications in Japanese patients with non-insulin-dependent diabetes mellitus: A randomized prospective 6-year study. *Diabetes Res Clin Pract* 1995; 28(2): 103–17. Epub May 1.

56 Duckworth W, Abraira C, Moritz T et al. Glucose control and vascular complications in veterans with type 2 diabetes. *New Eng J Med* 2009; 360(2): 129–39. Epub December 19, 2008.

57 Gerstein HC, Miller ME, Byington RP et al. Effects of intensive glucose lowering in type 2 diabetes. *New Eng J Med* 2008; 358(24): 2545–59. Epub June 10.

58 Foley RN, Murray AM, Li S et al. Chronic kidney disease and the risk for cardiovascular disease, renal replacement, and death in the United States Medicare population, 1998 to 1999. *J Am Soc Nephrol* 2005; 16(2): 489–95. Epub December 14, 2004.

59 Abaterusso C, Lupo A, Ortalda V et al. Treating elderly people with diabetes and stages 3 and 4 chronic kidney disease. *Clin J Am Soc Nephrol* 2008; 3(4): 1185–94. Epub April 18.

60 Kemfang Ngowa JD, Yomi J, Kasia JM, Mawamba Y, Ekortarh AC, Vlastos G. Breast cancer profile in a group of patients followed up at the Radiation Therapy Unit of the Yaounde General Hospital, Cameroon. *Obstet Gynecol Int* 2011; 2011: 143506. Epub July 26.

61 Inzucchi SE, Bergenstal RM, Buse JB, Diamant M, Ferrannini E, Nauck M, et al. Management of hyperglycemia in type 2 diabetes: a patient-centered approach: position statement of the American Diabetes Association (ADA) and the European Association for the Study of Diabetes (EASD). *Diabetes care.* 2012;35(6):1364-79. Epub 2012/04/21.

62 Fonseca VA. Incretin-based therapies in complex patients: Practical implications and opportunities for maximizing clinical outcomes: A discussion with Dr. Vivian A. Fonseca. *Am J Med* 2011; 124(1 Suppl): S54–61. Epub January 14.

63 Sharif A. Current and emerging antiglycaemic pharmacological therapies: The renal perspective. *Nephrology (Carlton)* 2011; 16(5): 468–75. Epub April 5.

64 Abe M, Okada K, Soma M. Antidiabetic agents in patients with chronic kidney disease and end-stage renal disease on dialysis: Metabolism and clinical practice. Curr Drug Metab 2011; 12(1): 57–69. Epub February 10.

65 Groop PH, Cooper M, Perkovic, V et al. Linagliptin lowers albuminuria on top of recommended standard treatment in patients with type 2 diabetes and renal dysfunction. *Diabetes Care* (In press). 2012.

66 KDOQI Clinical Practice Guidelines and Clinical Practice Recommendations for Diabetes and Chronic Kidney Disease. *Am J Kidney Dis* 2007; 49(2 Suppl 2): S12–154. Epub February 6.

67 Yu L, Lu S, Lin Y, Zeng S. Carboxyl-glucuronidation of mitiglinide by human UDP-glucuronosyltransferases. *Biochem Pharmacol* 2007; 73(11): 1842–51. Epub March 16.

68 Abe M, Kikuchi F, Kaizu K, Matsumoto K. Combination therapy of pioglitazone with voglibose improves glycemic control safely and rapidly in Japanese type 2-diabetic patients on hemodialysis. *Clin Nephrol* 2007; 68(5): 287–94. Epub November 30.

69 Scheen AJ. Pharmacokinetics of dipeptidylpeptidase-4 inhibitors. *Diabetes Obes Metab* 2010; 12(8): 648–58. Epub July 2.

70 Jacobsen LV, Hindsberger C, Robson R, Zdravkovic M. Effect of renal impairment on the pharmacokinetics of the GLP-1 analogue liraglutide. *Brit J Clin Pharmacol* 2009; 68(6): 898–905. Epub December 17.

71 Lv J, Neal B, Ehteshami P et al. Effects of intensive blood pressure lowering on cardiovascular and renal outcomes: A systematic review and meta-analysis. *PLoS Med* 2012; 9(8): e1001293. Epub August 29.

72 Lv J, Perkovic V, Foote CV, Craig ME, Craig JC, Strippoli GF. Antihypertensive agents for preventing diabetic kidney disease. *Cochrane Database Syst Rev* 2012; 12: CD004136. Epub December 14.

73 de Galan BE, Perkovic V, Ninomiya T et al. Lowering blood pressure reduces renal events in type 2 diabetes. *J Am Soc Nephrol* 2009; 20(4): 883–92. Epub February 20.

74 Joint British recommendations on prevention of coronary heart disease in clinical practice: Summary. British Cardiac Society, British Hyperlipidaemia Association, British Hypertension Society, British Diabetic Association. *Brit Med J* 2000; 320: 705–8.

75 Lewis EJ, Hunsicker LG, Bain RP, Rohde RD. The effect of angiotensin-converting-enzyme inhibition on diabetic nephropathy. The Collaborative Study Group. *New Eng J Med* 1993; 329(20): 1456–62. Epub November 11.

76 Strippoli GF, Craig M, Deeks JJ, Schena FP, Craig JC. Effects of angiotensin converting enzyme inhibitors and angiotensin II receptor antagonists on mortality and renal outcomes in diabetic nephropathy: Systematic review. *Brit Med J* 2004; 329(7470): 828. Epub October 2.

77 Maione A, Navaneethan SD, Graziano G et al. Angiotensin-converting enzyme inhibitors, angiotensin receptor blockers and combined therapy in patients with micro- and macroalbuminuria and other cardiovascular risk factors: A systematic review of randomized controlled trials. *Nephrol Dial Transplant* 2011; 26(9): 2827–47. Epub March 5.

78 Harel Z, Gilbert C, Wald R et al. The effect of combination treatment with aliskiren and blockers of the renin-angiotensin system on hyperkalaemia and acute kidney injury: Systematic review and meta-analysis. *Brit Med J* 2012; 344: e42. Epub January 11.

79 Strippoli GF, Navaneethan SD, Johnson DW et al. Effects of statins in patients with chronic kidney disease: Meta-analysis and meta-regression of randomised controlled trials. *Brit Med J* 2008; 336(7645): 645–51. Epub February 27.

80 Collins R, Armitage J, Parish S, Sleigh P, Peto R. MRC/BHF Heart Protection Study of cholesterol-lowering with simvastatin in 5963 people with diabetes: A randomised placebo-controlled trial. *Lancet* 2003; 361(9374): 2005–16. Epub June 20.

81 Colhoun HM, Betteridge DJ, Durrington PN et al. Effects of atorvastatin on kidney outcomes and cardiovascular disease in patients with diabetes: An analysis from the Collaborative Atorvastatin Diabetes Study (CARDS). *Am J Kidney Dis* 2009; 54(5): 810–19. Epub June 23.

82 Ansquer JC, Foucher C, Rattier S, Taskinen MR, Steiner G. Fenofibrate reduces progression to microalbuminuria over 3 years in a placebo-controlled study in type 2 diabetes: Results from the Diabetes Atherosclerosis Intervention Study (DAIS). *Am J Kidney Dis* 2005; 45(3): 485–93. Epub March 9.

83 Tonelli M, Moye L, Sacks FM, Cole T, Curhan GC. Effect of pravastatin on loss of renal function in people with moderate chronic renal insufficiency and cardiovascular disease. *J Am Soc Nephrol* 2003; 14(6): 1605–13. Epub May 23.

84 Baigent C, Landray MJ, Reith C et al. The effects of lowering LDL cholesterol with simvastatin plus ezetimibe in patients with chronic kidney disease (Study of Heart and Renal Protection): A randomised placebo-controlled trial. *Lancet* 2011; 377(9784): 2181–92. Epub June 15.

85 Park CW, Zhang Y, Zhang X et al. PPARalpha agonist fenofibrate improves diabetic nephropathy in db/db mice. *Kidney Int* 2006; 69(9): 1511–17. Epub May 5

86 Okopien B, Krysiak R, Herman ZS. Effects of short-term fenofibrate treatment on circulating markers of inflammation and hemostasis in patients with impaired glucose tolerance. *J Clin Endocrinol Metab* 2006; 91(5): 1770–8. Epub February 24.

87 Keech A, Simes RJ, Barter P et al. Effects of long-term fenofibrate therapy on cardiovascular events in 9795 people with type 2 diabetes mellitus (the FIELD study): Randomised controlled trial. *Lancet* 2005; 366(9500): 1849–61. Epub November 29.

88 Jun M, Zhu B, Tonelli M et al. Effects of fibrates in kidney disease: A systematic review and meta-analysis. *J Am Coll Cardiol* 2012; 60(20): 2061–71. Epub October 23.

89 Gaede P, Vedel P, Parving HH, Pedersen O. Intensified multifactorial intervention in patients with type 2 diabetes mellitus and microalbuminuria: The Steno type 2 randomised study. *Lancet* 1999; 353(9153): 617–22. Epub February 25.

90 Gaede P, Vedel P, Larsen N, Jensen GV, Parving HH, Pedersen O. Multifactorial intervention and cardiovascular disease in patients with type 2 diabetes. *New Engl J Med* 2003; 348(5): 383–93. Epub January 31.

91 Manto A, Cotroneo P, Marra G et al. Effect of intensive treatment on diabetic nephropathy in patients with type I diabetes. *Kidney Int* 1995; 47(1): 231–5. Epub January 1.

Answers to Multiple-Choice Questions For Case Study 1

1 C

Diabetic kidney disease usually has an insidious onset and is clinically asymptomatic at the early phase. Its diagnosis is usually made based on the presence of micro- or macro-albuminuria and reduced kidney function in the setting of diabetes, after excluding other causes of chronic kidney disease. While definitive diagnosis requires a kidney biopsy, this is uncommonly undertaken in a patient presenting with typical clinical features.

2 A, B, E

Treatment requires a multidisciplinary approach. Optimization of blood glucose and blood pressure control, as well as lifestyle modification, are the key treatment strategies. Reno-protective agents targeting the renin-angiotensin-aldosterone system, either angiotensin-converting enzyme inhibitor (ACEI) or angiotensin receptor blocker (ARB), are the first-line therapy of choice.

Answers to Multiple-Choice Questions For Case Study 2

1 C

This woman presented with kidney failure in the setting of long-standing type 2 diabetes mellitus. She was likely to have acute on chronic kidney failure, which was aggravated by sepsis (community-acquired pneumonia) and dehydration. She had lactic acidosis likely secondary to use of Metformin in the context of renal impairment.

2 B, D

Diabetic kidney disease increases the risk of both acute and chronic kidney failure requiring renal replacement therapy (RRT). People with diabetes should undergo regular surveillance in order to diagnose diabetic kidney disease early. Metformin needs to be used with caution in people with diabetes and reduced kidney function.

Her urine ACR was 12 mg/g and 24-hour urine protein excretion was 1 g/day. The urine sediment was inactive. The blood tests were negative for other secondary causes of kidney disease, including vasculitis, hepatitis, and hematological disorders. She underwent renal biopsy, which showed mesangial expansion, glomerular basement membrane thickening, and glomerular sclerosis.

She was diagnosed with diabetic kidney disease and was commenced on insulin therapy. Perindopril was recommended, and nephrologist follow-up was organized.

CHAPTER 4

Vascular Imaging

Kiyoko Uno[1], Jordan Andrews[2] and Stephen J. Nicholls[2]
[1] *Cleveland Clinic, Cleveland, OH, USA*
[2] *South Australian Health & Medical Research Institute, Adelaide, SA, Australia*

Key Points

- Artery wall imaging permits visualization of the full burden of atherosclerotic disease.
- Imaging demonstrates greater disease burden and progression in the patient with diabetes.
- There is impaired compensatory remodeling of the vessel wall in diabetes.
- Targeting metabolic risk factors has a favorable impact on disease progression.
- The impact of imaging in the clinical evaluation of the patient with diabetes remains to be determined.

Introduction

The ability of vascular imaging to characterize atherosclerotic disease within the artery wall permits greater understanding of the atherosclerotic disease process and its influence by clinical and pharmacological factors. Diabetic patients demonstrate the same risk of cardiovascular disease (CVD) associated mortality as nondiabetic patients with a prior history of myocardial infarction [1]. Pathological studies have demonstrated diffuse atherosclerotic disease in patients with diabetes, in contrast to the more localized involvement often seen in nondiabetic individuals [2]. Symptoms of myocardial ischemia are often absent or atypical in diabetic patients, and CVD is frequently detected at an advanced stage, characterized by extensive atherosclerotic obstructive disease [3, 4]. Considering these findings, the role of vascular imaging in diabetic patients on risk stratification, early detection, and evaluation of current severity is potentially of great importance in clinical practice.

Noninvasive imaging techniques can be used as markers of atherosclerosis in individuals with atherogenic risk factors, including asymptomatic diabetic patients [5]. These imaging techniques are most likely to be

---

Managing Cardiovascular Complications in Diabetes, First Edition.
Edited by D. John Betteridge and Stephen Nicholls.

useful for early detection and risk stratification during the early stage of atherosclerotic disease [6, 7]. Meanwhile, the widespread clinical use of invasive imaging techniques, including coronary angiography, permits the establishment of revascularization strategies [8]. The relative ease of its use in clinical trials also allows for a standardized approach for image acquisition and analysis. However, the requirement for an invasive procedure limits its use to patients who require cardiac catheterization for a clinical indication. Invasive techniques are normally justified in individuals with a strong clinical suspicion of advanced CVD. Furthermore, the current notion that inflammation and immune response may contribute to the development of plaque rupture has garnered increased interest in imaging vulnerable plaques. In both noninvasive and invasive, novel imaging techniques have shown the possibility of visually characterizing the components of plaque. According to patients' clinical stages and requirements, clinicians need to choose the appropriate imaging modality.

Vascular imaging is also being utilized in the development of new treatment strategies to reduce cardiovascular risks [9]. Given that background therapy will include a greater number of established medial therapies (statins, aspirin, antihypertensive agents), it is likely that the placebo event rate in clinical trials will continue to decline. As a result, future clinical trials are likely to require larger cohorts of patients who are followed for longer periods of time to demonstrate efficacy. In order to evaluate the efficacy of medical therapies in clinical trials, there has been an increased interest in using surrogate markers for clinical events. These surrogate markers will be modified by experimental therapies and reflect stages in the pathological pathways leading to clinical events. Accordingly, vascular imaging has been increasingly employed in risk assessment and the evaluation of novel anti-atherosclerotic therapies.

This chapter summarizes the imaging modalities currently available, their findings in relation to diabetes, and their potential role in clinical settings. There is a summary in Table 4.1.

Vascular Imaging Modalities and Findings in Relation to Diabetes

Noninvasive Imaging Techniques
Carotid Ultrasound

Measuring carotid intima-media thickness (CIMT) and identifying carotid plaque with B-mode ultrasound is a noninvasive, sensitive, and reproducible technique for identifying and quantifying subclinical vascular

Table 4.1 Major artery wall-imaging modalities.

Modality	Images	Invasive	Radiation	Advantages	Disadvantages
Carotid IMT	• Early artery wall thickening • Established plaque	No	No	• Can apply in clinical practice and trials • Associates with plaque burden and outcome	• Operator dependent • IMT is not plaque • Resolution
CT coronary angiography	• Coronary calcium • Plaque burden • Luminal stenosis • Plaque composition	No	Yes	• High negative predictive value in intermediate-risk patients • Potential role in acute evaluation of chest pain	• Need for contrast • Need to slow heart rate • Variable image quality • No evidence of benefit of clinical use
Magnetic resonance	• Plaque burden • Plaque composition	No	No	• Characterize burden, composition, and functional activity of plaque	• Coronary resolution poor • Limited to large arteries • Access to scanner
Coronary angiography	• Luminal stenosis • Calcium	Yes	Yes	• Widely used and standardized	• Invasive • Does not image plaque
Intravascular ultrasound	• Plaque burden • Plaque composition with radiofrequency analysis • Lumen size • Thrombus	Yes	No	• High-resolution imaging of full thickness of vessel wall • Measures plaque burden	• Invasive • Suboptimal composition assessment
Optical coherence tomography	• Lumen size and integrity • Fibrous cap thickness • Lipid and macrophage pools • Cholesterol crystals • Thrombus	Yes	No	• High-resolution imaging • Measures fibrous cap thickness • Detects artery wall dissections • Evaluates stent apposition and in-stent restenosis	• Invasive • Limited vessel wall penetration
Near-infrared spectroscopy	• Chemical composition	Yes	No	• Provides chemical fingerprint of plaque	• Invasive • Requires ongoing validation • Clinical utility remains to be determined

CT, computed tomography. IMT, intima-media thickness.

disease and for evaluating cardiovascular risk (Figure 4.1). Using this approach, it has been well established that increasing CIMT is associated with a greater prevalence of cardiovascular risk factors and the presence of atherosclerotic plaque within various vascular territories. Studies of large population cohorts have demonstrated that increasing CIMT provides additional prognostic information to that of conventional risk factors. The finding that therapies that slow the progression of CIMT also prevent cardiovascular events supports the use of carotid ultrasonic imaging in the evaluation of anti-atherosclerotic therapies [10].

Meanwhile, it is also important to recognize that CIMT is not a pre-atherosclerotic stage of the disease process. There is no evidence to suggest that plaque develops in the region where increasing CIMT is detected. Rather, it appears to be a systemic barometer of the presence of atherosclerosis throughout the arterial tree. The main predictors of medial hypertrophy or intimal thickening of common carotid arteries are age and hypertension, which do not necessarily reflect the atherosclerotic process. In contrast, carotid plaque, defined as the presence of focal wall thickening, is suggested as associated with the development of atherosclerotic

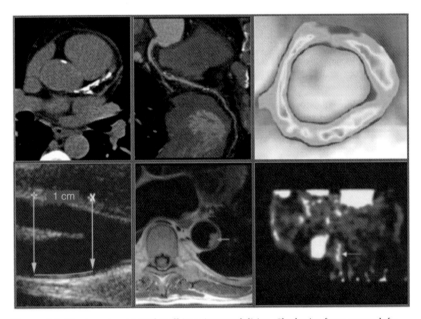

Figure 4.1 Noninvasive arterial wall imaging modalities. Clockwise from upper left: computed tomography calcium scoring, computed tomography coronary angiography, molecular imaging of vascular cell adhesion molecule-1 (VCAM-1) in plaque, fluorodeoxyglucose (FDG) positron emission tomography (PET) imaging of plaque inflammation, magnetic resonance imaging, and carotid intima-medial thickness evaluation on B-mode ultrasound. (Color plate 4.1)

disease [11]. Carotid plaque predominantly occurs at sites of nonlaminar turbulent flow such as in the bifurcation of carotid artery, but rarely in the common carotid artery except in advanced atherosclerotic disease.

The presence of CIMT greater than or equal to the 75th percentile for the patient's age, sex, and ethnicity, or carotid plaque, is indicative of increased CVD risk and may signify the need for more aggressive risk-reduction interventions.

Carotid Ultrasound in Diabetes

Numerous cross-sectional studies have continuously reported increased CIMT in patients with diabetes or even a prediabetic state compared with those without [12, 13]. In a report from the Atherosclerotic Risk In Communities (ARIC) cohort, CIMT was 0.07 mm thicker in patients with diabetes compared to those without. Mean common CIMT in middle-aged individuals is reported to range from 0.71–0.98 mm in diabetic patients vs. 0.66–0.85 mm in nondiabetic populations. In diabetic individuals without a history of myocardial infarction, CIMT is similar to that in nondiabetic individuals with a history of myocardial infarction [14]. In a meta-analysis of 21 clinical studies from 1995 to 2004 including 4,019 diabetic and 1,110 impaired glucose tolerance (IGT) patients, both type 2 diabetes (T2DM) and IGT demonstrated thicker CIMT compared with control subjects at 0.13 (95% CI 0.12–0.14) mm and 0.04 (95% CI 0.01–0.07) mm, respectively. Additional risk factors including age, gender, obesity, hypertension, increase of LDL cholesterol, and decrease of HDL cholesterol have been reported to accelerate the increase in CIMT. A longer duration of diabetes and an increase of urinary albumin excretion are also indicated as determinants of an increase in CIMT [15].

The prediabetic state has not been consistently associated with increased CIMT. In the prediabetic population, postprandial glucose levels have been suggested to be more strongly associated with CIMT than levels of fasting glucose and HbA1c [16]. It is likely that postprandial glucose elevation is associated with a clustering of standard risk factors. Consequently, postprandial hypertriglyceridemia, which could be induced by postprandial hyperglycemia, was closely associated with increased CIMT despite normal levels of fasting triglycerides [17].

Accelerated progression of CIMT has also been reported in diabetic patients. In the ARIC study, mean annual CIMT increases were greater by 3–10 μm/y in the patients with diabetes compared with those without [18]. The Insulin Resistance Atherosclerosis Study (IRAS) compared CIMT in CCA and ICA by a range of glucose tolerance at a five-year interval. The rate of CIMT progression was 3.8 μm/y in CCA and 17.7 μm/y in ICA in the normal glucose tolerance group, and both progression rates were approximately two times greater than in the patients with diabetes.

Furthermore, the patients who were diagnosed as diabetic at the time of enrollment showed a greater progression of CIMT in ICA than the patients with known diabetes (33.9 µm/y vs. 26.6 µm/y) [19]. This emphasizes the importance of early identification of diabetes and risk-factor control to reduce atherosclerotic change.

In patients with diabetes, CIMT was reported as an independent predictor of cardiovascular events [20]. In a prospective study with 229 T2DM patients free of any cardiovascular complication with at least one additional cardiovascular risk factor, the predictive value of increased CIMT, thicker than the median value of 0.835 mm, was similar to Framingham scores after a five-year follow-up. The addition of CIMT on Framingham scores showed further improvement of the risk-prediction value. CIMT was found to have a predictive value for future coronary events in combination with several other novel risk factors in the ARIC cohort, which included 1,500 diabetic participants [21].

A number of small studies have reported the effects of medical interventions on CIMT in diabetes, particularly with peroxisome proliferation activated receptor (PPAR-γ) agonists. The largest of these studies, the Carotid Intima-Media Thickness in Atherosclerosis Using Pioglitazone (CHICAGO) trial, directly compared the impact of two glucose-lowering strategies, the PPAR-γ agonist poiglitazone and the sulphonylurea glymepiride. Raising HDL-C and lowering both tryglycerides and CRP, in addition to improving glycemic control, were associated with halting of CIMT progression with pioglitazone [22]. Subsequent analysis revealed that raising HDL-C was the strongest independent predictor of the ability of pioglitazone to slow CIMT progression. A meta-analysis of five randomized controlled trials, which included four Japanese and 1 German study, examined the effect of alpha-glucosidase inhibitors on CIMT progression and suggested a beneficial impact. Significant increase of HDL-C was observed in the patients treated with alpha-glucosidase [23].

The Stop Atherosclerosis in Native Diabetics Study (SANDS) examined the effects of intensive lipid and blood pressure modifications on the progression of CIMT compared with the standard treatments in the patients with diabetes; target levels of LDL-C below 70 mg/dL and systolic blood pressure below 115 mmHg. After a three-year follow-up, CIMT showed regression in the intensive treatment group in comparison with progression in the standard treatment group (−0.012 mm vs. 0.038 mm; $P<0.001$). Adverse events related to blood pressure medications were observed more in the intensive treatment group, but clinical event rates did not differ significantly between groups [24]. Subsequently, several subanalyses of the SANDS data have been reported [25]. In the assessment of the additional effects of ezetimibe on statins within the aggressive treatment group, no difference was observed in the progression of CIMT between the statins plus ezetimibe and the statins alone groups. While a significant increase of arterial mass, calculated as the common carotid artery cross-sectional area, was observed in the whole cohort, it decreased in the association with achieved intensive target levels of LDL-C and systolic blood pressure [26]. In a recent analysis, HbA1 levels were negatively associated with the achievement of target levels, yet no relationship was observed between HbA1c and treatment-associated changes in CIMT [27].

The noninvasive CIMT measurement is a well-established technique for early detection of atherosclerosis or risk management in asymptomatic younger patients with type 1 diabetes (T1DM) [28]. Meanwhile, the evidence for increased CIMT seems to be weaker in T1DM patients compared to other conventional risk factors, including obesity, dyslipidemia, and hypertension [28]. A Japanese study showed a significant increase of CIMT related to T1DM in the older generation, 10–19 years old, and a not significant but greater increase in the younger generation, 4–9 years old. In a recent systematic review of CIMT measurements in children and adolescent patients, 6 out of 14 studies examining CIMT in association with T1DM did not show a significant increase of CIMT compared with the control group [29].

Similarly, in a larger study examining T1DM patients, the Epidemiology of Diabetes Interventions and Complications (EDIC) study, CIMT in T1DM did not show a difference between age- and sex-matched nondiabetic subjects, except in ICA among men [30, 31]. The EDIC study further extended its observations and measured CIMT at 1, 6, and 12 years after enrollment in combination with the long-term follow-up of the Diabetes Control and Complications Trial (DCCT) study, which compared the effects of intensive glycemic control on CIMT progression for 6 years [32]. The initial cohort was enrolled between 1983 and 1989, as 13 to 39 years old, had T1DM for 1 to 15 years, and was in generally good health at baseline. While there was no difference in the CIMT between the matched T1DM and nondiabetic population 1 year after enrollment ended, greater CIMT was observed after 6 years. During the DCCT study, CIMT progression was 0.019 mm less in the intensive glycemic control group with HbA1c target by 7.2% than in the standard glycemic control group with HbA1c target by 9%. This beneficial effect of intensive glycemic control was still evident 6 years after the DCCT study ended, but did not have an effect on the CIMT progression between 6 and 12 years [32]. This finding supports early and continued intensive glycemic control in T1DM to retard subclinical atherosclerotic changes.

Studies also showed a presence of more carotid plaques in patients with diabetes compared to those without [33]. In 738 Japanese subjects with normal fasting glucose and normal glucose tolerance, higher insulin resistance calculated as HOMA-IR showed a positive association with the presence of carotid plaque, with an odds ratio of 1.19 (95% CI 1.00-1.41).

Carotid plaque is shown as a predictor of cardiovascular events, especially associated with stroke, which supports the identification of carotid plaques for risk stratification [34]. Meanwhile, the evaluations of carotid plaque are usually cross-sectional in middle-aged or older subjects. To detect early atherosclerotic change and evaluate disease progression, combined use with CIMT is recommended.

The assessment of plaque echogenicity has been suggested to be useful in evaluating plaque vulnerability. Echolucent plaques, indicating proneness to rupture, were detected more in the patients with diabetes [35]. By using integrated backscatter (IBS), a Japanese group suggested an increase of echogenicity in carotid plaque due to treatment with poiglitazone in patients with acute coronary syndrome [36]. However, these studies are performed in a relatively small number of patients. Plaque characterization with carotid ultrasound requires standardized measuring methods and needs further investigation.

Computed Tomography

Multiple population studies have reported that calculation of a coronary artery calcium (CAC) score, measured in computed tomography (CT), is an independent predictor of cardiovascular events, even after controlling for risk factors. Without a requirement for contrast administration, CT imaging of the coronary arteries can detect calcification, defined as a hyperattenuating lesion exceeding a threshold of 130 Hounsfield units (HU) with an area of at least three adjacent pixels [37]. Agatston et al. developed a CAC scoring algorithm, based on calcification volume and density, that is now widely used in clinical practice [38]. Statin therapy in patients with a CAC score above 400 showed a reduction in coronary events.

The application of multislice computed tomography (MSCT) scanners for noninvasive coronary angiography has developed rapidly in recent years. Employment of more than 16-row systems have demonstrated a sensitivity ranging from 88% to 95% and a specificity of between 90% and 96% compared with intravascular ultrasound (IVUS) [39]. Since CT angiography has a high negative predictive value of 99% on average, the technique is currently most suited to exclude coronary artery disease. Plaque can be classified as noncalcified, mixed, or calcified. Compared to IVUS, sensitivity and specificity in coronary artery plaque diagnosis were 93% (84–97%) and 98% (96–99%) for calcified plaque; 88% (81–93%) and 92% (89–95%) for noncalcified plaque. Initial comparisons have shown that calcification may represent the duration of atherosclerosis, whereas noncalcified and mixed lesions are more frequently observed in patients with an acute coronary syndrome. Meanwhile, MSCT is subject to a number of limitations, including exposure to a relatively high dose of radiation, currently in the range of 9–12 mSv, lower accuracy in the presence of severe calcification and movement artifacts, and limited application possibilities in cases with irregular heart rate. Taking the radiation exposure and the high negative predictive value of MSCT angiography into consideration, this technique is recommended for excluding CVD in patients of intermediate risk.

Computed Tomography in Diabetes

Studies with CT continuously show the presence of extensive calcification in diabetic coronary arteries compared with nondiabetic. Furthermore, the association between CAC and future cardiovascular events has been observed particularly in patients with diabetes [40]. Raggi et al. followed 10,377 patients (903 with diabetes) for five years after CAC evaluations by CT. There was a significant interaction of CAC scores with diabetes even after adjusting for other risk factors. Mortality increased with increasing baseline CAC scores for both diabetic and nondiabetic individuals, and diabetic patients had a greater increase in mortality than nondiabetic patients for every increase in CAC scores. However, the study examined CAC scores in 269 diabetic patients and did not find a relationship between CAC scores and coronary events during a six-year follow-up [41]. Meanwhile, a recent study, the Diabetes Heart Study (DHS), showed an increase of mortality with increasing levels of CAC in 1,051 diabetic patients. Overall, a greater CAC score may increase the risk of CVD events in the diabetic population [42].

Serial observation of T2DM without prior coronary disease showed the progression of CAC in 30% of subjects after a 2.5-year follow-up in association with a higher baseline CAC score and suboptimal glycemic control. In the EDIC/DCCT study with a type 1 diabetes cohort, prior intensive glycemic control correlated with a lower CAC score in the subjects without retinopathy or microalbuminuria in association with reduced levels of HbA1c. These studies implicate intensive glycemic control as having beneficial impacts on CAC progression. However, it is not known whether the reduction in the prevalence of CAC can be translated into a reduction in the incidence of coronary artery disease. Other than the effects of glycemic control, the effects of statin use on CAC progression have also been reported. However, their results are not consistent. The different severities of diabetes and atherosclerosis in each cohort may cause this inconsistency.

In an evaluation of the diagnostic accuracy of CT angiography, there were no statistically significant differences observed between the diabetic and nondiabetic individuals with 85% sensitivity and 98% specificity compared with coronary angiography. The evidence for the prognostic value of CT angiography in the diabetic population is currently emerging. A small study examining a cohort of 49 diabetics and 49 matched nondiabetics showed that event-free survival was lower in the diabetic patients in association with the presence of coronary artery disease identified on CT.

In the patients who underwent CT angiography for recurrent chest pain, diabetic patients showed more diseased coronary segments than nondiabetic patients, with more nonobstructive (<50% luminal narrowing) plaques. In addition, diabetic patients demonstrated relatively more noncalcified (28% vs. 19%) and calcified (49% vs. 43%), and less mixed (23% vs. 38%) plaques. These observations were confirmed in a smaller population undergoing an invasive evaluation using virtual histology intravascular ultrasound (VH-IVUS) in addition to CT angiography. Furthermore, in asymptomatic T2DM patients, Scholte et al. showed a high prevalence of coronary artery disease in asymptomatic diabetic patients. In a total of 70 patients, 54% had nonobstructive and 26% obstructive (at least one significant ≥50% stenosis) coronary artery disease, and 55% patients had a calcium score greater than 10. These studies indicate the usefulness of noninvasive CT angiography to screen for coronary artery disease in the diabetic population.

Magnetic Resonance Imaging

Magnetic resonance imaging (MRI) of the artery wall has been developed in parallel to its potential in characterizing cardiac structure and function [43]. Early validation studies in animal models and human subjects demonstrated the ability of MRI not only to quantify the extent of disease, but also to provide a characterization of its individual components. These findings, in addition to the potential to assess pathological pathways within the plaque in a noninvasive fashion, suggest that MRI has considerable potential as a tool to evaluate novel anti-atherosclerotic agents. This is also supported by observations that the composition of plaque within the carotid artery on MRI correlated with a likelihood of cerebrovascular events [44]. A number of reports have demonstrated that statin therapy has a beneficial impact on disease progression within the carotid arteries and aorta. It is important to note that in each of the studies, areas containing relatively bulky disease were selected for evaluation, potentially limiting the findings of these studies to these areas. Imaging resolution currently limits this technique to larger arteries.

MRI in Diabetes

An MRI plaque-imaging study in carotid arteries showed overexpression of high-risk lesions in the patients with diabetes, characterized by a lipid or necrotic core surrounded by fibrous tissue with possible calcification (Types IV–V) or a complex plaque with possible surface defect, hemorrhage, or thrombus (Type VI), compared with the patients without diabetes [45]. This suggests a higher risk of carotid plaque rupture in patients with diabetes.

In a study by Kwong et al., MRI showed myocardial scar and delayed gadolinium enhancement in 28% of DM patients who had no known history of myocardial infarction. In this study, the presence of delayed gadolinium enhancement was a strong independent predictor of future major adverse cardiovascular events and death [46].

Fluorodeoxyglucose (FDG) PET/CT

FDG PET is a molecular imaging technique that is highly sensitive to metabolically active processes that use glucose as a fuel, such as tumors and inflamed lesions. The increased uptake of FDG was suggested to be secondary to macrophage accumulation. Macrophages are reliant on external glucose for metabolism because they are unable to store glycogen, have glycolytic activity five- to twentyfold higher than background tissues, and can increase fiftyfold further when activated. Studies have demonstrated FDG uptake in balloon-injured arteries in an animal model and in human atherosclerotic arteries. Imaging on a combination of PET/CT systems enables localization of F-FDG uptakes to the vascular tree with anatomical information. Clinical studies showed the feasibility of FDG-PET/CT to assess coronary FDG uptake. Retrospective studies with the images obtained for tumor staging showed the FDG uptake in a noncalcified plaque in the left main coronary artery. A recent study in patients with recent acute coronary syndrome reported the increase of FDG uptake in the culprit lesion as well as in the ascending aorta and the left main coronary artery compared to the patients with stable angina.

While it was thought that FDG uptake might reflect inflammatory activation of plaque macrophages, the mechanism that produces the FDG signal in association with atherosclerotic plaques was not clear. A recent study by Folco using cells in pro-atherogenic conditions demonstrated interesting results. In this study, smooth muscle cells, but not macrophages, increased glucose uptake when exposed to pro-inflammatory cytokines. In contrast, macrophages or foam cells, abundant constituents of inflamed human atheroma exposed to hypoxia, responded with a greatly increased rate of glucose uptake [47]. These findings suggest that FDG uptake signals in atherosclerotic lesions may reflect intraplaque hypoxia rather than inflammatory burden. This is an important issue and this report has raised caution for the interpretation of clinical trials that use FDG signals to monitor responses to interventions.

FDG-PET/CT in Diabetes

There have been a few studies investigating FDG uptake in relation to diabetes, in which higher FDG uptake was found in patients with diabetes compared with those without [48]. A recent study by Bucerius et al. measured FDG uptake in carotid arteries in patients with known or suspected CVD. It found a significant independent correlation between glucose-corrected values of FDG uptake and the presence of diabetes, despite the fact that these associations were not observed with nonglucose-corrected values [49]. The role of glucose correction of FDG uptake in the evaluation of atherosclerotic arteries has not been well understood. Whether to correct for fasting blood glucose is a matter of the glucose-utilization rate in the tissue being considered. Glycolytic activity is heterogeneous and glucose utilization varies among tissues. No data are yet available in vivo on glucose utilization in macrophage-induced inflammation, and further investigations are needed to better understand the use of FDG-PET in the assessment of atherosclerotic disease.

Additionally, the study by Bucerius et al. found an increase of FDG uptake in association with higher body mass index and alcohol intake [49]. A small study in Japan comparing the effects of piogitazone and glimepiride on FDG uptake in patients with diabetes or impaired glucose tolerance demonstrated a significant decrease of FDG uptake in the pioglitazone-treated patients. Also of interest is that it showed an inverse relationship between FDG uptake and levels of HDL cholesterol [50].

Myocardial Perfusion Imaging (MPI)

Stress perfusion imaging can detect heterogenous flow distribution due to decreased coronary flow reserve during exercise or pharmacological vasodilatation such as adenosine, dipyridamole, and dobutamine. The dimensions of the left ventricle and ejection fraction can also be determined. In a pooled analysis of 79 studies, stress testing combined with nuclear imaging has a sensitivity of 86% and a specificity of 74% to detect obstructive coronary artery disease ($\geq$50% stenosis) in the general population. With pharmacologically induced stress, sensitivity and specificity are 89% and 75%, respectively [51].

MPI in Diabetes

The study by Kang et al. showed comparable diagnostic accuracy of MPI in diabetic and nondiabetic patients with suspected coronary artery disease. Mean sensitivity and specificity were 86% and 56%, respectively, for $\geq$50% coronary stenosis, and 90% and 50% for $\geq$70% coronary stenosis [52].

Studies in asymptomatic diabetic patients reveal a high incidence of patients with silent ischemia [53]. Rajagoplan et al. performed stress MPI imaging in 1,427 asymptomatic diabetic patients without known coronary artery disease, in which 58% of patients showed some abnormalities at any level and 18% were diagnosed as high risk. In the high-risk patient group, 49% underwent coronary angiography, and 61% of them had angiographic coronary artery disease. Furthermore, a higher annual mortality rate was observed in this high-risk patient group [54]. In recent research, the Detection of Ischemia in Asymptomatic Diabetes (DIAD) study, 1,123 asymptomatic diabetic patients were randomly assigned to be screened with adenosine-stress radionuclide MPI or not to be screened; 6% of those who were screened demonstrated moderate or large perfusion defects (≥5% of left ventricle), which were significantly associated with a greater incidence of cardiac events (hazard ratio 6.3) during 4.8-year follow-up [55]. Microangiopathy or endothelial dysfunction in diabetic patients may cause the discrepancy in the results between MPI and coronary angiograms. Studies suggest the benefit of risk stratification by abnormal findings in MPI in asymptomatic diabetic patients [56, 57].

Catheter-Based Imaging Techniques
Coronary Angiography

For more than 50 years, angiography has served as the gold standard for the clinical detection and quantitation of obstructive disease within the coronary arteries (Figure 4.2) Accordingly, coronary angiography has become an essential tool in clinical practice for the triage of patients to a range of medical and revascularization strategies. Early studies in the era demonstrated that the extent and progression of coronary artery disease, measured by quantitative coronary arteriography (QCA) on angiography, correlated with clinical outcome. Meanwhile, angiography is a lumen-based approach, generating a two-dimensional silhouette of the arterial lumen containing contrast. The degree of stenosis is defined in relation to a reference segment judged to be "normal." The observation that artery walls change their size and shape, termed remodeling, in response to the accumulation of plaque is likely to cause "normal" or "minimally diseased" appearance on angiography despite considerable atherosclerosis in the vessel wall. In addition, it is likely that the apparent reference segment used

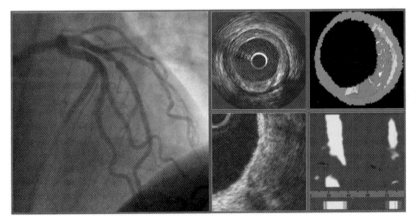

Figure 4.2 Invasive arterial wall imaging modalities. Clockwise from left: coronary angiography, intravascular ultrasound, ultrasound radiofrequency plaque composition analysis, near-infrared spectroscopy, and optical coherence tomography. (Color plate 4.2).

in this quantitative technique contains substantial disease and will not be "normal" at all.

Angiography in Diabetes

A number of small studies have compared angiographically determined coronary disease in diabetic patients and matched nondiabetic patients [58]. The results are controversial. While an early study did not find any differences in the angiographical findings between T2DM and nondiabetic patients with similar disease severity [59], most of the other studies demonstrated more extensive coronary artery disease in both type 1 and type 2 diabetic patients. Left main artery and multivessel disease are likely to be more common in diabetic patients. In a recent study comparing angiographic disease severity according to insulin resistance in nondiabetic patients, a severe degree of insulin resistance was associated with more severe, extensive, and distal types of coronary artery disease [60].

Very few studies employed serial evaluation of quantitative coronary angiography to assess therapies in diabetic patients. The most compelling evidence of benefit was observed in the Diabetes Atherosclerosis Intervention Study (DAIS). In subjects with relatively good glycemic control (mean hemoglobin A1c 7.5%), who had mild dyslipidemia and at least one visible coronary lesion, fenofibrate slowed the progression of lumen stenosis in this study [61]. In-stent restenosis quantitated with QCA was examined in association with rosiglitazone treatment. An early small study showed significant reduction of in-stent restenosis in the patients treated with rosiglitazone, one of the thiazolidinediones (TZD) [62].

Currently, angiography is more likely to be used for the evaluation of revascularization effects. With simple measurements of lumen diameter and with or without restenosis ($\geq$50% diameter stenosis at follow-up) in angiography, West et al. demonstrated more restenosis after stent deployment in diabetic patients compared to nondiabetic patients (31% vs. 21%). Smaller lumen diameter and greater stented length of vessel were revealed as predictors of restenosis in this diabetic cohort [63]. The diabetes and drug-eluting stent (DiabeDES) study, a Danish multicenter randomized trial, compared angiographical in-stent lumen loss between sirolimus-eluting Cypher stent (SES) and paclitaxel-eluting stens (PES). The primary endpoint, angiographic in-stent lumen loss, calculated with minimal luminal diameter in the stent and in the reference segments, was reduced in the SES-treated group compared to the PES-treated group [64]. In the DiabeDES III study, angiographic in-stent lumen loss was reduced and minimum lumen diameter in the stent was higher in the SES as compared to the zotarolimus-eluting Endeavor stent at 10-month follow-up [65].

Intravascular Ultrasound (IVUS)

Technological advances in ultrasound have permitted the placement of high-frequency (20–45 MHz) transducers on the tips of catheters within the coronary arteries. The application of IVUS generates high-resolution imaging of the entire thickness of the arterial wall within coronary vasculature. While IVUS has been employed for plaque progression/regression analysis, it is important to recognize that IVUS is a useful technique in the detection of vulnerable plaques associated with positive remodeling. However, conventional ultrasonic imaging within the coronary artery walls provides a suboptimal assessment of plaque composition. The study of plaque morphology regarding vessel remodeling showed that inflammation and medial thinning are primary determinants of expansive remodeling, which supports the link between expansive remodeling and vulnerable plaque. Serial evaluation of statin treatments in animals showed the relationship between fibrous-cap thickening and constrictive negative remodeling, suggesting that the constrictive negative remodeling may indicate arterial wall stabilization according to plaque volume regression and plaque stabilization by anti-atherosclerotic treatments. Serial IVUS studies with statins demonstrated constrictive remodeling of the arterial wall by using a remodeling index. The grayscale images that are generated permit a very broad classification of plaque components as echolucent, echodense, and calcific.

The ability of IVUS to image atherosclerosis burden within the artery wall in a serial fashion permits assessment of the impact of anti-atherosclerotic therapies on the natural history of coronary atherosclerosis. Subsequently, serial IVUS measurements have been widely employed to examine the effects of anti-atherosclerotic treatments on the rate of progression of coronary atherosclerosis, and contributed to the establishment of the current anti-atherosclerotic treatment strategy. A recent pooled analysis of six clinical IVUS trials demonstrated a direct relationship between the burden of coronary atherosclerosis, its progression, and adverse cardiovascular events. This supports the importance of using atheroma progression/regression analysis with IVUS in the evaluation of novel anti-atherosclerotic therapies.

Furthermore, IVUS is also a useful tool for coronary revascularization. Vessel remodeling is commonly observed in the atherosclerotic lesion site, which has been suggested to cause a larger reference diameter compared to the diameter measured in angiography. The group in Denmark compared the accumulated cost following the procedure and major adverse cardiac events between IVUS-guided and conventional revascularization strategies. In their study, IVUS-guided groups resulted in continued improvement of clinical outcome during 2.5-year follow-up, with lower repeated revascularization, hospitalization, and cumulative costs in the IVUS-guided group.

IVUS in Diabetes

IVUS has revealed the natural history of atherosclerotic plaque in patients with diabetes. (Figure 4.3). Several early IVUS studies showed that diabetes was characterized by diffuse atherosclerosis, with a predilection for involvement of distal segments in relatively small vessels. Another early study examined restenosis after revascularization demonstrated the increased risk of restenosis with intimal hyperplasia in both stented

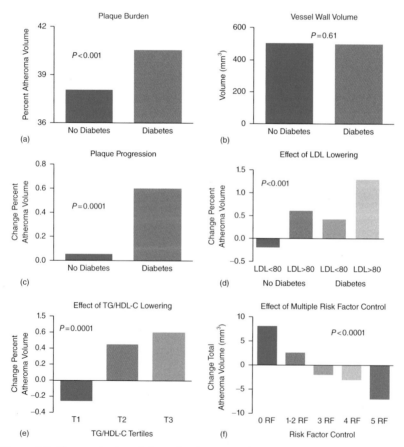

Figure 4.3 Characterization of plaque burden, arterial wall remodeling, and disease progression in patients with diabetes. Patients with diabetes harbor more extensive plaque (a), but similar vessel volumes suggest impaired arterial wall remodeling (b) and greater plaque progression (c). Slowing of disease progression is observed with lowering low-density lipoprotein cholesterol (LDL-C (d)), the triglyceride/high-density lipoprotein cholesterol ratio (TG/HDL-C (e)), and multiple metabolic risk factors (f).

and nonstented lesions in diabetic patients compared with nondiabetic patients [66]. Subsequently, a pooled analysis of five serial IVUS studies demonstrated more extensive atherosclerosis and inadequate compensatory remodeling in diabetic patients compared to nondiabetic patients. Inadequate compensatory remodeling, which shows a smaller lumen volume but no difference in vessel volume, was significantly observed in insulin-treated patients. Despite the use of anti-atherosclerotic treatments, an accelerated increase in coronary plaque volume was observed in this diabetic cohort. In another study with 45 diabetic patients, higher glycated hemoglobin, insulin requirements, hypertension, multivessel disease, and prior revascularization history were associated with smaller vessel size.

While intensively lowering LDL cholesterol slowed disease progression, it was evident that diabetic patients continue to demonstrate an increase in plaque burden, suggesting the need for additional therapeutic strategies to arrest disease progression. The Pioglitazone Effect on Regression of Intravascular Sonographic Coronary Obstruction Prospective Evaluation (PERISCOPE) study involved the comparison of pioglitazone vs. glimepiride on the progression of coronary atherosclerosis. While marked disease progression was observed in patients treated with glimepiride, no increase in plaque burden was found in pioglitazone-treated patients. This finding suggests that changing the triglyceride/HDL cholesterol ratio predicts the benefit of pioglitazone in slowing dyslipidemia in promoting cardiovascular risk in patients with diabetes. In the combined population of normoglycemic, impaired fasting glucose, and diabetes, Berry et al. suggested the association between glycemic controls and the severity and progression of coronary atherosclerosis [67]. Further analysis of diabetic patients who participated in serial IVUS studies demonstrated greater slowing of disease progression in association with achieving optimal control of increasing numbers of risk factors, including atherogenic lipids, blood pressure, glycemic control, and inflammation. This highlights the multifactorial nature of influences on cardiovascular risk in diabetic patients.

In the Assessment on the Prevention of Progression by Rosiglitazone on Atherosclerosis in Diabetes Patients with Cardiovascular History (APPROACH) study, rosiglitazone did not significantly decrease the primary endpoint of the progression of percentage atheroma compared with glipizide. The secondary endpoint of normalized total atheroma volume was significantly reduced by rosiglitazone compared with glipizide [68].

IVUS studies have also demonstrated the characteristics in diabetic coronary arteries regarding their revascularization strategies. While patients with diabetes showed less favorable outcomes after coronary interventions with balloon or bare-metal stents (BMS) than those without diabetes, the revascularization strategy with drug-eluting stent (DES) started showing similar benefits in reducing in-stent restenosis in patients with and without diabetes. In a serial IVUS study evaluating the effects of PES stents on in-stent neointima formation, diabetic patients treated with BMS showed greater intimal hyperplasia volume compared to the nondiabetic patients treated with BMS; those treated with PES demonstrated similar intimal hyperplasia volume to nondiabetic patients [69]. Another IVUS observation of plaque prolapse after stent deployment in diabetic patient coronary arteries was that lumen volume after plaque prolapse remained high in the lesions treated with DES compared to those treated with BMS. These findings support the benefit of using DES in diabetic coronary artery diseases. With 130 diabetic patients, the DiabeDES study compared neointimal hyperplasia after coronary artery stenting with SES and PES. After eight-month follow-up, neointimal hyperplasia was significantly reduced, including less involvement of the stent edges, in the SES- compared to the PES-treated coronary arteries [70]. The subanalysis of the DiabeDES study demonstrated less of an increase in peri-stent plaque volume and less expansion of external elastic membrane volume in SES- than PES-treated coronary arteries.

A multicenter randomized trial used angiography and IVUS to evaluate the effect of pioglitazone on in-stent neointimal hyperplasia after revascularization with BMS stents. Despite the fact that risk factor modifications were similar in both groups, including glycemic control during six-month follow-up, a significantly smaller in-stent neointimal index (neointimal volume/stent volume) was observed in the pioglitazone group than in the control group in IVUS. A small angiographic lumen diameter showed a trend toward larger diameters in the pioglitazone group than in the control group ($p = 0.08$). The frequency of binary restenosis was 17% in the pioglitazone group and 35% in the control group ($p = 0.06$). This suggests the beneficial impacts of pioglitazone treatment on in-stent neointimal proliferation. Meanwhile, in the study comparing the effects of rosiglitazone and glipizide on in-stent restenosis, no significant difference was observed in both angiographic and IVUS measurements.

Ultrasonic Radiofrequency Evaluation

Advances in analysis of the ultrasonic backscatter signal that returns from tissue to the transducer permit the opportunity to generate a tissue map of spectral radiofrequency. Given that different components of plaque emit different radiofrequencies, this approach has been demonstrated in ex vivo studies to have a positive correlation with histological findings in the artery wall. Virtual histology (VH)-IVUS uses an electronic catheter that acquires electrocardiogram-gated data. VH-IVUS feeds the spectra that are obtained from the radiofrequency data using autoregressive models into a classification tree that has reported diagnostic accuracies of over 90% of each plaque component as compared to histology, which identifies the four basic plaque compositions, fibrous, fibro-fatty, dense calcium, and necrotic core.

Several serial VH-IVUS clinical trials demonstrated the change in plaque components according to anti-atherosclerotic treatment. Statin treatment demonstrated an increase of calcium and fibrous volumes, and a reduction of the necrotic core. Meanwhile, a recent report assessing necrotic core size in porcine coronary arteries demonstrated no correlation between histology and VH-IVUS. A multicenter trial showed the differences in VH-IVUS assessments between different European IVUS centers. A recent study examining the accuracy of plaque classification by VH-IVUS showed a small but significant difference in border correction performed in different centers. VH-IVUS plaque classification is dependent on cross-sectional area rather than volumetric compositional analysis. This caused the greater differences in multi-center volumetric analysis of the entire diseased plaque segments in plaque volume components than for the cross-sectional areas of single frames. These factors reduce the use of VH-IVUS plaque classification to guide intervention in a live clinical setting, and also affect the comparison of diagnostic accuracy and natural history of plaques between studies. Studies have raised caution about interpreting the results in different studies.

VH-IVUS in Diabetes

Hong et al. performed grayscale IVUS and VH-IVUS in culprit lesions of patients with acute coronary syndrome. Multivessel disease, greater plaque burden, more plaque ruptures, and thrombus were more common in diabetic patients associated with higher sensitivity levels. In VH-IVUS, a greater volume of necrotic core and multiple TCFAs were observed in the diabetic coronary arteries [71]. Ogita et al. performed VH-IVUS in nonculprit lesion of stable angina pectoris. Compared to nondiabetic patients, there was no significant difference in plaque composition except for the percentage of dense calcium in diabetic patients. Within the diabetic patients, a higher percentage of necrotic core was observed in the patients with lower renal function [72]. Lindsey et al. performed IVUS and VH-IVUS in the most diseased 10 mm segment of a single coronary artery in patients undergoing diagnostic coronary angiography. A longer duration of diabetes was associated with greater plaque burden and TCFAs [73]. In a recent study by Zheng et al. characterizing VH-IVUS features in a three-vessel pre-intervention cohort, diabetes was associated with a larger plaque burden, higher necrotic core ratio, and more frequent VH-TCFA [74]. In the prospective multinational registry examining IVUS and VH-IVUS in the most diseased 10 mm segment of a single coronary artery in patients with clinical indication of cardiac catheterization, diabetic patients also showed a greater proportion of TCFA.

Recently, a serial integrated backscatter (IB)-IVUS evaluation in diabetic patients was reported. Nonculprit 20 mm coronary segments with mild to moderate stenosis were examined with IB-IVUS in 42 diabetic and 48 nondiabetic patients undergoing percutaneous coronary intervention. Greater progression of total plaque volume and total lipid volume was observed in diabetic patients. The increase in total lipid volume was blunted in diabetic patients who achieved an HbA1c level of less than 6.5%. Ogasawara et al. reported the significant reduction of necrotic core in VH-IVUS after a six-month treatment with pioglitazone compared to controls in association with improved blood sugar, high-sensitivity CRP, and adiponectine levels [75].

Optical Coherence Tomography

Optical coherence tomography (OCT) involves the use of light, in contrast to sound waves with ultrasound, to image tissues. Catheter-based OCT applications permit high-resolution imaging of the coronary artery wall. Unlike ultrasound, light can penetrate calcified plaques. Coronary OCT has a unique capacity in the volumetric quantification of calcium and produces high-quality imaging at the level of the lumen surface and potentially below the level of the fibrous cap. On the other hand, the increase in imaging resolution is accompanied by poor tissue penetration. The low penetration depth is the limitation of OCT, which hinders studying large vessels or remodeling. As a result, the major interest in the development of OCT has been stimulated by its potential to evaluate apposition and the endothelial overgrowth of stents [76]. This approach will also be able to detect early neointimal hyperplasia within stented regions with great precision.

The ability of OCT to image the superficial aspects of the atherosclerotic plaque with high resolution provides the opportunity to assess thin-cap fibroatheroma (TCFA), accumulation of lipid, macrophages, and hemorrhage below the endothelial surface. In a series of more than 200 sudden death cases, approximately 60% of acute thrombi resulted from rupture of TCFA. OCT also has a potential role to assess vasa vasorum. Proliferation of vasa vasorum is thought to link with intraplaque hemorrhage and inflammation, and suggest the development and destabilization of atherosclerotic plaque [77]. The serial evaluation of vasa vasorum may provide information regarding plaque stabilization by anti-atherosclerotic treatments. Meanwhile, the diagnosis of those features is based on subjective evaluation. Quantitative methods remain to be established.

OCT in Diabetes

A few studies have reported the findings of OCT imaging related to diabetes. A study examining patients with unstable angina pectoris demonstrated a higher presence of OCT-evaluated calcification and dissection in diabetic compared with nondiabetic patients [78]. Meanwhile, a small study comparing 19 diabetic and 63 nondiabetic patients characterized coronary plaques by OCT, and did not find any differences in frequency of lipid-rich plaques and TCFA, and minimum fibrous cap thickness in culprit lesions [79]. OCT has emerged as a powerful tool for stent assessment in revascularization. The study evaluating vascular response in nonrestenotic lesions nine months after SES implantation showed greater neointimal coverage and thickness in diabetic compared with nondiabetic patients.

Role of Vascular Imaging in Clinical Settings

In all patients with diabetes, annual evaluation of cardiovascular risk factors is required [80, 81, 82]. These risk factors include dyslipidemia, hypertension, smoking, a positive family history of premature coronary disease, and the presence of micro- or macroalbuminuria. While vascular-imaging studies have revealed a higher prevalence of cardiovascular disease in asymptomatic diabetic patients, the benefit of routine use of vascular imaging beyond risk stratification remains controversial. In diabetic patients, considering that symptoms of myocardial ischemia are often absent or atypical, screening with noninvasive imaging techniques to determine whether or not to perform further assessment becomes significant [3].

Measuring CIMT and identifying carotid plaque is considered to be useful for refining CVD risk assessment in patients at intermediate CVD risk; that is, Framingham risk score 6%–20% without established CVD. Patients with the following clinical circumstances are also considered for this screening test: (1) family history of premature CVD; (2) younger than 60 years old with severe abnormalities in a single risk factor who otherwise would not be candidates for pharmacotherapy; or (3) women younger than 60 years old with at least two CVD risk factors. Carotid vascular ultrasound is considered if the required level of aggressive medical treatment is uncertain and additional information about the burden of subclinical atherosclerotic disease or future CVD risk is needed. Carotid vascular ultrasound can reclassify patients at intermediate risk, discriminate between patients with and without prevalent CVD, and predict major adverse CVD events.

Noninvasive coronary imaging techniques including CAC score, CT angiography, and stress MPI test can be used as a pre-examination of coronary angiography. With those tests, clinicians can evaluate the need to perform further invasive examinations. According to the guidelines, CAC evaluation with CT is considered appropriate in asymptomatic individuals at intermediate risk or at low risk with family history of premature coronary artery disease. CAC score is deemed inappropriate in asymptomatic individuals at low risk and of uncertain appropriateness in individuals at high risk. Meanwhile, the presence of CAC, regardless of severity, is not considered as an indication for coronary angiography. CT angiography is stated as inappropriate in asymptomatic individuals at low or moderate risk and of uncertain appropriateness in those at high risk. While there is no certain appropriate indication for CT angiography, suspicious obstructive disease ($\geq$50% stenosis) in symptomatic patients and a suspicious left main lesion in both symptomatic and asymptomatic patients in CT angiography are the indications of coronary angiography. Stress MPI is considered appropriate in asymptomatic patients at high risk or its equivalent who have specific comorbidities such as LV dysfunction or ventricular tachycardia, and inappropriate in those at low or intermediate risk. Therefore, asymptomatic patients at intermediate risk would undergo CAC evaluations with CT, and those at high risk would undergo stress MPI examinations for screening of coronary artery disease. In symptomatic patients, CT angiography or stress MPI tests will be considered, with an exception for primary intervention cases.

With intermediate- or high-risk findings for coronary artery disease in those pre-examinations, symptomatic patients are considered appropriate to undergo coronary angiography. While invasive imaging modalities should be performed in patients with definite or suspected coronary artery disease, the images in those invasive imaging techniques provide valuable information for clinical decision-making, especially related to revascularization. Furthermore, novel imaging techniques have demonstrated the possibility of imaging plaque characteristics in association with greater CVD events. This supports the establishment of more effective treatment strategies with the guidance of those imaging modalities.

Conclusion

Subsequent to the pathological findings, vascular imaging continuously provides information regarding the atherosclerotic disease process in relation to diabetes. Carotid ultrasound demonstrated the presence of subclinical atherosclerotic change in the early stage of diabetes, which was shown as a risk for future cardiovascular events. Noninvasive coronary artery-imaging studies including CT, MPI, and FDG-PET/CT revealed the high prevalence of coronary artery disease in asymptomatic diabetic patients. Invasive imaging techniques provided anatomically precise images for revascularization. Furthermore, the findings regarding the effects of medical interventions on atherosclerotic disease progression have contributed to the establishment of disease management strategies. The worldwide increased prevalence of diabetes and the associated increased cardiovascular risk requires comprehensive disease management in diabetes to be addressed. A better understanding is required of the features of each imaging technique, and the strategy for using them effectively.

Case Study 1

A 61-year-old male with poorly controlled type 2 diabetes for the past eight years presents for coronary angiography to investigate ischemic chest pain. His angiogram revealed three-vessel coronary artery disease with mild left ventricular systolic dysfunction. His blood pressure is 135/80 mmHg and his LDL cholesterol is 2.4 mmol/L. He is currently treated with atorvastatin 20 mg daily.

Multiple-Choice Questions

1 The most appropriate type of management is:
   A Medical management
   B Coronary artery bypass grafting
   C Percutaneous coronary intervention

2 The most appropriate option for management of his LDL cholesterol is:
   A Addition of fibric acid derivative
   B Addition of ezetimibe
   C No change to management, he is at goal
   D Increase statin dose aiming for a LDL cholesterol less than
       1.8 mmol/L

3 The diabetic medication that has been demonstrated to have a
   beneficial impact on atherosclerosis progression is:
   A Insulin
   B Metformin
   C Pioglitazone
   D Sitagliptin
   E Glibenclamide

Answers provided after the References

Case Study 2

A 55-year-old woman with a history of type 2 diabetes for six years and no known clinical atherosclerotic disease presents for an annual check-up.

Multiple-Choice Questions

1 The best option for noninvasive evaluation of atherosclerotic burden is:
   A Coronary angiography
   B Near-infrared spectroscopy

    C Magnetic resonance imaging
    D Carotid ultrasound
    E Optical coherence tomography

2 In the setting of optimal LDL cholesterol lowering, the factor that most strongly associates with disease progression is:
    A High-sensitivity C-reactive protein
    B Triglyceride/HDL cholesterol ratio
    C Blood pressure
    D Glycemic control
    E Smoking

Answers provided after the References

Guidelines and Web Links

http://www.escardio.org/guidelines-surveys/esc-guidelines/GuidelinesDocuments
   /guidelines-dyslipidemias-addenda.pdf
Guidelines for the management of dyslipidemia.

References

1 Chen K, Lindsey JB, Khera A et al. Independent associations between metabolic syndrome, diabetes mellitus and atherosclerosis: Observations from the dallas heart study. *Diabetes Vasc Dis Res* 2008; 5: 96–101.

2 Shaw JA, White AJ, Reddy R et al. Evaluation of differences in coronary plaque mechanical behavior in individuals with and without type 2 diabetes mellitus. *Arterioscler Thromb Vasc Biol* 2006; 26: 2826–7.

3 Bax JJ, Young LH, Frye RL, Bonow RO, Steinberg HO, Barrett EJ. Screening for coronary artery disease in patients with diabetes. *Diabetes Care* 2007; 30: 2729–36.

4 Raggi P, Bellasi A, Ratti C. Ischemia imaging and plaque imaging in diabetes: Complementary tools to improve cardiovascular risk management. *Diabetes Care* 2005; 28: 2787–94.

5 Van de Veire NR, Djaberi R, Schuijf JD, Bax JJ. Non-invasive imaging: Non-invasive assessment of coronary artery disease in diabetes. *Heart* 2010; 96: 560–72.

6 Berry C, Tardif JC, Bourassa MG. Coronary heart disease in patients with diabetes: Part I: Recent advances in prevention and noninvasive management. *J Am Coll Cardiol* 2007; 49: 631–42.

7 Berry C, Tardif JC, Bourassa MG. Coronary heart disease in patients with diabetes: Part II: Recent advances in coronary revascularization. *J Am Coll Cardiol* 2007; 49: 643–56.

8 Fallow GD, Singh J. The prevalence, type and severity of cardiovascular disease in diabetic and non-diabetic patients: A matched-paired retrospective analysis using coronary angiography as the diagnostic tool. *Mol Cell Biochem* 2004; 261: 263–9.

9 Owen AR, Roditi GH. Peripheral arterial disease: The evolving role of non-invasive imaging. *Postgrad Med J* 2011; 87: 189–98.

10 Taylor AJ, Villines TC, Stanek EJ et al.Extended-release niacin or ezetimibe and carotid intima-media thickness. *New Eng J Med* 2009; 361: 2113–22.

11 Inaba Y, Chen JA, Bergmann SR. Carotid plaque, compared with carotid intima-media thickness, more accurately predicts coronary artery disease events: A meta-analysis. *Atherosclerosis* 2012; 220: 128–33.

12 Lamotte C, Iliescu C, Libersa C, Gottrand F. Increased intima-media thickness of the carotid artery in childhood: A systematic review of observational studies. *Eur J Pediatr* 2011; 170: 719–29.

13 Bonora E, Tessari R, Micciolo R et al.Intimal-medial thickness of the carotid artery in nondiabetic and niddm patients: Relationship with insulin resistance. *Diabetes Care* 1997; 20: 627–31.

14 Chambless LE, Folsom AR, Davis V et al. Risk factors for progression of common carotid atherosclerosis: The atherosclerosis risk in communities study, 1987–1998. *Am J Epidemiol* 2002; 155: 38–47.

15 Distiller LA, Joffe BI, Melville V, Welman T, Distiller GB. Carotid artery intima-media complex thickening in patients with relatively long-surviving type 1 diabetes mellitus. *J Diabetes Complications* 2006; 20: 280–84.

16 Hanefeld M, Koehler C, Schaper F, Fuecker K, Henkel E, Temelkova-Kurktschiev T. Postprandial plasma glucose is an independent risk factor for increased carotid intima-media thickness in non-diabetic individuals. *Atherosclerosis* 1999; 144: 229–35.

17 Hanefeld M, Koehler C, Henkel E, Fuecker K, Schaper F, Temelkova-Kurktschiev T. Post-challenge hyperglycaemia relates more strongly than fasting hyperglycaemia with carotid intima-media thickness: The RIAD study. Risk factors in impaired glucose tolerance for atherosclerosis and diabetes. *Diabet Med* 2000; 17: 835–40.

18 Folsom AR, Eckfeldt JH, Weitzman S et al. Relation of carotid artery wall thickness to diabetes mellitus, fasting glucose and insulin, body size, and physical activity. Atherosclerosis Risk in Communities (ARIC) study investigators. *Stroke* 1994; 25: 66–73.

19 Wagenknecht LE, D'Agostino R, Jr., Savage PJ, O'Leary DH, Saad MF, Haffner SM. Duration of diabetes and carotid wall thickness. The Insulin Resistance Atherosclerosis Study (IRAS). *Stroke* 1997; 28: 999–1005.

20 Lee EJ, Kim HJ, Bae JM et al. Relevance of common carotid intima-media thickness and carotid plaque as risk factors for ischemic stroke in patients with type 2 diabetes mellitus. *Am J Neuroradiol* 2007; 28: 916–19.

21 Folsom AR, Chambless LE, Duncan BB, Gilbert AC, Pankow JS. Prediction of coronary heart disease in middle-aged adults with diabetes. *Diabetes Care* 2003; 26: 2777–84.

22 Mazzone T, Meyer PM, Feinstein SB et al. Effect of pioglitazone compared with glimepiride on carotid intima-media thickness in type 2 diabetes: A randomized trial. *JAMA* 2006; 296: 2572–81.

23 Geng DF, Jin DM, Wu W, Fang C, Wang JF. Effect of alpha-glucosidase inhibitors on the progression of carotid intima-media thickness: A meta-analysis of randomized controlled trials. *Atherosclerosis* 2011; 218: 214–19.

24 Fleg JL, Mete M, Howard BV et al. Effect of statins alone versus statins plus ezetimibe on carotid atherosclerosis in type 2 diabetes: The SANDS (Stop Atherosclerosis in Native Diabetics study) trial. *J Am Coll Cardiol* 2008; 52: 2198–2205.

25 Howard BV, Roman MJ, Devereux RB et al. Effect of lower targets for blood pressure and LDL cholesterol on atherosclerosis in diabetes: The SANDS randomized trial. *JAMA* 2008; 299: 1678–89.

26 Russell M, Fleg JL, Galloway WJ et al. Examination of lower targets for low-density lipoprotein cholesterol and blood pressure in diabetes: The Stop Atherosclerosis in Native Diabetics study (SANDS). *Am Heart J* 2006; 152: 867–75.

27 Mete M, Wilson C, Lee ET et al. Relationship of glycemia control to lipid and blood pressure lowering and atherosclerosis: The SANDS experience. *J Diabetes Complications* 2011; 25: 362–7.

28 Schwab KO, Doerfer J, Krebs A et al. Early atherosclerosis in childhood type 1 diabetes: Role of raised systolic blood pressure in the absence of dyslipidaemia. *Eur J Pediatr* 2007; 166: 541–8.

29 Jarvisalo MJ, Putto-Laurila A, Jartti L et al. Carotid artery intima-media thickness in children with type 1 diabetes. *Diabetes* 2002; 51: 493–8.

30 Effect of intensive diabetes treatment on carotid artery wall thickness in the epidemiology of diabetes interventions and complications. Epidemiology of Diabetes Interventions and Complications (EDIC) research group. *Diabetes* 1999; 48: 383–90.

31 Nathan DM, Lachin J, Cleary P et al. Intensive diabetes therapy and carotid intima-media thickness in type 1 diabetes mellitus. *New Eng J Med* 2003; 348: 2294–303.

32 Polak JF, Backlund JY, Cleary PA et al. Progression of carotid artery intima-media thickness during 12 years in the diabetes control and complications trial/epidemiology of diabetes interventions and complications (dcct/edic) study. *Diabetes* 2011; 60: 607–13.

33 Pollex RL, Spence JD, House AA et al. A comparison of ultrasound measurements to assess carotid atherosclerosis development in subjects with and without type 2 diabetes. *Cardiovasc Ultrasound* 2005; 3: 15.

34 Ishizaka N, Ishizaka Y, Takahashi E et al. Association between insulin resistance and carotid arteriosclerosis in subjects with normal fasting glucose and normal glucose tolerance. *Arterioscler Thromb Vasc Biol* 2003; 23: 295–301.

35 Ostling G, Hedblad B, Berglund G, Goncalves I. Increased echolucency of carotid plaques in patients with type 2 diabetes. *Stroke* 2007; 38: 2074–8.

36 Hirano M, Nakamura T, Kitta Y et al. Rapid improvement of carotid plaque echogenicity within 1 month of pioglitazone treatment in patients with acute coronary syndrome. *Atherosclerosis* 2009; 203: 483–8.

37 Achenbach S, Raggi P. Imaging of coronary atherosclerosis by computed tomography. *Eur Heart J* 2010; 31: 1442–8.

38 Agatston AS, Janowitz WR, Hildner FJ, Zusmer NR, Viamonte M, Jr., Detrano R. Quantification of coronary artery calcium using ultrafast computed tomography. *J Am Coll Cardiol* 1990; 15: 827–32.

39 Gao D, Ning N, Guo Y, Ning W, Niu X, Yang J. Computed tomography for detecting coronary artery plaques: A meta-analysis. *Atherosclerosis* 2011; 219: 603–9.

40 Perrone-Filardi P, Achenbach S, Mohlenkamp S et al. Cardiac computed tomography and myocardial perfusion scintigraphy for risk stratification in asymptomatic individuals without known cardiovascular disease: A position statement of the Working Group on Nuclear Cardiology and Cardiac CT of the European Society of Cardiology. *Eur Heart J* 2011; 32: 1986–93.

41 Raggi P, Shaw LJ, Berman DS, Callister TQ. Prognostic value of coronary artery calcium screening in subjects with and without diabetes. *J Am Coll Cardiol* 2004; 43: 1663–9.

42 Agarwal S, Morgan T, Herrington DM et al. Coronary calcium score and prediction of all-cause mortality in diabetes: The diabetes heart study. *Diabetes Care* 2011; 34: 1219–24.

43 Beaussier H, Naggara O, Calvet D et al. Mechanical and structural characteristics of carotid plaques by combined analysis with echotracking system and MR imaging. *JACC Cardiovasc Imaging* 2011; 4: 468–77.

44 Wasserman BA, Sharrett AR, Lai S et al. Risk factor associations with the presence of a lipid core in carotid plaque of asymptomatic individuals using high-resolution MRI: The Multi-Ethnic Study of Atherosclerosis (MESA). *Stroke* 2008; 39: 329–35.

45 Esposito L, Saam T, Heider P et al. MRI plaque imaging reveals high-risk carotid plaques especially in diabetic patients irrespective of the degree of stenosis. *BMC Med Imaging* 2010; 10: 27.

46 Kwong RY, Sattar H, Wu H et al. Incidence and prognostic implication of unrecognized myocardial scar characterized by cardiac magnetic resonance in diabetic patients without clinical evidence of myocardial infarction. *Circulation* 2008; 118: 1011–20.

47 Folco EJ, Sheikine Y, Rocha VZ et al. Hypoxia but not inflammation augments glucose uptake in human macrophages: Implications for imaging atherosclerosis with 18fluorine-labeled 2-deoxy-d-glucose positron emission tomography. *J Am Coll Cardiol* 2011; 58: 603–14.

48 Prior JO. Diabetes and vascular (18)f-fluorodeoxyglucose positron emission tomography uptake: Another step toward understanding inflammation in atherosclerosis. *J Am Coll Cardiol* 2012; 59: 2089–90.

49 Bucerius J, Mani V, Moncrieff C et al. Impact of noninsulin-dependent type 2 diabetes on carotid wall 18f-fluorodeoxyglucose positron emission tomography uptake. *J Am Coll Cardiol* 2012; 59: 2080–88.

50 Mizoguchi M, Tahara N, Tahara A et al. Pioglitazone attenuates atherosclerotic plaque inflammation in patients with impaired glucose tolerance or diabetes: A prospective, randomized, comparator-controlled study using serial FDG PET/CT imaging study of carotid artery and ascending aorta. *JACC Cardiovasc Imaging* 2011; 4: 1110–18.

51 Miyamoto MI, Vernotico SL, Majmundar H, Thomas GS. Pharmacologic stress myocardial perfusion imaging: A practical approach. *J Nucl Cardiol* 2007; 14: 250–55.

52 Kang X, Berman DS, Lewin H et al. Comparative ability of myocardial perfusion single-photon emission computed tomography to detect coronary artery disease in patients with and without diabetes mellitus. *Am Heart J* 1999; 137: 949–57.

53 Moralidis E, Didangelos T, Arsos G, Athyros V, Mikhailidis DP. Myocardial perfusion scintigraphy in asymptomatic diabetic patients: A critical review. *Diabetes Metab Res Rev* 2010; 26: 336–47.

54 Rajagopalan N, Miller TD, Hodge DO, Frye RL, Gibbons RJ. Identifying high-risk asymptomatic diabetic patients who are candidates for screening stress single-photon emission computed tomography imaging. *J Am Coll Cardiol* 2005; 45: 43–9.

55 Young LH, Wackers FJ, Chyun DA et al. Cardiac outcomes after screening for asymptomatic coronary artery disease in patients with type 2 diabetes: The DIAD study: A randomized controlled trial. *JAMA* 2009; 301: 1547–55.

56 Prior JO, Monbaron D, Koehli M, Calcagni ML, Ruiz J, Bischof Delaloye A. Prevalence of symptomatic and silent stress-induced perfusion defects in diabetic patients with suspected coronary artery disease referred for myocardial perfusion scintigraphy. *Eur J Nucl Med Mol Imaging* 2005; 32: 60–69.

57 Giri S, Shaw LJ, Murthy DR et al. Impact of diabetes on the risk stratification using stress single-photon emission computed tomography myocardial perfusion imaging in patients with symptoms suggestive of coronary artery disease. *Circulation* 2002; 105: 32–40.

58 Gui MH, Qin GY, Ning G et al. The comparison of coronary angiographic profiles between diabetic and nondiabetic patients with coronary artery disease in a Chinese population. *Diabetes Res Clin Pract* 2009; 85: 213–19.

59 Pajunen P, Nieminen MS, Taskinen MR, Syvanne M. Quantitative comparison of angiographic characteristics of coronary artery disease in patients with

noninsulin-dependent diabetes mellitus compared with matched nondiabetic control subjects. *Am J Cardiol* 1997; 80: 550–56.

60 Graner M, Syvanne M, Kahri J, Nieminen MS, Taskinen MR. Insulin resistance as predictor of the angiographic severity and extent of coronary artery disease. *Ann Med* 2007; 39: 137–44.

61 Effect of fenofibrate on progression of coronary-artery disease in type 2 diabetes: The Diabetes Atherosclerosis Intervention study, a randomised study. *Lancet* 2001; 357: 905–10.

62 Choi D, Kim SK, Choi SH et al. Preventative effects of rosiglitazone on restenosis after coronary stent implantation in patients with type 2 diabetes. *Diabetes Care* 2004; 27: 2654–60.

63 West NE, Ruygrok PN, Disco CM et al. Clinical and angiographic predictors of restenosis after stent deployment in diabetic patients. *Circulation* 2004; 109: 867–73.

64 Maeng M, Jensen LO, Galloe AM et al. Comparison of the sirolimus-eluting versus paclitaxel-eluting coronary stent in patients with diabetes mellitus: The Diabetes and Drug-Eluting Stent (DIABEDES) randomized angiography trial. *Am J Cardiol* 2009; 103: 345–9.

65 Jensen LO, Maeng M, Thayssen P et al. Late lumen loss and intima hyperplasia after sirolimus-eluting and zotarolimus-eluting stent implantation in diabetic patients: The Diabetes and Drug-Eluting Stent (DIABEDES III) angiography and intravascular ultrasound trial. *EuroIntervention* 2011; 7: 323–31.

66 Kornowski R, Mintz GS, Abizaid A, Leon MB. Intravascular ultrasound observations of atherosclerotic lesion formation and restenosis in patients with diabetes mellitus. *Int J Cardiovasc Intervent* 1999; 2: 13–20.

67 Berry C, Noble S, Gregoire JC et al. Glycaemic status influences the nature and severity of coronary artery disease. *Diabetologia* 2010; 53: 652–8.

68 Gerstein HC, Ratner RE, Cannon CP et al. Effect of rosiglitazone on progression of coronary atherosclerosis in patients with type 2 diabetes mellitus and coronary artery disease: The assessment on the prevention of progression by rosiglitazone on atherosclerosis in diabetes patients with cardiovascular history trial. *Circulation* 2010; 121: 1176–87.

69 Jensen LO, Maeng M, Mintz GS et al. Intravascular ultrasound assessment of expansion of the sirolimus-eluting (cypher select) and paclitaxel-eluting (taxus express-2) stent in patients with diabetes mellitus. *Am J Cardiol* 2008; 102: 19–26.

70 Jensen LO, Maeng M, Thayssen P et al. Neointimal hyperplasia after sirolimus-eluting and paclitaxel-eluting stent implantation in diabetic patients: The randomized Diabetes and Drug-Eluting Stent (DIABEDES) intravascular ultrasound trial. *Eur Heart J* 2008; 29: 2733–41.

71 Hong YJ, Jeong MH, Choi YH et al. Plaque characteristics in culprit lesions and inflammatory status in diabetic acute coronary syndrome patients. *JACC Cardiovasc Imaging* 2009; 2: 339–49.

72 Ogita M, Funayama H, Nakamura T et al. Plaque characterization of non-culprit lesions by virtual histology intravascular ultrasound in diabetic patients: Impact of renal function. *J Cardiol* 2009; 54: 59–65.

73 Lindsey JB, House JA, Kennedy KF, Marso SP. Diabetes duration is associated with increased thin-cap fibroatheroma detected by intravascular ultrasound with virtual histology. *Circ Cardiovasc Interv* 2009; 2: 543–8.

74 Zheng M, Choi SY, Tahk SJ et al. The relationship between volumetric plaque components and classical cardiovascular risk factors and the metabolic syndrome: A 3-vessel coronary artery virtual histology-intravascular ultrasound analysis. *JACC Cardiovasc Interv* 2011; 4: 503–10.

75 Ogasawara D, Shite J, Shinke T et al. Pioglitazone reduces the necrotic-core component in coronary plaque in association with enhanced plasma adiponectin in patients with type 2 diabetes mellitus. *Circulation* 2009; 73: 343–51.

76 Mehanna EA, Attizzani GF, Kyono H, Hake M, Bezerra HG. Assessment of coronary stent by optical coherence tomography, methodology and definitions. *Int J Cardiovasc Imaging* 2011; 27: 259–69.

77 Cheng KH, Sun C, Vuong B et al. Endovascular optical coherence tomography intensity kurtosis: Visualization of vasa vasorum in porcine carotid artery. *Biomed Opt Express* 2012; 3: 388–99.

78 Feng T, Yundai C, Lian C et al. Assessment of coronary plaque characteristics by optical coherence tomography in patients with diabetes mellitus complicated with unstable angina pectoris. *Atherosclerosis* 2010; 213: 482–5.

79 Chia S, Raffel OC, Takano M, Tearney GJ, Bouma BE, Jang IK. Comparison of coronary plaque characteristics between diabetic and non-diabetic subjects: An in vivo optical coherence tomography study. *Diabetes Res Clin Pract* 2008; 81: 155–60.

80 Standards of medical care in diabetes – 2011. *Diabetes Care* 2011; 34(Suppl 1): S11–S61.

81 Executive summary: Standards of medical care in diabetes – 2011. *Diabetes Care.* 2011; 34(Suppl 1): S4–S10.

82 Webster MW. Clinical practice and implications of recent diabetes trials. *Current Opin Cardiol* 2011; 26: 288–93.

Answers to Multiple-Choice Questions for Case Study 1

1 B

2 D

3 C

Answers to Multiple-Choice Questions for Case Study 2

1 D

2 B

CHAPTER 5

Glycemia and CVD and Its Management

Jeffrey W. Stephens[1], Akhila Mallipedhi[2] and Stephen C. Bain[1]
[1] *Swansea University College of Medicine, Swansea, UK*
[2] *Morriston Hospital, Swansea, UK*

Key Points

- Hyperglycemia (fasting, postprandial glucose, and elevated HBA1c) is associated with increased cardiovascular risk, independently of other risk factors.
- Impaired fasting glycemia and impaired glucose tolerance are associated with increased CVD risk.
- Hyperglycemia increases CVD risk through oxidative and inflammatory mechanisms.
- The aggressive treatment of plasma glucose is associated with hypoglycemia and increased CVD risk.
- All novel therapeutic agents targeting glucose control are subject to clinical trials examining cardiovascular safety.
- The target range for HBA1c should be tailored according to the patient's risk of hypoglycemia.
- The current treatment algorithms include the use of newer therapies (GLP-1 analogs and DPP-IV inhibitors) that are associated with a lower risk of hypoglycemia-associated complications.

Diabetes, Glucose and Cardiovascular Disease

Cardiovascular disease (CVD) including coronary heart disease (CHD) is the major cause of mortality in patients with diabetes [1, 2, 3]. In patients without diabetes several well-studied environmental and physiological factors are now documented for CVD. These include hypercholesterolemia, hypertension, age, cigarette smoking, and obesity. Patients with diabetes are at a considerably higher risk [4] than those without and there are additive effects of other risk factors [5]. Of interest is that no more than 25% of the excess CHD risk in diabetes can be accounted for by established risk factors [6]. This illustrates the complexity of CVD, particularly in high-risk

---

Managing Cardiovascular Complications in Diabetes, First Edition.
Edited by D. John Betteridge and Stephen Nicholls.
© 2014 John Wiley & Sons, Ltd. Published 2014 by John Wiley & Sons, Ltd.

states such as diabetes, and may explain the inaccuracy of methods such as the Framingham equation and the PROCAM calculation to predict CHD risk in diabetes [7]. Until recently, the contribution of fluctuations and changes in glucose levels to CVD risk was relatively ignored. It should be noted that many of the CVD risk-prediction tools do not take into account glycemic control or fluctuations in glucose excursions. Our understanding of the direct and indirect effects of glucose on vascular dysfunction has grown over the past decade and basic scientific, epidemiological and clinical research has now demonstrated an independent association between glucose and CVD risk. For example, glucose-mediated oxidative stress is an important mediator of endothelial dysfunction [7]. Recent epidemiological data has confirmed associations between plasma glucose and CVD risk [3].

In recent years, there has been evidence to suggest that not only hyperglycemia contributes to CVD risk, but also hypoglycemia. As a result, guidelines relating to the therapeutic targets of glucose control have been under revision. Furthermore, some of the oral hypoglycemic therapies have come under scrutiny as they have been associated with increased CVD outcomes. As a result, all newer therapies have also been subject to intensive CVD evaluation to ensure CVD safety. Newer therapies targeting hyperglycemia with lower risks of hypoglycemia have also emerged.

This chapter will examine the role of glucose in the etiology and pathophysiology of CVD in diabetes. It will also explore some of the current controversies relating to plasma glucose and CVD risk and will describe the current guidance and evidence relating to the role of current glucose-lowering therapies and their effects on CVD risk.

Epidemiological Evidence for a Causal Role of Hyperglycemia in Cardiovascular Disease

Hyperglycemia as a risk factor for CVD has been established for many years. Mortality from CVD accounts for more than 60% of deaths in patients with type 2 diabetes mellitus and clearly accounts for this ultimate complication of diabetes [3, 8]. The association between differing degrees of hyperglycemia and CVD risk has been an area of debate. The United Kingdom Prospective Diabetes Study (UKPDS) demonstrated that the incidence of myocardial infarction rose by 14% per 1% rise in HBA1c [9]. This is in line with other studies showing that glucose is a continuous risk factor in people with both type 1 and type 2 diabetes.

Excess CVD risk is also observed in subjects with impaired glucose tolerance. The Bedford survey [10], the Whitehall study [11, 12, 13], and others [14, 15] have shown an increased mortality at the upper end of the blood glucose distribution before type 2 diabetes becomes apparent.

Furthermore, differing associations have been observed along the spectrum of impaired fasting glycemia (IFG) and impaired glucose tolerance (IGT) in relation to CVD risk. In the Japanese Funagata Diabetes Study [16], survival analysis concluded that IGT and not IFG was associated with CVD outcome. Within this sample of approximately 2,500 subjects, IGT was associated with a doubling of CVD events relative to subjects with normoglycemia. The Diabetes Epidemiology: Collaborative Analysis of Diagnostic Criteria in Europe (DECODE) study jointly analyzed data from more than 10 prospective European cohort studies and included more than 22,000 subjects [17]. Death rates from all causes, cardiovascular and CHD, were higher in subjects with diabetes diagnosed by the two-hour postload plasma glucose than in those who did not meet these criteria. Significant increase in mortality was also observed in patients with IGT, whereas there was no difference in mortality between subjects with IFG and normal fasting glucose. In the recently published Emerging Risk Factor Collaboration study [3], a fasting plasma glucose greater than 5.6 mmol/L (100 mg/dL) was associated with increased mortality.

Other evidence supporting the role of hyperglycemia as a causative factor for CVD comes from studies where CVD risk has changed as a result of intensive treatment. As previously described in the UKPDS [18] of type 2 diabetes there was a 16% reduction in CVD (combined fatal or nonfatal MI and sudden death) in the intensive glycemic control arm ($P = 0.052$). In the Diabetes Control and Complications Trial (DCCT) there was a trend toward lower CVD risk with intensive control (risk reduction 41%), but the number of events was small [19]. In a nine-year post-DCCT study, follow-up of the cohort participants previously randomized to the intensive arm had a 42% reduction ($P = 0.02$) in CVD outcomes and a 57% reduction ($P = 0.02$) in the risk of nonfatal myocardial infarction, stroke, or CVD death compared with those in the standard arm [1].

While the above discussion demonstrates a causative association between hyperglycemia and CVD risk, debate also exists on the role of postprandial hyperglycemia versus fasting hyperglycemia to CVD risk. In Western society only a small amount of time is spent fasting and a far greater proportion of the day is spent in the postprandial state. Thus, it is not surprising that postprandial hyperglycemia is a greater contributor to blood glucose control than fasting glucose concentration [20]. The importance of the postprandial state also becomes apparent from the observation that therapies used to target postprandial glucose are more effective at lowering HBA1c than those aimed at lowering fasting glucose [21]. Several studies provide evidence supporting the suggestion that postprandial glucose levels are more closely associated with CVD risk than HBA1c or fasting glucose [22]. This has been observed in the DECODE study, described above [23], and by Bonora et al. [24]. In the latter, a cohort of 1,121 patients were followed for a mean of

52 months, with plasma glucose being assessed two hours after breakfast or lunch. It was observed that postprandial glucose was able to predict the onset of CVD, even after adjusting for other risk factors. Other studies such as the Hoorn study [25], the Honolulu Heart study [26], and the Chicago Heart study [27] have also shown that plasma glucose two hours after oral challenge is a powerful predictor of CVD risk.

To conclude, there is sufficient evidence to support the role of hyperglycemia in relation to CVD risk. Later in the chapter we will explore the effects of glucose variability and fluctuations on CVD risk and the underlying pathophysiological mechanisms by which these changes are brought about.

Glucose Fluctuations and Cardiovascular Risk

There is considerable evidence showing a link between postprandial hyperglycemia and cardiovascular risk [25, 27, 28, 29]. Furthermore, two-hour postprandial glucose is a better predictor of mortality in diabetes than is HBA1c [22, 25]. Later in this chapter, we will discuss the role that oxidative stress related to hyperglycemia plays in diabetes-related cardiovascular risk. There is also evidence that glucose fluctuations (the highs and lows) are associated with increased oxidative stress [30, 31]. Of interest is that postprandial glucose control with a short-acting insulin secretagogue (repaglinide v glibenclamide) is observed to result in regression of carotid artery intima-media thickness [32]. Similarly, the reduction of postmeal glucose excursions with a premeal bolus of a rapid insulin analog (aspart) is associated with a decrease in plasma markers of oxidative stress [33]. This provides direct evidence for a link with acute rather than chronic hyperglycemia. An increase in postprandial glucose is usually the major contributor of glucose variability; however, downward fluctuations are also important. For example, urinary markers of oxidative stress are associated with the mean amplitude of glycemic excursions [31]. Furthermore, in a study in which episodes of symptomatic angina were recorded in the presence of continuous glucose monitoring and a holter cardiac monitor, sudden changes in glucose levels (100 mg/dL/hr or 5.5 mmol/L/hr) were associated with more episodes of angina [34].

Important Physiological Mechanisms of Glucose-Mediated Cardiovascular Risk

In this section we will discuss the mechanisms of glucose-mediated CVD risk, focusing on the three areas of oxidative stress, autonomic dysfunction, and hypoglycemia.

Oxidative Stress, Advanced Glycosylation End Products, and Endothelial Dysfunction

Considerable interest has developed in the role of free radical-mediated damage in many chronic disorders, in particular CVD, diabetes, and cancer [30, 35]. Free radicals are atoms or molecules that have one or more unpaired electrons in their atomic structure and are therefore highly reactive. Oxygen is the most ubiquitous of all biologically important chemical species and is a major source of reactive oxygen species (ROS). Increased oxidative stress results from an imbalance between oxidant production and antioxidant defenses [36]. Diabetes mellitus, obesity, micro- and macrovascular complications have been consistently associated with increased oxidative stress [37, 38, 39] and several studies have demonstrated that hyperglycemia per se is associated with increased oxidative stress [39, 40]. Furthermore, increased biomarkers of oxidative stress are independently associated with future CVD risk [41]. Possible mechanisms [36, 42] by which hyperglycemia may induce ROS formations are shown in Figure 5.1. As shown, hyperglycemia may result in the glucose-mediated nonenzymatic glycosylation of proteins (the Maillard reaction). The result of this is the formation of advanced glycosylation end products (AGEs). These not only increase ROS production but may also initiate a cascade of events which have harmful effects on the vascular system and are important in the etiology of both micro- and macrovascular complications relating to diabetes. Alternatively, glucose may undergo auto-oxidation to form a highly reactive enendiol radical. This may catalyze the conversion of molecular oxygen to $O_2{}^{\cdot-}$ (and hence increase ROS).

There is also an important direct mitochondrial mechanism that increases ROS [42] as a result of excess energy substrate (typically glucose and free fatty acids) entering into the citric acid cycle. The mitochondria of the endothelial cells of the vasculature may be particularly affected by "overfeeding," as these cells are not dependent on insulin for glucose uptake and therefore take up glucose freely in the setting of hyperglycemia. As shown in Figure 5.2, increased OS is associated with many of the risk factors implicated in the pathophysiology of atherosclerosis [43]. All molecules are potential targets for ROS (proteins, lipids, and DNA), but because of their ubiquitous distribution within cell membranes, and their propensity to contain double bonds, unsaturated lipids are often targeted [42]. Increased oxidative stress is associated with the increased expression of cell adhesion molecules [44], important in the initiation of atherosclerosis [45]. Apart from the global effects associated with increased oxidative stress described above, more specific effects also occur. Low-density lipoprotein (LDL) is an important target of oxidation, and oxidative modification of LDL is a key step in the pathogenesis of atherosclerosis [46]. Elevated levels of oxidized LDL (Ox-LDL) are independently associated with increased

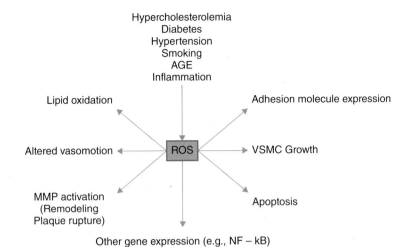

Figure 5.1 Causes and consequences of oxidative stress. ROS, Reactive oxygen species; MMP, Matrix metalloproteinases; VSMC, Vascular smooth muscle cell; HR, Hazard ratio. (Source: Stephens et al. 2009 [30]. Reproduced with permission of Elsevier.)

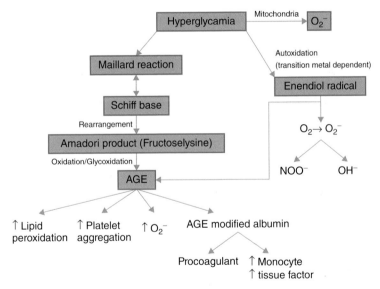

Figure 5.2 Hyperglycemia-induced oxidative stress. AGE, Advanced glycosylation end products; $O_2^{\cdot-}$, Superoxide radical; $NOO^{\cdot}$, Peroxynitrite radical. (Source: Stephens et al. 2009 [30]. Reproduced with permission of Elsevier.)

atherosclerotic burden and increased CHD risk [47, 48, 49]. It is now clear that Ox-LDL, with its many oxidatively modified lipids and degradation products, contributes to the pathophysiology of both the initiation and progression of atherosclerosis.

Autonomic Dysfunction

Both cardiac and noncardiac autonomic neuropathy are risk factors for CVD in patients with diabetes [50]. These are associated with poor glycemic control and duration of diabetes [51, 52]. Of interest is that a hyperactive sympathetic system and a hypoactive parasympathetic system have been associated with CVD in subjects with diabetes [53]. Furthermore, in vitro studies suggest that hyperglycemia has an effect on postganglionic sympathetic neurons, resulting in functional changes in the perivascular sympathetic nerves due to changes in norepinephrine release [54]. This effect may partly be related to oxidative stress; however, hyperglycemia also has a direct inhibitory effect on ATP-sensitive potassium channels [55], which depolarize neuronal tissue and alter norepinephrine release [56]. There remains uncertainty on the underlying mechanisms relating to autonomic dysfunction, diabetes, and CVD risk. Recent studies suggest that adipokines such as leptin and tumour necrosis factor-alpha influence autonomic function [57]. Cardiac autonomic neuropathy is associated with multiple risk factors including duration of diabetes, severity of hyperglycemia, and the presence of coronary artery disease, but the precise contribution to CVD risk is difficult to ascertain. Nevertheless, recent analysis in the Action to Control Cardiovascular Risk in Diabetes (ACCORD) study participants shows that cardiac autonomic neuropathy predicts all-cause and CVD mortality independently of baseline CVD, diabetes duration, and multiple other important CVD risk factors [42].

Hypoglycemia

Hypoglycemia is also associated with increased cardiovascular mortality [58, 59], although the mechanisms behind this remain unclear. A decrease in myocardial blood flow reserve during hypoglycemia may be a possible mechanism [60]. Alternatively, in vivo studies have demonstrated that acute hypoglycemia is associated with an increase in the concentration of a potent vasoconstrictor, Endothelin-1 [61]. As well as being associated with increased oxidative stress [62], hypoglycemia also has pro-inflammatory effects on the vasculature. These include increased neutrophil numbers and elevated neutrophil elastase [63]. These changes contribute to a hypercoagulable state associated with increased platelet aggregation and plasma concentrations of coagulation factors [29, 64]. Acute hypoglycemia has also been associated with long QT syndrome, which is associated with an increased risk of sudden cardiac death [65]. This may be related to sudden changes in catecholamine levels. Prolonged hypoglycemia may also have a direct detrimental effect on cardiac function because of the inability of the heart to utilize glucose, the preferred substrate instead of fatty acids (during acute myocardial ischemia), after exhaustion of myocardial glycogen reserves [66].

The Controversy of Intensive Glucose Management and Cardiovascular Risk

Intensive Glucose Control and Cardiovascular Mortality in the Action to Control Cardiovascular Risk in Diabetes (ACCORD) Study

Previously, several studies [67, 68] have clearly shown a direct relationship between HBA1c and CVD risk; however, the role of intensive glycemic control in reducing CVD events has not been well demonstrated. In the Diabetes Control and Complications Trial (DCCT) there was a trend toward a lower CVD risk with intensive control (risk reduction 41%), but the number of events was small [19]. In a nine-year post-DCCT study, follow-up of the cohort participants previously randomized to the intensive arm had a 42% reduction ($P = 0.02$) in CVD outcomes and a 57% reduction ($P = 0.02$) in the risk of nonfatal myocardial infarction, stroke, or CVD death compared with those in the standard arm [1]. In the UKPDS study [18], there was a 16% reduction in CVD (combined fatal or nonfatal MI and sudden death) in the intensive glycemic control arm ($P = 0.052$). However, further analysis showed a continuous association such that for every percentage point of lower median on-study HBA1c, there was a statistically significant 18% reduction in CVD events, again with no glycemic threshold.

In 2008, two studies (Table 5.1) – namely, the Action in Diabetes and Vascular Disease–Preterax and Diamicron Modified Release Controlled Evaluation (ADVANCE) [69] and the Veterans Affairs Diabetes Trial (VADT) [70] – were published that showed no significant reduction in CVD outcomes with intensive glycemic control. Another trial, the Action to Control Cardiovascular Risk in Diabetes (ACCORD) [71], terminated prematurely due to the finding of increased mortality in participants randomized to intensive glycemic control with a target HBA1c <6%. The ACCORD trial was designed to examine the hypothesis that reducing blood glucose concentrations to near-normal levels in adults with type 2 diabetes at high risk of a CVD event would result in a reduction in nonfatal and fatal CVD. The participants were randomly assigned to receive therapy for intensive glycemia control (HBA1c <6.0%) or therapy for standard glycaemia control (HBA1c 7.0–7.9%). As stated, the ACCORD intensive glycemia control intervention was stopped early, after 3.5 years, because

Table 5.1 Comparison of ACCORD, ADVANCE, and VADT

	ACCORD	ADVANCE	VADT
Number recruited	10,251	11,140	1,791
Median HBA1c (%)	8.1	7.2	9.4
HBA1c target (%) Intensive vs. standard	<6.0 vs. 7.0–7.9	≤6.5 vs. local guidelines	<6.0 (action if >6.5) vs. planned separation of 1.5
Median follow-up (years)	3.5 (terminated)	5	5.6
Median HBA1c (%) Intensive vs. standard	6.4 vs. 7.5	6.3 vs. 7.0	6.9 vs. 8.5
Primary outcome	Nonfatal MI, nonfatal stroke, CVD death	Microvascular plus macrovascular (nonfatal MI, nonfatal stroke, CVD death)	Nonfatal MI, nonfatal stroke, CVD death, hospitalization for heart failure, revascularization
HR for primary outcome	0.90 (0.78–1.04)	0.90 (0.82–0.98) macrovascular 0.94 (0.84–1.06)	0.88 (0.74–1.05)
HR for mortality	1.22 (1.01–1.46)	0.93 (0.83–1.06)	1.07 (0.81–1.42)
Reference	[71]	[69]	[70]

of higher mortality in this study arm (1.42% of patients died each year compared with 1.14% a year in the standard intervention arm; hazard ratio 1.22 [1.01–1.46]; $P = 0.04$) [71]. This increase in mortality was initially thought to be related to intensive-treatment-associated hypoglycemia. However, subsequent analysis of the ACCORD data suggests that this is not the case [72]. The later study showed that symptomatic hypoglycemia did not differ between the two groups and did not account for the difference in mortality between the two study arms.

Another study examined the ACCORD data to examine whether on-treatment HBA1c itself had an independent relationship with mortality [73]. This study found no evidence to suggest that lower average HBA1c was associated with higher mortality, which would have been the case if hypoglycemia had been the cause of death. Of interest is that a higher mortality rate was observed in both the intensive and standard therapy arms for individuals with a higher average and last HBA1c. This result was statistically significant in the intensive treatment arm only where a linear relationship was observed between HBA1c and mortality for an HBA1c between 6.0% and 9.0%.

The evidence for a cardiovascular benefit of intensive glycemic control remains strongest for those patients with type 1 diabetes. In a recent review, Skyler et al. [74] suggest that subset analyses of ACCORD, ADVANCE, and

VADT support the hypothesis that patients with a shorter duration of type 2 diabetes and without established atherosclerosis might gain CVD benefit from intensive glycemic control. Conversely, it is possible that the potential risks of intensive glycemic control may outweigh the benefits in other patients, such as those with a very long duration of diabetes, known history of severe hypoglycemia, advanced atherosclerosis, and advanced age. There has led to the recommendation that care providers should be vigilant in preventing severe hypoglycemia in patients with advanced disease, and should not aggressively attempt to achieve near-normal HBA1c levels in patients in whom such a target cannot be reasonably easily and safely achieved.

HBA1c: The U-Shaped Curve and Cardiovascular Outcomes

A U-shaped curve has previously been described with respect to serum cholesterol [75] and blood pressure [76] measurements in relation to mortality. A recent publication by Currie et al. suggests that a U-shaped curve also exists between HBA1c and all-cause mortality and CVD events in patients with type 2 diabetes [77]. This study is contradictory to others [78]. However, Currie et al. examined 27,000 patients retrospectively within a UK General Practice Research Database. Compared to the HBA1c decile with the lowest hazard (median HBA1c 7.5%, IQR 7.5–7.6), the adjusted hazard ratio of all-cause mortality in the lowest HBA1c decile (6.4%, 6.1–6.6) was 1.52 (95% CI 1.32–1.76), and in the highest HBA1c decile (median 10·5%, IQR 10.1–11.2) was 1.79 (95% CI 1.56–2.06). There was a U-shaped association, with the lowest risk at an HBA1c of 7.5%. There was also an increase in all-cause mortality (1.49 [95% CI 1.39–1.59]) in patients treated with insulin (2,834 deaths) compared to those given combination oral agents (2,035 deaths). This is in line with the ACCORD study findings described above. Furthermore, Johnstone et al. have also reported hypoglycemia to be associated with acute CVD events in a retrospective study of 860,845 patients [79]. Within this study, patients with hypoglycemic episodes had a 79% higher risk of events compared to those without hypoglycemia, which was independent of age.

Glucose-Lowering Medication and the Risk of Cardiovascular Disease

The management of CVD risk in patients with diabetes requires a multifactorial approach and, clearly, all CVD risk factors need to be addressed. The intensive management of each CVD risk factor (e.g., HBA1c, cholesterol, systolic blood pressure) additively reduces CVD risk [5]. An interesting observation was made in a follow-up study of the UKPDS cohort [80, 81].

Within the cohort, the difference in HBA1c was lost after the first year, but within the initial intensively treated glycemic arm after ten years' follow-up, there was a lower incidence of complications. These included a 21% reduction in any diabetes-related endpoint ($P = 0.01$), a 33% reduction in myocardial infarction ($P = 0.005$), and a 27% reduction in death from any cause ($P = 0.002$). Therefore, there was a "legacy" effect of intensive early glycemic control that was associated with benefits late on. Within this section we will briefly examine the associations between different glucose-lowering therapies and CVD outcome.

Metformin

Metformin is generally accepted as the first-line agent for the treatment of type 2 diabetes when not satisfactory controlled by lifestyle alone. Metformin has no adverse effects on CVD risk factors and furthermore may be associated with weight reduction and has a low risk of hypoglycemia [82]. Within the UKPDS, early improved glycemic control with metformin in overweight patients with type 2 diabetes was associated with a reduction in the risk of CVD events [18]. The use of metformin was associated with a 39% reduction in myocardial infarction ($P = 0.01$). Patients with established CVD may also have coexisting renal (creatinine >150 μmol/L [1.97 mg/dL] or eGFR <30), hepatic, and cardiac impairment, and current guidance should be followed in relation to the use of metformin in these circumstances.

Sulfonylurea and Insulin

Within the UKPDS, intensive blood glucose control by either sulfonylureas or insulin substantially decreases the risk of microvascular complications, but not macrovascular disease in patients with type 2 diabetes [83]. Treatment with sulfonylurea and insulin was also associated with weight gain and increased risk of hypoglycemia. Sulfonylureas act by binding to specific sulfonylurea-ATP-sensitive K+ channels/receptors. Since these agents reduce hyperglycemia and hence glucose-mediated oxidative stress and endothelial dysfunction, they should also reduce CVD risk. During 10 years of UKPDS post-trial follow-up, a risk reduction in myocardial infarction and all-cause mortality emerged in patients treated with sulfonylureas or insulin [80, 83].

Interest has also focused on whether short-acting postprandial glucose-regulator drugs (e.g., repaglinide) may have different benefits in relation to CVD risk compared to longer-acting sulfonylureas (e.g., glibenclamide). The rationale behind this is that the postprandial regulators are typically administered with meals and act to reduce the postmeal glucose fluctuation. This may also influence postprandial changes in oxidative stress, which may be associated with CVD risk. Mazella et al. demonstrated in a small sample of 16 patients with type 2 diabetes treated with diet alone and poor glucose control that repaglinide was associated with a significant reduction in two-hour plasma glucose levels, plasma markers of total antioxidant status and brachial reactivity, which was not observed when treated with glibenclamide [84]. A similar postprandial reduction in plasma total antioxidant status was also observed in a previous study by Tankova et al. [85], but not by Stephens et al. [86].

Glitazones

In recent years, the glitazones have had a troubled time with respect to CVD. They are associated with increased risk of heart failure and controversy exists on the effect of these agents on acute coronary events. Previously, rosiglitazone has been associated with a reduction in stent restenosis rate [87] and improvements in cardiovascular risk factors [88, 89, 90]. However, in a meta-analysis of 42 studies in a sample of patients with type 2 diabetes with a mean age of 57 years, the use of rosiglitazone was associated with an increased risk of myocardial infarction and death from CVD [91]. While this study was open to criticisms and limitations, the manuscript led to a series of studies exploring this association and eventually led to the removal of rosiglitazone from routine use on the advice of the FDA and MHRA. Of interest is that in a subsequent paper [92], an increase in CVD risk was not observed. The prospective pioglitazone clinical trial in macrovascular events (PROACTIVE) study examined the risk of CVD events associated with pioglitazone. This showed that pioglitazone reduces the composite of all-cause mortality, nonfatal myocardial infarction, and stroke in patients with type 2 diabetes who have a high risk of macrovascular events [93]. Despite the continued use of pioglitazone, caution is often practiced, especially in patients with a history of acute coronary syndrome and heart failure.

DPP-IV Inhibitors and GLP-1 Analogues

DPP-IV inhibitors are a relatively new treatment choice for the management of type 2 diabetes. These agents benefit from a low risk of hypoglycemia and no weight gain. To date, short-term and cross-sectional studies have raised no concerns in relation to CVD risk. In fact, a recent meta-analysis [94] of 53 trials enrolling 20,312 and 13,569 patients for DPP-IV and comparators respectively showed a significant reduction in major CV events (OR 0.689 [0.528–0.899], $P = 0.006$). With respect to CVD outcome, ongoing studies are currently underway, as shown in Table 5.2. These studies will clarify the long-term cardiovascular safety of the agents.

With respect to GLP-1 analogs, long-term safety evaluations are underway: the Liraglutide Effect and Action in Diabetes: Evaluation of Cardiovascular Outcome Results (LEADER) study and the Exenatide Study

Table 5.2 Summary of long-term cardiovascular outcome studies underway for linagliptin, sitagliptin, saxagliptin, and alogliptin

Study	CAROLINA	TECOS	SAVOR-TIMI53	EXAMINE
DPP-4 inhibitor	Linagliptin	Sitagliptin	Saxagliptin	Alogliptin
Comparator	SU (Active)	Placebo	Placebo	Placebo
Number of patients	6,000	14,000	16,500	5,400
Trial initiation	Oct 2010	Nov 2008	May 2010	Sept 2009
Expected diabetes disease stage	Early	Advanced	Advanced	All, but limited to CV events

of Cardiovascular Event Lowering (EXSCEL) study. At present, no harmful cardiovascular signal has been reported, and preclinical data and effects on risk markers suggest a potential for benefit [95]. Both exenatide [96, 97] and liraglutide [98, 99] have been associated with mild reductions in both systolic and diastolic blood pressure, which appear to be independent of weight loss and improvements in lipid parameters. Animal studies have also shown that exenatide improves recovery from ischemic-reperfusion injury and improves survival in dilated cardiomyopathy. At present, no long-term cardiovascular outcome studies have been completed for any of the GLP-1 receptor agonists. There is a post hoc analysis of exenatide exposure in the ACCORD trial, which showed a relative reduction in cardiovascular events and morbidity [71]. Another meta-analysis [100] showed a reduction in cardiovascular events associated with exenatide performed on data from 12 randomized trials.

Current Practice Guidance for Glucose Management in Relation to Cardiovascular Disease

As emphasized in this chapter, diabetes is an independent risk factor for CVD and a linear association exists between rising HBA1c and CVD events. For this reason, previous guidelines relating to glycemic control argued for the aggressive lowering of HBA1c levels in patients with established vascular disease (e.g., National Institute of Clinical Excellence [NICE] 2002 guidelines for the management of type 2 diabetes). However, the ADVANCE [69], VADT [70], and ACCORD [71] trials demonstrated that the evidence for intensive glycemic control preventing cardiovascular complications in type 2 diabetes mellitus was not robust, and in particular that the ACCORD trial was associated with an increase in CVD in the intensive glycemic control arm. The impact of these randomized controlled trials, along with observational data from routinely collected data sets [77], has been profound. First, it has halted the continual lowering of HBA1c targets in type 2 diabetes, previously led by key opinion leaders, such that it is unusual to find a guideline advocating an HBA1c lower than 6.5% (ACCORD aimed for <6.0%). Second, in the UK there has actually been a relaxation of HBA1c targets, with the primary care general medical services (GMS) target rising from <7.0% to <7.5%. The NICE guideline in the UK for glycemic management of patients with type 2 diabetes, published in 2009, also advocates an HBA1c target of less than 7.5% when patients are prescribed more than two hypoglycemic agents.

In relation to the use of specific hypoglycemic therapies, there is a lack of consensus in relation to the choice of agents with respect to CVD outcome. However, all guidelines are consistent in the primary role of metformin as first-line therapy for patients with type 2 diabetes not controlled by diet and lifestyle alone. As already discussed, metformin is the only hypoglycemic agent to have shown a cardiovascular mortality benefit [18]. However, a recent meta-analysis pointed out that this is the only study that has shown such an impact [101], and the small cohort size plus an increased cardiovascular risk of metformin when used with a sulfonylurea in the same study must cast some doubt. It is likely that the low acquisition cost of metformin is at least partly responsible for its popularity.

After metformin, the guidelines are highly variable in their recommendations. In the UK, the NICE guidance advocates the use of a sulfonylurea (with options of pioglitazone and/or gliptins in some groups). Thereafter, the use of triple oral therapy regimes comes into play, as well as insulin or the use of GLP-1 analogs. However, the National Health Service QIPP agenda (Quality, Innovation, Productivity, and Prevention), currently being pursued in the UK, strongly promotes the sequential use of metformin and sulfonylurea followed by human intermediate-acting insulin. The well-established side effects of weight gain and hypoglycemia (and their potential effects on cardiovascular risk) are underplayed, along with any specific cardiovascular safety concerns that have previously been raised with both sulfonylureas and insulin.

The most recent joint position statement from the American Diabetes Association (ADA) and European Association of Specialist Diabetologists (EASD) in relation to the management of type 2 diabetes advocates a much more "patient-centered approach" [102]. In the consensus document, the second-line therapy after metformin monotherapy failure can be any one of five combinations, which include both GLP-1 analogs and insulin. Triple therapy combinations of all of those drugs licensed for such use then forms the third-line option. Although the newer classes of hypoglycemic drugs are acknowledged to have the potential to reduce cardiovascular risk, this has little impact on their recommendation. Similarly, the PROACTIVE study, which showed reduced cardiovascular events with pioglitazone, is effectively ignored [93].

One area where cardiovascular risk has certainly influenced the development of diabetes therapies is in the increased amount of safety data needed to achieve a license for the use of new drugs. The European withdrawal of rosiglitazone in 2010, ten years after launch, followed a controversy over whether it increased the risk of myocardial infarction in patients with type 2 diabetes [91]. This is a controversial topic but, nevertheless, the debate has altered the way in which the Food and Drug Administration (FDA) in the United States and the European Medicines Agency (EMA) assess new hypoglycemic agents. The FDA issued guidance for industry in 2008 stating, "To establish the safety of a new antidiabetic therapy to treat type 2 diabetes, sponsors should demonstrate that the therapy will not result in an unacceptable increase in cardiovascular risk." The methodology by which this was to be achieved was to compare the incidence of cardiovascular events occurring with the investigational agent to the incidence of the same types of events occurring with the control group, noting that these would inevitably be short-term studies in relatively small cohorts of patients (and thus have very low rates of cardiovascular events). If such analyses could not show that the upper bound of the 95% confidence interval is less than 1.8, then license would be delayed pending the conduct of a randomized controlled trial (typically placebo control) to demonstrate safety. If the premarketing application contained data showing that the upper bound of the 95% confidence interval is between 1.3 and 1.8, then a postmarketing cardiovascular trial would typically be needed, once again with placebo control.

Case Study 1

A 48-year-old man with type 2 diabetes of 20 years' duration attends for his annual diabetes review. He had an acute myocardial infarction six months ago. He is unable to lose weight and claims to walk for 30 minutes on three occasions per week. His current therapy consists of metformin 1 g BD, aspirin 75 mg OD, simvastatin 40 mg OD, ramipril 10 mg OD and atenolol 50 mg OD. On review he has a BMI of 37 kg/m², HBA1c 8.0%, Creatinine 120 μmol/L, eGFR 60 ml/min, ACR 10, total cholesterol of 3.2 mmol/L (123.4 mg/dL). His blood pressure is 110/70 mmHg.

Multiple-Choice Questions

1 Which *one* of the following therapeutic strategies would be the best option to improve his glycaemic control?

   A Make no change

   B Commence basal insulin therapy in addition to his current medication

C Commence a GLP-1 analog

D Commence rosiglitazone

E Commence a sulfonylurea (e.g., glibenclamide or gliclazide)

2 During the subsequent consultation his wife also attends the clinic. She is in good health and informs you that she has been diagnosed with impaired glucose tolerance. She asks if she is at higher risk of ischemic heart disease. Which *one* of the following would be the best answer?

A She is at no higher risk than a person without diabetes

B She is at the same risk as a patient with diabetes

C She is at an intermediate risk between that of a patient without diabetes and one with diabetes

D She is at a higher cardiovascular risk than someone with impaired fasting glycemia

E She is at an intermediate risk between that of a patient without diabetes and one with diabetes, but more information and assessment are required to assess her risk accurately

Answers provided after the References

Case Study 2

A 73-year-old woman with unstable angina and a recent forearm fracture following an accidental fall is noted to have highly variable home glucose values ranging from 2.7–16.6 mmol/L (48.6–298.8 mg/dL). On several occasions her husband has been woken at night to find her in an agitated state with a low capillary glucose measurement. Her eating habits are erratic and she misses meals frequently. Her current medication consists of glibenclamide 10 mg OD, metformin 1 g BD, ramipril 10 mg OD, aspirin 75 mg OD and amlodipine 5 mg OD. She has background retinopathy, suffers with distal symmetrical sensory loss in both feet, and occasionally complains of dizziness on standing. She rarely measures her home blood glucose and will not have insulin therapy. She has an HBA1c of 10.0% (86 mmol/mol), BP 160/100 mmHg, creatinine 185 μmol/L (2.10 mg/dL), eGFR 25 ml/min, ACR 10.

Multiple-Choice Questions

1 Which of the following risk factors would predispose to further cardiovascular events in this case? (There can be more than one option.)

A Hypoglycemia

B Peripheral and autonomic neuropathy

C Erratic glucose fluctuations

D Hypertension

E Impaired renal function

2 She subsequently agrees to insulin therapy and to monitor her home glucose capillary readings. She is commenced on a premixed insulin at

a total daily dose of 40 units. She is well and has home glucose values ranging from 4.1–10.2 mmol/L (73.8–183.6 mg/dL). Her HBA1c is 9.5% (80 mmol/mol). What would be the target HBA1c?

A 6.0% (42 mmol/mol)

B 6.5% (48 mmol/mol)

C 7.0% (53 mmol/mol)

D 8.0% (64 mmol/mol)

E 9.0% (75 mmol/mol)

Answers provided after the References

Guidelines and Web Links

guidance.nice.org.uk/cg87
**www.fda.gov/downloads/Drugs/GuidanceComplianceRegulatoryInformation/
    Guidances/ucm071627.pdf**
Guidance for Industry. Diabetes Mellitus – Evaluating Cardiovascular Risk in New Antidi-
    abetic Therapies to Treat Type 2 Diabetes. U.S. Department of Health and Human
    Services. Food and Drug Administration. Center for Drug Evaluation and Research
    (CDER).
Type 2 diabetes: The management of type 2 diabetes. Issued May 2009, last modified
    March 2010. NICE clinical guideline 87.

References

1 Nathan DM, Cleary PA, Backlund JY et al. Intensive diabetes treatment and cardio-
    vascular disease in patients with type 1 diabetes. *N Engl J Med* 2005; 353: 2643–53.
2 Amos AF, McCarty DJ, Zimmet P. The rising global burden of diabetes and its com-
    plications: Estimates and projections to the year 2010. *Diabet Med* 1997; 14(Suppl 5):
    S1–S85.
3 Seshasai SR, Kaptoge S, Thompson A et al. Diabetes mellitus, fasting glucose, and
    risk of cause-specific death. *N Engl J Med* 364: 829–41.
4 Haffner SM, Lehto S, Ronnemaa T, Pyorala K, Laakso M. Mortality from coronary
    heart disease in subjects with type 2 diabetes and in nondiabetic subjects with and
    without prior myocardial infarction. *N Engl J Med* 1998; 339: 229–34.
5 Gaede P, Vedel P, Larsen N, Jensen GV, Parving HH, Pedersen O. Multifactorial inter-
    vention and cardiovascular disease in patients with type 2 diabetes. *N Engl J Med*
    2003; 348: 383–93.
6 Pyorala K, Laakso M, Uusitupa M. Diabetes and atherosclerosis: An epidemiologic
    view. *Diabetes Metab Rev* 1987; 3: 463–524.
7 Stephens JW, Ambler G, Vallance P, Betteridge DJ, Humphries SE, Hurel SJ. Car-
    diovascular risk and diabetes: Are the methods of risk prediction satisfactory? *Eur J
    Cardiovasc Prev Rehabil* 2004; 11: 521–8.
8 Duckworth W, Abraira C, Moritz T et al. Glucose control and vascular complications
    in veterans with type 2 diabetes. *N Engl J Med* 2009; 360: 129–39.
9 Stratton IM, Adler AI, Neil HA et al. Association of glycaemia with macrovascular
    and microvascular complications of type 2 diabetes (UKPDS 35): Prospective obser-
    vational study. *Brit Med J* 2000; 321: 405–12.

10 Keen H, Jarrett RJ, McCartney P. The ten-year follow-up of the Bedford survey (1962–1972): Glucose tolerance and diabetes. *Diabetologia* 1982; 22: 73–8.

11 Fuller JH, McCartney P, Jarrett RJ et al. Hyperglycaemia and coronary heart disease: The Whitehall study. *J Chronic Dis* 1979; 32: 721–8.

12 Fuller JH, Shipley MJ, Rose G, Jarrett RJ, Keen H. Coronary-heart-disease risk and impaired glucose tolerance: The Whitehall study. *Lancet* 1980; 1: 1373–6.

13 Fuller JH, Shipley MJ, Rose G, Jarrett RJ, Keen H. Mortality from coronary heart disease and stroke in relation to degree of glycaemia: The Whitehall study. *Br Med J (Clin Res Ed)* 1983; 287: 867–70.

14 Eschwege E, Richard JL, Thibult N et al. Coronary heart disease mortality in relation with diabetes, blood glucose and plasma insulin levels: The Paris Prospective Study, ten years later. *Horm Metab Res Suppl* 1985; 15: 41–6.

15 Kuusisto J, Mykkanen L, Pyorala K, Laakso M. NIDDM and its metabolic control predict coronary heart disease in elderly subjects. *Diabetes* 1994; 43: 960–67.

16 Tominaga M, Eguchi H, Manaka H, Igarashi K, Kato T, Sekikawa A. Impaired glucose tolerance is a risk factor for cardiovascular disease, but not impaired fasting glucose: The Funagata Diabetes Study. *Diabetes Care* 1999; 22: 920–24.

17 Glucose tolerance and mortality: Comparison of WHO and American Diabetes Association diagnostic criteria. The DECODE study group. European Diabetes Epidemiology Group. Diabetes Epidemiology: Collaborative analysis of Diagnostic criteria in Europe. *Lancet* 1999; 354: 617–21.

18 Effect of intensive blood-glucose control with metformin on complications in overweight patients with type 2 diabetes (UKPDS 34). UK Prospective Diabetes Study (UKPDS) Group. *Lancet* 1998; 352: 854–65.

19 The effect of intensive treatment of diabetes on the development and progression of long-term complications in insulin-dependent diabetes mellitus. The Diabetes Control and Complications Trial Research Group. *N Engl J Med* 1993; 329: 977–86.

20 Avignon A, Radauceanu A, Monnier L. Nonfasting plasma glucose is a better marker of diabetic control than fasting plasma glucose in type 2 diabetes. *Diabetes Care* 1997; 20: 1822–6.

21 Bastyr EJ, III,, Stuart CA, Brodows RG et al. Therapy focused on lowering postprandial glucose, not fasting glucose, may be superior for lowering HBA1c. IOEZ Study Group. *Diabetes Care* 2000; 23: 1236–41.

22 Hanefeld M, Fischer S, Julius U et al. Risk factors for myocardial infarction and death in newly detected NIDDM: The Diabetes Intervention Study, 11-year follow-up. *Diabetologia* 1996; 39: 1577–83.

23 Glucose tolerance and cardiovascular mortality: Comparison of fasting and 2-hour diagnostic criteria. *Arch Intern Med* 2001; 161: 397–405.

24 Bonora E, Muggeo M. Postprandial blood glucose as a risk factor for cardiovascular disease in Type II diabetes: The epidemiological evidence. *Diabetologia* 2001; 44: 2107–14.

25 de Vegt F, Dekker JM, Ruhe HG et al. Hyperglycaemia is associated with all-cause and cardiovascular mortality in the Hoorn population: The Hoorn Study. *Diabetologia* 1999; 42: 926–31.

26 Donahue RP, Abbott RD, Reed DM, Yano K. Postchallenge glucose concentration and coronary heart disease in men of Japanese ancestry. Honolulu Heart Program. *Diabetes* 1987; 36: 689–92.

27 Lowe LP, Liu K, Greenland P, Metzger BE, Dyer AR, Stamler J. Diabetes, asymptomatic hyperglycemia, and 22-year mortality in black and white men. The Chicago Heart Association Detection Project in Industry Study. *Diabetes Care* 1997; 20: 163–9.

28 Qiao Q, Hu G, Tuomilehto J et al. Age- and sex-specific prevalence of diabetes and impaired glucose regulation in 11 Asian cohorts. *Diabetes Care* 2003; 26: 1770–80.

29 Trovati M, Anfossi G, Cavalot F et al. Studies on mechanisms involved in hypoglycemia-induced platelet activation. *Diabetes* 1986; 35: 818–25.

30 Stephens JW, Khanolkar MP, Bain SC. The biological relevance and measurement of plasma markers of oxidative stress in diabetes and cardiovascular disease. *Atherosclerosis* 2009; 202: 321–9.

31 Monnier L, Mas E, Ginet C et al. Activation of oxidative stress by acute glucose fluctuations compared with sustained chronic hyperglycemia in patients with type 2 diabetes. *JAMA* 2006; 295: 1681–7.

32 Ceriello A, Quagliaro L, Piconi L et al. Effect of postprandial hypertriglyceridemia and hyperglycemia on circulating adhesion molecules and oxidative stress generation and the possible role of simvastatin treatment. *Diabetes* 2004; 53: 701–10.

33 Ceriello A, Quagliaro L, Catone B et al. Role of hyperglycemia in nitrotyrosine postprandial generation. *Diabetes Care* 2002; 25: 1439–43.

34 Desouza C, Salazar H, Cheong B, Murgo J, Fonseca V. Association of hypoglycemia and cardiac ischemia: A study based on continuous monitoring. *Diabetes Care* 2003; 26: 1485–9.

35 Baynes JW. Role of oxidative stress in development of complications in diabetes. *Diabetes* 1991; 40: 405–12.

36 Maritim AC, Sanders RA, Watkins JB, III,. Diabetes, oxidative stress, and antioxidants: A review. *J Biochem Mol Toxicol* 2003; 17: 24–38.

37 Cai H, Harrison DG. Endothelial dysfunction in cardiovascular diseases: The role of oxidant stress. *Circ Res* 2000; 87: 840–44.

38 Brownlee M. Biochemistry and molecular cell biology of diabetic complications. *Nature* 2001; 414: 813–20.

39 Sampson MJ, Gopaul N, Davies IR, Hughes DA, Carrier MJ. Plasma F2 isoprostanes: Direct evidence of increased free radical damage during acute hyperglycemia in type 2 diabetes. *Diabetes Care* 2002; 25: 537–41.

40 Nourooz-Zadeh J, Tajaddini-Sarmadi J, McCarthy S, Betteridge DJ, Wolff SP. Elevated levels of authentic plasma hydroperoxides in NIDDM. *Diabetes* 1995; 44: 1054–8.

41 Stephens JW, Gable DR, Hurel SJ, Miller GJ, Cooper JA, Humphries SE. Increased plasma markers of oxidative stress are associated with coronary heart disease in males with diabetes mellitus and with 10-year risk in a prospective sample of males. *Clin Chem* 2006; 52(3): 446–52.

42 Pop-Busui R, Evans GW, Gerstein HC et al. Effects of cardiac autonomic dysfunction on mortality risk in the Action to Control Cardiovascular Risk in Diabetes (ACCORD) trial. *Diabetes Care* 33: 1578–84.

43 Harrison D, Griendling KK, Landmesser U, Hornig B, Drexler H. Role of oxidative stress in atherosclerosis. *Am J Cardiol* 2003; 91: 7A–11A.

44 Jang Y, Lincoff AM, Plow EF, Topol EJ. Cell adhesion molecules in coronary artery disease. *J Am Coll Cardiol* 1994; 24: 1591–601.

45 Ross R. The pathogenesis of atherosclerosis: A perspective for the 1990s. *Nature* 1993; 362: 801–9.

46 Witztum JL, Steinberg D. The oxidative modification hypothesis of atherosclerosis: Does it hold for humans? *Trends Cardiovasc Med* 2001; 11: 93–102.

47 Toshima S, Hasegawa A, Kurabayashi M et al. Circulating oxidized low density lipoprotein levels: A biochemical risk marker for coronary heart disease. *Arterioscler Thromb Vasc Biol* 2000; 20: 2243–7.

48 Ehara S, Ueda M, Naruko T et al. Elevated levels of oxidized low density lipoprotein show a positive relationship with the severity of acute coronary syndromes. *Circulation* 2001; 103: 1955–60.

49 Weinbrenner T, Cladellas M, Isabel Covas M et al. High oxidative stress in patients with stable coronary heart disease. *Atherosclerosis* 2003; 168: 99–106.

50 Vinik AI, Ziegler D. Diabetic cardiovascular autonomic neuropathy. *Circulation* 2007; 115: 387–97.

51 Toyry JP, Niskanen LK, Mantysaari MJ, Lansimies EA, Uusitupa MI. Occurrence, predictors, and clinical significance of autonomic neuropathy in NIDDM: Ten-year follow-up from the diagnosis. *Diabetes* 1996; 45: 308–15.

52 Laitinen T, Lindstrom J, Eriksson J et al. Cardiovascular autonomic dysfunction is associated with central obesity in persons with impaired glucose tolerance. *Diabet Med* 28: 699–704.

53 Gerritsen J, Dekker JM, TenVoorde BJ et al. Impaired autonomic function is associated with increased mortality, especially in subjects with diabetes, hypertension, or a history of cardiovascular disease: The Hoorn Study. *Diabetes Care* 2001; 24: 1793–8.

54 Damon DH. Vascular-dependent effects of elevated glucose on postganglionic sympathetic neurons. *Am J Physiol Heart Circ Physiol* 300: H1386–92.

55 Minami K, Miki T, Kadowaki T, Seino S. Roles of ATP-sensitive K+ channels as metabolic sensors: Studies of Kir6.x null mice. *Diabetes* 2004; 53 Suppl 3: S176–80.

56 Burgdorf C, Dendorfer A, Kurz T et al. Role of neuronal KATP channels and extraneuronal monoamine transporter on norepinephrine overflow in a model of myocardial low flow ischemia. *J Pharmacol Exp Ther* 2004; 309: 42–8.

57 Jung CH, Kim BY, Kim CH, Kang SK, Jung SH, Mok JO. Association of serum adipocytokine levels with cardiac autonomic neuropathy in type 2 diabetic patients. *Cardiovasc Diabetol* 11: 24.

58 Wei M, Gibbons LW, Mitchell TL, Kampert JB, Stern MP, Blair SN. Low fasting plasma glucose level as a predictor of cardiovascular disease and all-cause mortality. *Circulation* 2000; 101: 2047–52.

59 Kosiborod M, Inzucchi SE, Goyal A et al. Relationship between spontaneous and iatrogenic hypoglycemia and mortality in patients hospitalized with acute myocardial infarction. *JAMA* 2009; 301: 1556–64.

60 Rana O, Byrne CD, Kerr D et al. Acute hypoglycemia decreases myocardial blood flow reserve in patients with type 1 diabetes mellitus and in healthy humans. *Circulation* 124: 1548–56.

61 Yanagisawa M, Kurihara H, Kimura S et al. A novel potent vasoconstrictor peptide produced by vascular endothelial cells. *Nature* 1988; 332: 411–15.

62 Wang J, Alexanian A, Ying R et al. Acute exposure to low glucose rapidly induces endothelial dysfunction and mitochondrial oxidative stress: Role for AMP kinase. *Arterioscler Thromb Vasc Biol* 32: 712–20.

63 Collier A, Patrick AW, Hepburn DA et al. Leucocyte mobilization and release of neutrophil elastase following acute insulin-induced hypoglycaemia in normal humans. *Diabet Med* 1990; 7: 506–9.

64 Hilsted J, Madsbad S, Nielsen JD, Krarup T, Sestoft L, Gormsen J. Hypoglycemia and hemostatic parameters in juvenile-onset diabetes. *Diabetes Care* 1980; 3: 675–8.

65 Marques JL, George E, Peacey SR et al. Altered ventricular repolarization during hypoglycaemia in patients with diabetes. *Diabet Med* 1997; 14: 648–54.

66 Depre C, Vanoverschelde JL, Taegtmeyer H. Glucose for the heart. *Circulation* 1999; 99: 578–88.

67 Selvin E, Marinopoulos S, Berkenblit G et al. Meta-analysis: Glycosylated hemoglobin and cardiovascular disease in diabetes mellitus. *Ann Intern Med* 2004; 141: 421–31.

68 Stettler C, Allemann S, Juni P et al. Glycemic control and macrovascular disease in types 1 and 2 diabetes mellitus: Meta-analysis of randomized trials. *Am Heart J* 2006; 152: 27–38.

69 Patel A, MacMahon S, Chalmers J et al. Intensive blood glucose control and vascular outcomes in patients with type 2 diabetes. *N Engl J Med* 2008; 358: 2560–72.

70 Reaven PD, Moritz TE, Schwenke DC et al. Intensive glucose-lowering therapy reduces cardiovascular disease events in veterans affairs diabetes trial participants with lower calcified coronary atherosclerosis. *Diabetes* 2009; 58: 2642–8.

71 Gerstein HC, Miller ME, Byington RP et al. Effects of intensive glucose lowering in type 2 diabetes. *N Engl J Med* 2008; 358: 2545–59.

72 Bonds DE, Miller ME, Bergenstal RM et al. The association between symptomatic, severe hypoglycaemia and mortality in type 2 diabetes: Retrospective epidemiological analysis of the ACCORD study. *Brit Med J* 340: b4909.

73 Riddle MC, Ambrosius WT, Brillon DJ et al. Epidemiologic relationships between A1C and all-cause mortality during a median 3.4-year follow-up of glycemic treatment in the ACCORD trial. *Diabetes Care* 33: 983–90.

74 Skyler JS, Bergenstal R, Bonow RO et al. Intensive glycemic control and the prevention of cardiovascular events: Implications of the ACCORD, ADVANCE, and VA diabetes trials: A position statement of the American Diabetes Association and a scientific statement of the American College of Cardiology Foundation and the American Heart Association. *Diabetes Care* 2009; 32: 187–92.

75 Epstein FH. Relationship between low cholesterol and disease: Evidence from epidemiological studies and preventive trials. *Ann NY Acad Sci* 1995; 748: 482–90.

76 Samuelsson OG, Wilhelmsen LW, Pennert KM, Wedel H, Berglund GL. The J-shaped relationship between coronary heart disease and achieved blood pressure level in treated hypertension: Further analyses of 12 years of follow-up of treated hypertensives in the Primary Prevention Trial in Gothenburg, Sweden. *J Hypertens* 1990; 8: 547–55.

77 Currie CJ, Peters JR, Tynan A et al. Survival as a function of HbA(1c) in people with type 2 diabetes: A retrospective cohort study. *Lancet* 375: 481–9.

78 Eeg-Olofsson K, Cederholm J, Nilsson PM et al. New aspects of HBA1c as a risk factor for cardiovascular diseases in type 2 diabetes: An observational study from the Swedish National Diabetes Register (NDR). *J Intern Med* 268: 471–82.

79 Ma H, Hagen F, Stekel DJ et al. The fatal fungal outbreak on Vancouver Island is characterized by enhanced intracellular parasitism driven by mitochondrial regulation. *Proc Natl Acad Sci USA* 2009; 106: 12980–85.

80 Holman RR, Paul SK, Bethel MA, Matthews DR, Neil HA. 10-year follow-up of intensive glucose control in type 2 diabetes. *N Engl J Med* 2008; 359: 1577–89.

81 Holman RR, Paul SK, Bethel MA, Neil HA, Matthews DR. Long-term follow-up after tight control of blood pressure in type 2 diabetes. *N Engl J Med* 2008; 359: 1565–76.

82 UK prospective diabetes study 16. Overview of 6 years' therapy of type II diabetes: A progressive disease. UK Prospective Diabetes Study Group. *Diabetes* 1995; 44: 1249–58.

83 Intensive blood-glucose control with sulfonylureas or insulin compared with conventional treatment and risk of complications in patients with type 2 diabetes (UKPDS 33). UK Prospective Diabetes Study (UKPDS) Group. *Lancet* 1998; 352: 837–53.

84 Manzella D, Grella R, Abbatecola AM, Paolisso G. Repaglinide administration improves brachial reactivity in type 2 diabetic patients. *Diabetes Care* 2005; 28: 366–71.

85 Tankova T, Koev D, Dakovska L, Kirilov G. The effect of repaglinide on insulin secretion and oxidative stress in type 2 diabetic patients. *Diabetes Res Clin Pract* 2003; 59: 43–9.

86 Stephens JW, Bodvarsdottir TB, Wareham K et al. Effects of short-term therapy with glibenclamide and repaglinide on incretin hormones and oxidative damage associated with postprandial hyperglycaemia in people with type 2 diabetes mellitus. *Diabetes Res Clin Pract* 94: 199–206.

87 Choi D, Kim SK, Choi SH et al. Preventative effects of rosiglitazone on restenosis after coronary stent implantation in patients with type 2 diabetes. *Diabetes Care* 2004; 27: 2654–60.

88 St. John Sutton M, Rendell M, Dandona P et al. A comparison of the effects of rosiglitazone and glyburide on cardiovascular function and glycemic control in patients with type 2 diabetes. *Diabetes Care* 2002; 25: 2058–64.

89 Shargorodsky M, Wainstein J, Gavish D, Leibovitz E, Matas Z, Zimlichman R. Treatment with rosiglitazone reduces hyperinsulinemia and improves arterial elasticity in patients with type 2 diabetes mellitus. *Am J Hypertens* 2003; 16: 617–22.

90 Haffner SM, Greenberg AS, Weston WM, Chen H, Williams K, Freed MI. Effect of rosiglitazone treatment on nontraditional markers of cardiovascular disease in patients with type 2 diabetes mellitus. *Circulation* 2002; 106: 679–84.

91 Nissen SE, Wolski K. Effect of rosiglitazone on the risk of myocardial infarction and death from cardiovascular causes. *N Engl J Med* 2007; 356: 2457–71.

92 Home PD, Pocock SJ, Beck-Nielsen H et al. Rosiglitazone evaluated for cardiovascular outcomes: An interim analysis. *N Engl J Med* 2007; 357: 28–38.

93 Dormandy JA, Charbonnel B, Eckland DJ et al. Secondary prevention of macrovascular events in patients with type 2 diabetes in the PROactive Study (PROspective pioglitAzone Clinical Trial In macroVascular Events): A randomised controlled trial. *Lancet* 2005; 366: 1279–89.

94 Monami M, Dicembrini I, Martelli D, Mannucci E. Safety of dipeptidyl peptidase-4 inhibitors: A meta-analysis of randomized clinical trials. *Curr Med Res Opin* 2011; 27(Suppl 3): 57–64.

95 Aroda VR, Ratner R. The safety and tolerability of GLP-1 receptor agonists in the treatment of type 2 diabetes: A review. *Diabetes Metab Res Rev* 2011; 27: 528–42.

96 Drucker DJ, Buse JB, Taylor K et al. Exenatide once weekly versus twice daily for the treatment of type 2 diabetes: A randomised, open-label, non-inferiority study. *Lancet* 2008; 372: 1240–50.

97 Sonne DP, Engstrom T, Treiman M. Protective effects of GLP-1 analogues exendin-4 and GLP-1(9-36) amide against ischemia-reperfusion injury in rat heart. *Regul Pept* 2008; 146: 243–9.

98 Nauck M, Frid A, Hermansen K et al. Efficacy and safety comparison of liraglutide, glimepiride, and placebo, all in combination with metformin, in type 2 diabetes: The LEAD (liraglutide effect and action in diabetes)-2 study. *Diabetes Care* 2009; 32: 84–90.

99 Buse JB, Rosenstock J, Sesti G et al. Liraglutide once a day versus exenatide twice a day for type 2 diabetes: A 26-week randomised, parallel-group, multinational, open-label trial (LEAD-6). *Lancet* 2009; 374: 39–47.

100 Ratner R, Han J, Nicewarner D, Yushmanova I, Hoogwerf BJ, Shen L. Cardiovascular safety of exenatide BID: An integrated analysis from controlled clinical trials in participants with type 2 diabetes. *Cardiovasc Diabetol* 10: 22.

101 Boussageon R, Supper I, Bejan-Angoulvant T, et al. Reappraisal of metformin effi-cacy in the treatment of type 2 diabetes: A meta-analysis of randomised controlled trials. *PLoS Med* 9: e1001204.

102 Inzucchi SE, Bergenstal RM, Buse JB et al. Management of hyperglycemia in type 2 diabetes: A patient-centered approach: Position statement of the American Diabetes Association (ADA) and the European Association for the Study of Diabetes (EASD). *Diabetes Care* 35: 1364–79.

Answers

The answers to these cases are debatable and the aim is to provoke discus-sion and thought for the reader. During the course of the chapter the ratio-nale for the answers will have become clear (but may remain for debate).

Answers to Multiple-Choice Questions for Case Study 1

1 C
This young obese male with CVD has suboptimal glycemic control (HBA1c of 8.0%) with satisfactory blood pressure and cholesterol levels. He is already prescribed a variety of agents for the secondary cardiovascular prevention of CVD. Rosiglitazone is no longer licensed for use in the treatment of type 2 diabetes and doing nothing would not be an option. Insulin or sulfonylurea therapies are options but (as described in this chapter) would be associated with weight gain and hypoglycemia risk. The use of a GLP-1 analog would be associated with an improvement in glycemia control and weight reduction. While these agents appear to be safe from a cardiovascular viewpoint, long-term studies examining this are not complete at present.

2 E
She is at an intermediate risk between that of a patient without diabetes and one with diabetes, but more information and assessment are required to assess her risk accurately. This should include the measurement of cholesterol, blood pressure, and so on. During the course of this chapter the cardiovascular glycemic risk associated with impaired fasting glycemia, impaired glucose tolerance, and diabetes is discussed.

Answers to Multiple-Choice Questions for Case Study 2

1 A, B, C, D, and E
This 73-year-old woman with a previous history of CVD has numerous cardiovascular risk factors in the setting of variable glucose control. Hypoglycemia, fluctuations in glucose levels, microvascular complications, peripheral and autonomic neuropathy, and chronic kidney disease would also increase the risk of subsequent cardiovascular events.

2 C

The HBA1c should be tailored to the patient. Clearly, the aim would be to control the blood glucose without precipitating hypoglycemia-associated complications. An HBA1c of 7% would be a reasonable target (American Diabetes Association, European Association of Specialist Diabetologists). Targeting the HBA1c below this level may result in increased morbidity and mortality and therefore caution would be required in a middle-aged patient already with complications resulting from diabetes and a previous cardiovascular history.

CHAPTER 6

Hypertension and Cardiovascular Disease and Its Management

José A. García-Donaire and Luis M. Ruilope

Hospital 12 de Octobre, Madrid, Spain

Key Points

- The increasing prevalence of diabetes mellitus worldwide is increasing global cardiovascular morbidity and mortality.

- Arterial hypertension occurs in more than 75% of diabetics.

- Optimal management of hypertensive diabetics needs to prevent and regress, if developed, cardio-renal and cerebrovascular damage.

- Management in this population is continuously being reevaluated based on the newest evidence from randomized controlled trials.

Introduction

The world's health authorities are warning about the global epidemic of diabetes mellitus (DM) [1, 2]. The increasing number of people at risk of glycemic abnormalities is directly related to the obesity pandemic in both developed and developing countries [3, 4, 5]. Millions of these people are not aware that they have or may have type 2 DM. The number of individuals with prediabetes is also quite alarming, corresponding to more than a third of adults older than 20; this is a condition that raises the risk of rather morbid complications, including microvascular and macrovascular disease (in particular kidney disease), retinopathy, blindness, amputation, and cardiovascular disease (CVD) [6, 7, 8, 9, 10]. The majority of people with type 2 DM are hypertensives, which gives them a two to four times greater probability of developing ischemic cardiomyopathy, kidney failure, cerebrovascular disease, and/or peripheral disease compared to patients without diabetes [11]. Hypertension may either precede or appear following type 2 DM; furthermore, the etiological factors linking diabetes and hypertension are not fully clear. Genetic factors, insulin resistance (IR),

---

Managing Cardiovascular Complications in Diabetes, First Edition.
Edited by D. John Betteridge and Stephen Nicholls.
© 2014 John Wiley & Sons, Ltd. Published 2014 by John Wiley & Sons, Ltd.

inflammation, the renin-angiotensin-aldosterone system (RAAS), sodium retention, and hyperglycemia are implicated [12, 13, 14]. The activation of the RAAS system and IR may trigger the production of reactive oxygen species and increased oxidative stress, which may lead to endothelial dysfunction and atherogenesis [12]. The macrovascular and microvascular complications are more common in type 2 diabetics with preexisting hypertension, with the RAAS emerging as a likely unifying mechanism.

Epidemiological studies have clearly shown a direct relationship between the levels of blood pressure (BP), glycemia and lipids, and the complications of diabetes [15, 16, 17]. Although "lower should be better," the results of recent clinical trials examining the benefits of normalizing risk-factor levels have been counter-intuitive and, sometimes, disconcerting, and have called into question this belief [18, 19]. This review focuses on patients with type 2 diabetes, arterial hypertension, its association with target organ damage, and its management; it aims to provide a clear interpretation of recent trials and guidelines to help clinicians set targets for CV risk factors in individual patients.

Interaction between Type 2 Diabetes and Hypertension

The closing years of the twentieth century were marked by a series of trials highlighting the importance, and potentially large benefits, of effective hypertension treatment in patients with type 2 DM. Reduction of BP in patients with hypertension and type 2 DM is known to reduce the risk of CV events. Importantly, baseline age, percentage of patients with previous CVD, and mean BP varied substantially across the studies. This important variation in baseline characteristics could explain some of the observed differences in long-term outcomes. Additionally, new risk-lowering treatments and therapy for vascular disease have emerged over that period, such as aspirin, statins, and RAAS inhibitors; these therapeutic developments, along with temporal changes in the disease such as the increasing prevalence of obesity have well-established effects on outcomes [20, 21].

Early Trials Including Hypertensive Diabetics

The UK Prospective Diabetes Study (UKPDS) was first regarded as a cornerstone trial, with several reports comparing the effects of tight BP control on macrovascular and microvascular diabetic complications in patients with recently diagnosed type 2 diabetes [22]. A total of 758 patients were randomized to a tight control group with a BP target of <150/85 mmHg to be achieved using either captopril (400 patients) or atenolol (358 patients), with other agents added if required. A further 390 patients were allocated to less tight control (target <180/105 mmHg) using treatments other than beta-blockers and angiotensin-converting-enzyme (ACE) inhibitors. After a median follow-up of 8.4 years, the achieved BP levels in both groups differed by less than their targets, being 144/82 mmHg and 154/87 mmHg in the tight and less tight control groups, respectively. However, the differences in outcome were striking, with a reduction of 32% in the risk of death related to diabetes in the tight control group, accompanied by reductions of 44% in stroke and 34% in all macrovascular diseases. By six years of follow-up, the risk of microalbuminuria (urinary albumin ≥50 mg/L) was reduced by 29%, and fewer patients showed deterioration in retinopathy in the tight control group. The study clearly showed the benefits of BP control in preventing vascular diabetic complications when using ACE inhibitors, and the authors concluded that management of BP should have a high priority in the treatment of type 2 diabetes. Interestingly, 29% of patients in the tight control group required three or more antihypertensive treatments to achieve the BP target. A subsequent analysis revealed no significant differences in any clinical endpoint between the captopril- and atenolol-based groups [23].

Soon after the UKPDS came the Captopril Prevention Project (CAPPP), in which 10,985 patients were randomized to receive either the ACE inhibitor captopril or conventional treatment with diuretics and beta-blockers. During 6.1 years of follow-up, captopril and conventional treatment did not differ in preventing CV morbidity and mortality [24]. However, in the relatively small subgroup of 572 patients with diabetes at baseline (4.9% of the overall patient sample), the primary composite endpoint of myocardial infarction, stroke, and CV death was substantially lower in the captopril group (relative risk 0.59), and total mortality was also significantly reduced (relative risk 0.54). In this trial, the differences in outcome could not be explained by differences in BP reductions; if anything, the achieved BP levels were slightly lower with conventional treatment than with captopril in diabetic patients [25]. What these studies had in common was a clear demonstration of the very considerable benefits in terms of CV morbidity and mortality that could be achieved by antihypertensive therapies such as ACE inhibitors in patients with diabetes. However, they also gave an early indication of the controversies to come relating to specific benefits of different classes of antihypertensive drug and their combinations, and of the difficulties of clinical trial design when many effective treatments are available and optimum treatment for many patients will involve combinations of two or more drugs.

January 2000 saw the publication of the hugely influential Heart Outcomes Prevention Evaluation (HOPE) study [26]. A total of 9,297 high-risk patients with a history of vascular disease or diabetes plus one other CV risk factor were randomized to receive the ACE inhibitor ramipril or placebo for approximately 4.5 years. Study drugs were given on top of usual CV medications, except for RAAS inhibitors, which were not allowed unless required by patients' clinical condition during the study. Ramipril reduced the incidence of the primary outcome – the composite of myocardial infarction, stroke, and CV death – by 22%, CV death by 26%, and all-cause death by 16%. An important finding was that the reduction in BP with ramipril, relative to placebo, was small (approximately 3/2 mmHg), which the authors argued was too small to account for the observed benefits. A further result was that the incidence of new-onset diabetes during the study was markedly lower in the ramipril group, with a relative risk of 0.66. There soon followed a subgroup analysis in the 3,577 patients with diabetes at baseline [27]. The BP reduction with ramipril was even smaller in this subgroup (2.4/1.0 mmHg), but the risk reductions tended to be slightly larger than in the full study population, with reductions in the primary outcome of 25%, CV death by 37%, and all-cause death by 24%. There was also a reduction in the incidence of overt nephropathy of 24%. A further analysis in patients with mild renal insufficiency [28] showed that such patients were at markedly increased risk of CV and all-cause mortality, and the relative risk reductions with ramipril were larger in patients with renal insufficiency (41% for both) than in those without (22% for CV and 10% for all-cause death).

This somewhat influential trial was soon followed by PROGRESS [29], which was primarily a study in the secondary prevention of stroke, but which had important implications for subsequent trial design, especially regarding combination therapies. Patients ($n = 6,105$) with history of stroke or transient ischemic attack were randomized to active treatment with perindopril, with or without the addition of the diuretic indapamide, or placebo, and mean follow-up was 3.9 years. Overall, active treatment produced a reduction of 28% in stroke and 26% in major vascular events; the benefits were similar in hypertensive and nonhypertensive patients. Approximately 42% of patients were treated with perindopril alone and 58% with the perindopril plus indapamide combination. BP was reduced by 5/3 mmHg by perindopril alone, and by 12/5 mmHg by the combination. Results in patients receiving the perindopril plus indapamide combination were dramatic, with risk reductions of 43% in stroke and 40% in major vascular events. Subsequent analysis in the 761 patients with diabetes at baseline indicated a nonsignificantly larger treatment effect in diabetic compared with nondiabetic patients, with risk reductions for stroke of 38% and 28%, respectively [30], and diabetic patients who received perindopril plus indapamide showed a dramatic 46% reduction in stroke risk.

Intensive versus Less-Intensive BP Goals

The Hypertension Optimal Treatment (HOT) study [31] and the above-mentioned UKPDS [22] were the first to assign patients randomly to less-intensive or more-intensive BP goals. The HOT study investigators randomly assigned patients to three different diastolic BP target groups ($\leq$90 mmHg, $\leq$85 mmHg, and $\leq$80 mmHg). In the cohort of HOT participants with diabetes ($n = 1,501$), those in the $\leq$80 mmHg target group had a 51% reduced risk of CV events and 70% reduced risk of CV-related mortality compared with those in the $\leq$90 mmHg group after four years of follow-up. Notably, patients randomly assigned to the $\leq$80 mmHg target group achieved a mean BP of 144/81 mmHg, whereas those in the $\leq$90 mmHg target group achieved a mean BP of 148/85 mmHg.

Investigators of the Appropriate Blood Pressure Control in Diabetes (ABCD) trial [32] randomly assigned patients with diabetes and high BP [33] (mean baseline diastolic BP $\geq$90 mmHg) or who were normotensive [34] (mean baseline diastolic BP 80–89 mmHg) to more-intense and less-intense diastolic BP goals. Patients with hypertension enrolled in the ABCD trial were randomly assigned to a diastolic BP goal of 75 mmHg (intense control) or 80–89 mmHg (less-intense control), whereas normotensive patients were randomly assigned to a 10 mmHg decrease in diastolic BP (intense control) or no intended change in diastolic BP (less-intense control). At five years, a significant 49% decrease in risk of all-cause mortality was observed in the population with hypertension in favour of intense BP control, although this risk was a secondary outcome. No difference was observed in the primary outcome, a change in 24-hour creatinine clearance. In the normotensive population, a significant 70% reduction in relative risk of stroke was seen, although this risk was also a secondary outcome, and only 17 strokes occurred during the five years of follow-up.

The Action to Control Cardiovascular Risk in Diabetes (ACCORD) trial [35, 36] investigators randomly assigned patients with hypertension and diabetes ($n = 4,733$) to antihypertensive therapy considered intensive (targeting a systolic BP of <120 mmHg) or standard (targeting a systolic BP of <140 mmHg). The risk of nonfatal MI, nonfatal stroke, or death from causes over a mean follow-up of 4.7 years was evaluated. ACCORD is the first large randomized trial that provides the opportunity to assess the effects of lower achieved systolic BP (<120 mmHg) in patients with diabetes. Patients randomly assigned to the intensive therapy group achieved a mean BP of 119/64 mmHg, whereas those in the standard therapy group achieved a mean BP of 134/71 mmHg. The therapeutical needing's to attain BP control in the two groups are depicted in Figure 6.2. No significant difference in risk of nonfatal MI or MI-related death was observed when comparing the intensive therapy and standard therapy groups. However, a significant 42% reduced risk of total stroke and 38% reduced risk of nonfatal stroke were seen, although the overall annual stroke rate was very low (0.32% and 0.53% in the intensive therapy and standard therapy groups, respectively). A significantly increased incidence of serious adverse events was also seen in the intensive therapy group, including hypotension, bradycardia, and arrhythmia, all of which are known to be associated with poor outcomes. The ACCORD investigators concluded that their results provide no evidence that intensive BP control reduces the rate of a composite of major events.

Although it may be surprising that significant reductions in the rate of events were not observed in ACCORD, it is important to note that patients in ACCORD had lower systolic BP at baseline than that achieved in the intense control groups of either HOT [31] or UKPDS [22]. This factor suggests that the benefit observed in the intense control groups of HOT and UKPDS was likely to be based on reducing systolic BP from a mean ≥160 mmHg at baseline to 144 mmHg, and that the benefit of reducing systolic BP from an average baseline value of 139 mmHg to 119 mmHg, as was observed in ACCORD, is smaller. The normotensive population in ABCD [32] is, among the patient groups studied in these trials, the one most similar to the ACCORD population, in factors such as BP, age, and percentage of patients with CVD at baseline. In both of these studies, a small, though significant, reduction in the risk of stroke was observed in the intense therapy groups.

Clinical Interpretation of Trials

The Irbesartan Diabetic Nephropathy Trial (IDNT) [37] offers the chance to assess the effects of achieved BP on outcomes in a diabetic hypertensive population with nephropathy who were followed for three years. Progressively lower achieved systolic BP to 120 mmHg predicted a decrease in related mortality and congestive heart failure, but not of MI. When patients were categorized according to achieved systolic BP of ≤120 mmHg ($n = 53$) or systolic BP >120 mmHg ($n = 1,537$), a significant increase in relative risk of all-cause mortality as well as related mortality was seen in the small group that achieved systolic BP of ≤120 mmHg. Achieving diastolic BP <85 mmHg was associated with a trend to increased all-cause mortality, a significant increase in risk of MI, but a decrease in risk of stroke. Although only 29% of IDNT participants had CVD at baseline, when categorized according to achieved systolic BP, a higher fraction of patients in the ≤120 mmHg group had a history of CVD or congestive heart failure at baseline compared with those in the >120 mmHg group [38].

The International Verapamil SR/Trandolapril (INVEST) study [39] also offers the opportunity to assess the influence of achieved systolic BP on CV outcomes in a unique population of patients with hypertension and diabetes ($n = 6,400$), all of whom had documented coronary artery disease at baseline and were followed for three years. INVEST participants were categorized according to achievement of a systolic BP <130 mmHg (tight control) or 130 mmHg to <140 mmHg (usual control). No difference was seen when comparing the tight control and usual control groups with regard to the rate of the primary outcome (first occurrence of all-cause death, nonfatal MI, or nonfatal stroke), nor was there any difference in the rates of nonfatal MI or nonfatal stroke when evaluated separately. However, a significant 8% increase was seen in the relative risk of all-cause mortality in the group with tight systolic control BP ($p = 0.04$). Extended follow-up of US participants in INVEST, using information from the National Death Index, revealed that over a total of 10 years patients in the tight systolic control BP group had a 15% excess risk of all-cause mortality compared with those in the usual systolic control BP group. This excess risk was concentrated among those with systolic BP <120 mmHg.

Available Data on Microvascular Endpoints

Some studies have also evaluated microvascular endpoints in patients with diabetes. In those receiving active treatment (perindopril and indapamide), ADVANCE investigators found a significant reduction in the development of microalbuminuria ($P < 0.0001$), and a borderline significant reduction in the rate of new or worsening nephropathy ($p = 0.055$) [40]. However, no difference between the active and control groups was found in the rate of new or worsening retinopathy, visual deterioration, or new or worsening neuropathy [41]. In UKPDS, patients in the tight control group had a 34% reduction in risk of deterioration of retinopathy ($p = 0.0004$), and a 47% reduction in risk of deterioration in visual acuity by three lines according to the Early Treatment of Diabetic Retinopathy Study vision chart ($p = 0.004$) [22], although these microvascular benefits were not sustained during UKPDS posttrial follow-up [42]. In those patients with normoalbuminuria or microalbuminuria enrolled in ABCD, BP lowering stabilized renal function in both groups; however, patients with overt albuminuria at baseline had a steady decline in creatinine clearance throughout the study regardless of BP reduction [33]. In ACCORD, patients in the intensive control group had a significantly lower estimated glomerular filtration rate ($P < 0.001$), more cases of elevated serum creatinine ($P < 0.001$), and more cases of estimated glomerular filtration rate <30 ml/min/1.73m^2 ($P < 0.001$), although significantly fewer cases of macroalbuminuria ($p = 0.009$) [35]. In a substudy of ACCORD on retinopathy, intensive BP lowering was not associated with a reduction in the rate of progression of diabetic retinopathy [43].

Renal Outcomes in Hypertensive Diabetics

Nephropathy has long been recognized as an important complication of diabetes, and diabetes and hypertension are the most common causes of chronic kidney disease (CKD) [44, 45]. Worsening renal disease carries a steeply increasing risk of CV death [46] (Figure 6.1), and the complex interactions between CV disease, CKD, and diabetes are becoming more

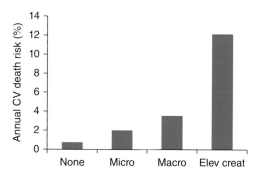

Figure 6.1 Annual risk of cardiovascular (CV) death in patients with type 2 diabetes mellitus and different degrees of nephropathy in the UKPDS. Micro: microalbuminuria; Macro: macroalbuminuria; Elev creat: elevated plasma creatinine or renal replacement therapy. (Source: Adler et al. 2003 [47]. Reproduced with permission of Nature Publishing Group.)

widely appreciated, if not fully understood [45, 47]. Blockade of the renin–angiotensin system is widely accepted as beneficial in terms of renal outcomes, and a series of meta-analyses have indicated that ACE inhibitors can prevent new-onset microalbuminuria and progression to macroalbuminuria, and reduce all-cause mortality in patients with diabetic nephropathy, and that angiotensin receptor blockers (ARB) have only renoprotective properties [48]. During the last 10 years, there has been a series of placebo-controlled, randomized trials of ARB in patient populations comprising or including patients with diabetes, with and without nephropathy. Characteristics of these trials are summarized in Table 6.1, including the total number of deaths that occurred in each study, as an indication of its likely power to detect a mortality benefit of active treatment, and the approximate mortality rate in the placebo group, as an indication of the risk status of the patient population. Full trial names are given in the footnote to Table 6.1, and the main results are summarized in Table 6.2.

The IDNT [37] and RENAAL [49] trials included patients with type 2 diabetes and nephropathy. In both trials, randomized treatments were given in addition to standard hypertensive therapy, which excluded ACE inhibitors, ARB, and, in the case of IDNT, calcium-channel blockers. In the IDNT trial, irbesartan treatment was associated with a 20% reduction, relative to placebo, in the primary renal endpoint (the composite of doubling of serum creatinine, end-stage renal disease, and all-cause death), mainly due to a 33% reduction in the doubling of serum creatinine (Table 6.2). End-stage renal disease was reduced by 23%, but the difference just failed to reach significance ($p = 0.07$). Renal outcomes in the amlodipine group were similar to placebo. The RENAAL trial was stopped early on ethical grounds due to the exclusion of ACE inhibitors from the permitted background therapies in the study design. During the mean 3.4 years of follow-up, losartan

Table 6.1 Characteristics of large randomized trials with renal endpoints including patients with diabetes mellitus.

Study	Patient characteristics	Treatments	Follow-up (years)	Baseline BP (mmHg)	BP difference vs. placebo (mmHg)	Total deaths (approximate rate)[a]
Monotherapy vs. placebo						
IDNT (n = 1,715) [37]	Type 2 DM + nephropathy	Irbesartan (n = 579) Placebo (n = 569) Amlodipine (n = 567)	2.6	159/87	−3.3	263 (55)
RENAAL (n = 1,513) [49]	Type 2 DM + nephropathy	Losartan (n = 751) Placebo (n = 762)	3.4	153/82	−2	313 (60)
IRMA 2 (n = 590) [51]	Type 2 DM + persistent microalbuminuria	Irbesartan 150 mg (n = 195) Irbesartan 300 mg (n = 195) Placebo (n = 201)	2.0	153/90	−3	4 (2.5)
TRANSCEND (n = 5,927) [55]	Cardiovascular disease or DM with end-organ damage	Telmisartan (n = 2,954) Placebo (n = 2,972)	4.7	141/82	−4	713 (25)
DIRECT-Renal (n = 5,231) [57]	Type 1 and type 2 DM, normoalbuminuria	Candesartan (n = 2,613) Placebo (n = 2,618)	4.7	118/73	−3.3	99 (4)
Combination therapy						
ONTARGET (n = 25,620) [69]	Cardiovascular disease or DM with end-organ damage	Ramipril (n = 8,576) Telmisartan (n = 8,542) Ramipril + telmisartan (n = 8,502)	4.7	142/82	−2.4 (Combination vs ramipril)	3,068 (25) (all groups)

Trial	Population	Treatment groups	Approximate death rate[a]	BP (mmHg)	BP difference	Deaths n (%)
ADVANCE (n = 11,140) [41]	Type 2 DM + cardiovascular disease or ≥1 risk factor	Perindopril + indapamide (n = 5,569) Placebo (n = 5,571)	4.3	145/81	−5.6	879 (18)
ACCOMPLISH (n = 11,506) [73]	Hypertension + cardiovascular disease or DM (in 60% of patients)	Benazepril + amlodipine (n = 5,744) Benazepril + hydrochlorothiazide (n = 5,762)	3.0	145/80	−1.1 (Ben + Am vs Ben + Hyd)	498 (14) (both groups)
Comparison of blood pressure targets						
ACCORD BP (n = 4,733) [35]	Type 2 DM at high risk for cardiovascular events	Target BP <120 mmHg systolic (n = 2,362) Target BP <140 mmHg systolic (n = 2,371)	5.0 (for mortality)	139/76	−14.2	249 (10)

Notes:

[a] Approximate rate given for placebo group unless stated, expressed as deaths per 1000 patient-years.

Am: amlodipine; Ben: benazepril; BP: blood pressure (systolic if available); DM: diabetes mellitus; Hyd: hydrochlorothiazide

Trial names:

IDNT: Irbesartan Diabetic Nephropathy Trial; RENAAL: Reduction of Endpoints in NIDDM with the Angiotensin II Antagonist Losartan Study; IRMA 2: Irbesartan in Patients with Type 2 Diabetes and Microalbuminuria Study; TRANSCEND: Telmisartan Randomised Assessment Study in ACE Intolerant Subjects with Cardiovascular Disease; DIRECT: Diabetic Retinopathy Candesartan Trials; ONTARGET: Ongoing Telmisartan Alone and in Combination with Ramipril Global Endpoint Trial; ADVANCE: Action in Diabetes and Vascular Disease: Preterax and Diamicron-MR Controlled Evaluation Trial; ACCOMPLISH: Avoiding Cardiovascular Events Through Combination Therapy in Patients Living with Systolic Hypertension; ACCORD BP: Action to Control Cardiovascular Risk in Diabetes blood pressure trial.

Table 6.2 Summary of results of large randomized trials with renal endpoints including patients with diabetes mellitus.

Study	Albuminuria New-onset	Progression	Renal endpoints			Cardiovascular		Mortality	
			Primary endpoint or renal events	Doubling of serum creatinine	ESRD or dialysis	All events	Stroke	All-cause	Cardiovascular
Monotherapy vs. placebo									
IDNT									
Irbesartan vs. placebo	–	–	–20% (p = 0.02)	–33% (p = 0.003)	–23% (NS)	–10% (NS)	+1% (NS)	–8% (NS)	+8% (NS)
Amlodipine vs. placebo	–	–	+4% (NS)	+6% (NS)	0% (NS)	0% (NS)	–35% (NS)	–12% (NS)	–21% (NS)
RENAAL									
Losartan vs. placebo	–	–35% in UACR (p = 0.001)	–16% (p = 0.02)	–25% (p = 0.006)	–28% (p = 0.002)	–10% (NS)	–	+2% (NS)	–
IRMA 2									
Irbesartan 300 mg vs. placebo	–	–38% in urine albumin (p < 0.001)	–70% (p < 0.001)	–	–	–	–	–	
TRANSCEND									
Telmisartan vs. placebo	–	–42% (p = 0.018)	+10% (NS)	+59% (p = 0.031)	–29% (NS)	–8% (NS)	–17% (NS)	+5% (NS)	+3% (NS)
DIRECT-Renal									
Candesartan vs. placebo	–5% (NS) (primary renal endpoint)	–	Also a –5.5% change in UAER (p = 0.024)	–	–	–	–	Candesartan: 51 Placebo: 48	–

Combination therapy

ONTARGET									
Telmisartan vs. ramipril		−6% (NS)	−17% (NS)	0% (NS)	+7% (NS)	+1% (NS)	−9% (NS)	−2% (NS)	0% (NS)
Combination vs. ramipril	−12% (p = 0.003)	−24% (p = 0.019)	+9% (p = 0.037)	+20% (NS)	+33% (NS)	−1% (NS)	−7% (NS)	+7% (NS)	+4% (NS)
ADVANCE									
Perindopril + indapamide vs. placebo		−22% (p = 0.001)	−21% (p < 0.0001)	+21% (NS)	+18% (NS)	−14% (p = 0.020)	−6% (NS)	−14% (p = 0.025)	−18% (p = 0.027)
ACCOMPLISH									
Benazepril + amlodipine vs. benazepril + hydrochlorothiazide		—	−48% (p < 0.0001)	−49% (p < 0.0001)	−47% (NS)	−17% (p = 0.002)	−16% (NS)	−10% (NS)	−20% (NS)
Comparison of blood pressure targets									
ACCORD BP									
Target <120 mmHg vs. target <140 mmHg systolic	30.2% vs. 32.3% (NS)	6.6% vs 8.7% (p = 0.009)	—	24% vs. 16% (p < 0.001) (Elevated serum creatinine only)	No significant difference	−13% (NS) (Nonfatal MI only)	−41% (p = 0.01)	+7% (NS)	+6% (NS)

MI: myocardial infarction; NS: not significant; UACR: urinary albumin-to-creatinine ratio; UAER: urinary albumin excretion rate.

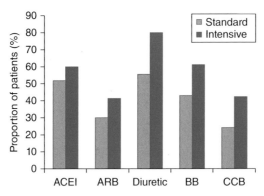

Figure 6.2   Main classes of antihypertensive drugs prescribed at the last study visit in patients in the intensive and standard treatment groups in the ACCORD trial. Alpha blockers, reserpine, and other antihypertensives were also prescribed in <25% of patients in either group. ACEI: angiotensin-converting-enzyme inhibitor; ARB: angiotensin-II receptor blocker; BB: beta-blocker; CCB: calcium channel blocker. (Source: Data from ACCORD Study Group (2010) [36].)

produced a significant 16% reduction in the primary renal endpoint (the same composite as in IDNT), with significant reductions in both doubling of serum creatinine and end-stage renal disease (Table 6.2). Losartan also led to an average reduction in the level of proteinuria (measured as urinary albumin to creatinine ratio) of 35% from baseline, while the ratio tended to increase in the placebo group ($p < 0.001$ for treatment effect). Despite the renal benefits in both trials, ARB treatment did not produce any substantial or significant improvement in the risk of all CV events or in all-cause or CV mortality. In the IDNT trial, irbesartan produced a significant reduction of 28% in heart failure, but no improvement in myocardial infarction, stroke, or all-cause or CV death (which actually increased by 8%). This may be contrasted with the effect of amlodipine, which produced a significant reduction of 42% in myocardial infarction, and non-significant reductions in stroke and CV death of 35% and 21%, respectively, despite no discernible benefit in renal endpoints [50].

IRMA 2 [51] was a smaller study, which compared two doses of irbesartan with placebo in patients with type 2 diabetes and persistent microalbuminuria, who could receive other antihypertensive drugs apart from ARB and ACE inhibitors. The primary efficacy endpoint was onset of overt nephropathy, defined as urinary albumin excretion rate >200 μg per minute and ≥30% higher than at baseline, and this endpoint was reached by 30 patients in the placebo group, compared with 19 in the irbesartan 150 mg group and 10 in the 300 mg group, corresponding to hazard ratios of 0.61 (NS) and 0.30 ($p < 0.001$), respectively. The level of urinary albumin excretion reduced by 38% in the irbesartan 300 mg group compared with a reduction of 2% in the placebo group ($p < 0.001$). The number of deaths was 8 in the irbesartan 300 mg group, versus 5 in the placebo group.

The publication of the renal outcome results from the ACCOMPLISH study confirmed the need for future hypertension trials to consider CV and renal outcomes jointly [52]. The study results showed that the combination of the ACE inhibitor benazepril and the calcium-channel blocker amlodipine was superior to benazepril and the diuretic hydrochlorothiazide in terms of both CV protection and slowing the progression of nephropathy to a greater extent in patients with hypertension at high risk of CV events. These results indicate that the mechanisms that facilitate the progression of CV disease have similarities to those that lead to the progression of renal disease. A subgroup of analysis of patients with diabetes in the ACCOMPLISH study, also published in 2010, showed that the combination of renin–angiotensin system suppression with amlodipine was superior to the combination of renin–angiotensin system suppression with hydrochlorothiazide in reducing CV events in the diabetic subgroup [53].

In contrast to the previous three trials, patients in the TRANSCEND study [54, 55] had either established CV disease or diabetes with end-organ damage, but without macroalbuminuria or heart failure. Intolerance of ACE inhibitors was an inclusion requirement; other antihypertensive drugs were allowed, including nonstudy ARB, although these were only taken by <10% of patients. The primary renal endpoint was the composite of dialysis, renal transplantation, doubling of serum creatinine, and death, and this occurred with similar incidence in the two groups. However, doubling of serum creatinine occurred significantly more frequently with telmisartan than with placebo (hazard ratio 1.59, $p = 0.031$), and significantly more patients experienced a reduction in estimated glomerular filtration rate with telmisartan. On the other hand, among patients with microalbuminuria at baseline, progression to macroalbuminuria was markedly reduced by 42% by telmisartan ($p = 0.018$). However, telmisartan had no significant effect on the main composite CV endpoint, or on all-cause or CV death. The authors concluded that ARB offer no renal benefit in ACE-intolerant people at high vascular risk but without macroalbuminuria [54].

The final study in this category is a combined analysis of renal endpoints in the three DIRECT trials, which were designed primarily to evaluate the effect of candesartan on the incidence and progression of retinopathy in normoalbuminuric patients with type 1 or type 2 diabetes [56, 57, 58]. The primary renal endpoint was development of microalbuminuria, with rate of change in urinary albumin excretion rate as a secondary endpoint. Similar numbers of patients in the candesartan and placebo groups developed microalbuminuria in each of the three studies, with a hazard ratio (candesartan vs. placebo) of 0.95 in the combined analysis

(p = 0.60). The annual rate of change in urinary albumin excretion rate was 5.5% lower with candesartan (p = 0.024); this corresponds to an absolute reduction of 0.11 µg/min, which the authors describe as modest and of uncertain clinical significance. However, it must be remembered that the study was not powered for a renal endpoint. The number of deaths was similar in the candesartan (51 deaths) and placebo (48 deaths) groups.

The studies considered in this section suggest that treatment with ARB can delay progression to macroalbuminuria, and reduce the incidence of manifestations of more severe renal disease such as doubling of serum creatinine and need for dialysis, although there were inconsistencies between different renal endpoints. However, none of the trials showed a significant benefit of ARB on mortality. The lack of significant effect might be expected in trials with relatively small numbers of deaths, such as IRMA 2 and DIRECT, but is of more concern for those trials that, due to their large size and/or the high-risk nature of their patients, involved substantial numbers of deaths. A recent analysis of 16 randomized trials in predominantly hypertensive patients since 2000 [59] indicated that only three trials (ASCOT-BPLA [60], ADVANCE [41], and HYVET [61]) showed a significant reduction in all-cause mortality. The successful treatments in these three studies were amlodipine (± perindopril), perindopril plus indapamide, and indapamide (± perindopril), respectively. The other 13 studies, individually and when pooled, showed no significant mortality benefit (odds ratio 0.996 for the pooled analysis).

Cerebrovascular Outcomes in Hypertensive Diabetics

There is no question about the need to treat hypertension in either the primary prevention or secondary prevention settings for cerebrovascular disease, irrespective of the presence of diabetes. A systematic review of the effects of different BP-lowering drug regimens in people with hypertension, diabetes, or vascular disease found that the relative risks of stroke and other major vascular outcomes were proportional to the BP reduction achieved [62]. However, as discussed above, there is a general consensus that ACE inhibitors or ARB are the first-line drugs of choice in both diabetes and metabolic syndrome. In primary prevention, the only question is the level of BP above which treatment is indicated. Observational studies have found no evidence of a threshold of systolic or diastolic BP (at least down as far as about 115/75 mmHg) below which there was no reduction in stroke [63]. The recommended threshold for treatment in primary prevention is currently under discussion in both diabetics and nondiabetics. Moreover, there is increasing uncertainty about the use of absolute thresholds of BP to determine the need for treatment, and there is a developing consensus that the need for treatment decisions should be based on the predicted absolute risks of CV events [64].

BP reduction is indicated in most people with a prior stroke or TIA, particularly among diabetics. A systematic review of nine randomized controlled trials in 6,753 people with a prior stroke or TIA found that antihypertensive treatment significantly reduced the risk of stroke (RR = 0.72, 95% CI 0.61–0.85) and major CV events (RR = 0.79, 95% CI 0.68–0.91) during follow-up [65]. However, there is evidence that stroke risk is increased at lower levels of systolic BP in patients with bilateral severe carotid stenosis, in whom cerebral perfusion is frequently impaired, particularly if systolic BP is <130 mmHg [66]. BP should be lowered cautiously in this group and endarterectomy may be necessary in order to allow proper control of BP.

The above mentioned PROGRESS trial, in 6,105 people with a prior stroke or TIA, compared four years of the ACE inhibitor perindopril plus indapamide (added at the discretion of the treating physician) versus placebo [29]. Active treatment reduced BP by 9/4 mmHg and reduced stroke (RR = 0.72, 95% CI 0.62–0.83) and major vascular events (RR = 0.74, 95% CI 0.66–0.84) compared with placebo. Relative risks were similar irrespective of baseline BP and the type of qualifying cerebrovascular event (ischemic or hemorrhagic). PROGRESS included 761 (14.2%) patients with diabetes. The overall reduction in BP with treatment in the diabetes group was 9.5/4.6 mmHg compared with 8.9/3.9 mmHg in nondiabetics and the relative reductions in the risk of stroke were 38% (95% CI 8–58%) and 28% (95% CI 16–39%), respectively. Since the absolute risk of ischemic stroke during follow-up was also higher in patients with diabetes (hazard ratio = 1.53, 95% CI 1.23–1.90), the RR with treatment was higher. The same pattern was reported in the HOPE trial, in which 9,297 people at high risk of vascular disease (1,013 with a prior stroke or TIA) were randomized to the ACE inhibitor ramipril, versus placebo. Ramipril reduced stroke (RR = 0.68, 95% CI 0.56–0.84) and major vascular events (RR = 0.78, 95% CI 0.70–0.86) at 4.5 years compared with placebo [26]. Subsequent analysis found that relative risks were similar in people with and without a prior stroke or TIA [67], and slightly greater in diabetics than nondiabetics. The absolute risk of stroke in the placebo group was again higher in diabetics than in nondiabetics (6.1 vs. 4.1%), and so the absolute benefit of treatment was also about 50% greater [27].

Combination Therapy in Hypertensive Diabetics

Many hypertensive patients in clinical practice receive more than one antihypertensive drug, and the use of combination therapy is widely recommended in hypertension guidelines. Combinations may be especially important for patients with diabetes, for whom recommended BP targets are challenging. It should be pointed out that in most large recent hypertension trials the study drug is given on top of the usual antihypertensive therapy, which is often left to the discretion of the investigator. Thus, most trials evaluate the efficacy of combinations of drugs, but the type and dose of the components other than the randomized study drug are not standardized. However, three large recent trials have explicitly studied specific combinations, with striking results.

First, the initial questions must be when to initiate pharmacological treatment and which should be the chosen drug. This issue seems to be clarified with recent concluding data that confirms that ACE-I and/or ARB are beneficial even in normotensive high-risk patients, supporting calls to base decisions about the prescription of these agents on each patient's CV risk rather than just their BP level [68].

In the very large ONTARGET trial [69], telmisartan and the combination of telmisartan and ramipril were compared with ramipril alone in patients with CV disease or diabetes with end-organ damage. There were no significant differences between the telmisartan and ramipril groups for any renal, CV, or mortality endpoint (Table 6.2). However, the comparison between the combination and ramipril revealed important differences.

The combination was more effective than ramipril alone in preventing new-onset microalbuminuria and progression of preexisting microalbuminuria, with hazard ratios of 0.88 ($p = 0.003$) and 0.76 ($p = 0.019$) respectively. On the other hand, the primary renal endpoint, the composite of doubling of serum creatinine, dialysis, or death, occurred significantly more frequently with the combination than with ramipril (hazard ratio 1.09, $p = 0.037$); each component was numerically more frequent with the combination, by 20%, 33%, and 7%, respectively. Declines in estimated glomerular filtration rate were greater with the combination than with ramipril ($p < 0.0001$). Rates of CV endpoints and mortality were similar in the combination and ramipril groups. Renal abnormalities were reported as adverse events in significantly more patients in the combination group than with ramipril (relative risk 1.33, $p < 0.0001$), and more patients stopped medication due to renal abnormalities with the combination than with ramipril (relative risk 1.58, $p < 0.005$). Thus, the addition of telmisartan to ramipril reduced the incidence of proteinuria, but caused a more rapid decline in glomerular filtration rate, increased the incidence of major renal events, and showed no benefit in terms of CV events or mortality. This may be one of the reasons guidelines do not recommend this association.

The ADVANCE trial is the largest trial performed in diabetics, involving 11,140 patients. It compared a fixed-dose combination of perindopril and the original diuretic indapamide with placebo in patients with type

2 diabetes and a history of major CV disease or at least one other CV risk factor [70]. Combination therapy reduced the composite renal end-point (new-onset microalbuminuria, new-onset nephropathy, doubling of serum creatinine, or end-stage renal disease) by 21% (hazard ratio 0.79, $p < 0.0001$). There were also significant reductions in new-onset microalbuminuria (21%) and progression from microalbuminuria to macroalbuminuria (31%). Later-stage renal events were infrequent in this population; end-stage renal disease occurred with similar frequency in the combination and placebo groups. In contrast to the trials of ARBs described in the previous section, the renal benefits of the perindopril plus indapamide combination were accompanied by significant reductions in all-cause mortality (by 14%, $p = 0.025$), CV death (by 18%, $p = 0.027$), and coronary events (by 14%, $p = 0.020$).

At least three further features of the ADVANCE trial are notable. First, almost all other antihypertensive treatments were allowed (including RAAS inhibitors in 73% of patients in the control group, a first in these trials), except that thiazide diuretics were not permitted. The effectiveness of the permitted treatments was illustrated by the fact that regression of albuminuria by at least one stage was observed in 50.2% of patients in the placebo group; nonetheless, active treatment provided a further benefit of 16% in the incidence of regression ($p = 0.0017$). Second, significant reductions in renal events were seen in all subgroups of patients defined by baseline BP, including those with starting BP below 125/75 mmHg. Indeed, the lowest risk for renal events was observed in patients with achieved BP levels below 110 mmHg systolic or 65 mmHg diastolic. Third, a recent analysis has shown that the relative risk of all-cause mortality was reduced to a similar extent in patients with or without nephropathy, and whatever their CKD stage at baseline [71]. One issue not resolved by ADVANCE was whether the observed benefits were independent of BP reduction, because the BP achieved was lower in the active treatment group by an average of 5.6 mmHg systolic and 2.2 mmHg diastolic. However, since the majority of diabetic patients with hypertension in clinical practice do not reach their target BP [72], the greater antihypertensive efficacy of the perindopril plus indapamide combination could be regarded as an additional positive result.

The third trial in this group is ACCOMPLISH [52, 73], which compared two fixed-dose combinations, benazepril plus amlodipine and benazepril plus hydrochlorothiazide, in patients with hypertension and a history of CV disease or diabetes; approximately 60% of randomized patients had diabetes. The primary endpoint was the composite of CV events and CV death, and the trial was halted prematurely due to a significant reduction in this endpoint in the benazepril plus amlodipine group (hazard ratio 0.80, $p < 0.001$). There was a significant reduction in the composite of all CV events (17%, $p = 0.002$), but the reductions in all-cause death (10%), CV death

(20%), and stroke (16%) did not reach significance. The primary renal end-point, the composite of doubling of serum creatinine and end-stage renal disease, was almost halved in the benazepril plus amlodipine group (hazard ratio 0.52, $p < 0.0001$), due mainly to a 49% reduction in doubling of serum creatinine ($p < 0.0001$). As in the ADVANCE trial, dialysis was infrequent, occurring in 7 patients in the benazepril plus amlodipine group and 13 patients in the benazepril plus hydrochlorothiazide group (NS). Despite the marked reduction in later-stage renal events with benazepril plus amlodipine, the proportion of patients with baseline microalbuminuria who regressed to normoalbuminuria was substantially lower in this group (41.7%) than with benazepril plus hydrochlorothiazide (68.3%, $p = 0.0016$). The systolic BP level in the two treatment groups differed by less than 1 mmHg.

Case Study 1

A 56-year-old women attends the Hypertension Unit as a periodic consultation. She has essential hypertension and type 2 diabetes mellitus since 2000, hypercholesterolemia since 2004, global and abdominal obesity since 20 years old, with no history of smoking, toxic habits, surgeries, or complications during her pregnancies. Her treatment is olmesartan 40 mg/day and simvastatin 20 mg/day. Her blood pressure control is 128/78 mmHg (office); 130/80 mmHg (home). Her current serum and urine analytics shows fasting glucose 158 mg/dl; Hb A1C 7.5%; potassium 5.1 mEq/, uric acid 7.8 mg/dl; total cholesterol 219 mg/dl; triglycerides 189 mg/dl; HDL-c 41 mg/dl; LDL-c 140 mg/dl; creatinine 1.2 mg/dl; glomerular filtration rate (MDRD-4) 49 ml/min; albumin to creatinine ratio 56 mg/g. The remaining values are normal.

Multiple-Choice Questions

1 These results can affirm that the glycemic status of the patient is:
   A Type 2 diabetes
   B Prediabetes. Abnormal fasting glucose
   C Prediabetes. Carbohydrate intolerance
   D Normoglycemia

2 The optimal management for the glycemic status of this patient should be:
   A Lifestyle counselling
   B Start metformin
   C Start a combination of metformin and sulfonylurea
   D Insulin

3 The lipid profile of this patient is out of goal range. Which objective for LDL-c is desirable?
   A <130 mg/dl
   B <100 mg/dl

C <70 mg/dl

D <50 mg/dl

4 The renal function of this patient can de considered as:

   A Normal

   B Chronic kidney disease stage 3 with albuminuria

   C Chronic kidney disease stage 3 without albuminuria

   D Chronic kidney disease stage 4

5 Her blood pressure levels should be considered as:

   A Adequate

   B Suboptimal. The goal is <120/80 mmHg

   C Suboptimal. The goal is <115/75 mmHg

   D Ambulatory blood pressure monitoring is needed to respond the question

Answers provided after the References

Guidelines and Web Links

http://eurheartj.oxfordjournals.org/content/28/12/1462.full.pdf

http://www.eshonline.org/

http://www.nice.org.uk/CG034

2007 Guidelines for the Management of Arterial Hypertension, European Society of Cardiology.

Guideline on the Management of Hypertension, NICE and the British Hypertension Society.

Website of the European Society of Hypertension.

References

1 Cheung BM, Ong KL, Cherny SS et al. Diabetes prevalence and therapeutic target achievement in the United States, 1999 to 2006. *Am J Med* 2009; 122: 443–53.

2 Agardh E, Allebeck P, Hallqvist J et al. Type 2 diabetes incidence and socio-economic position: A systematic review and meta-analysis. *Int J Epidemiol* 2011; 40: 3804–818.

3 Samaranayake NR, Ong KL, Leung RY, Cheung BM. Management of obesity in the National Health and Nutrition Examination Survey (NHANES), 2007–2008. *Ann Epidemiol* 2012; 22: 349–53.

4 Sowers JR, Whaley-Connell A, Hayden MR. The role of overweight and obesity in the cardiorenal syndrome. *Cardiorenal Med* 2011; 1: 5–12.

5 Sorof J, Daniels S. Obesity hypertension in children: A problem of epidemic proportions. *Hypertension* 2002; 40: 441–7.

6 Preis SR, Hwang SJ, Coady S et al. Trends in all-cause and cardiovascular disease mortality among women and men with and without diabetes mellitus in the Framingham Heart Study, 1950 to 2005. *Circulation* 2009; 119: 1728–35.

7 Kannel WB, McGee DL. Diabetes and glucose tolerance as risk factors for cardiovascular disease: The Framingham Study. *Diabetes Care* 1979; 2: 120–26.

8 Haffner SM, Lehto S, Rönnemaa T et al. Mortality from coronary heart disease in subjects with type 2 diabetes and in nondiabetic subjects with and without prior myocardial infarction. *N Engl J Med* 1998; 339: 229–34.

9 Kuusisto J, Mykkänen L, Pyörälä K, Laakso M. Non-insulin-dependent diabetes and its metabolic control are important predictors of stroke in elderly subjects. *Stroke* 1994; 25: 1157–64.

10 Kanaya AM, Grady D, Barrett-Connor E. Explaining the sex difference in coronary heart disease mortality among patients with type 2 diabetes mellitus: A meta-analysis. *Arch Intern Med* 2002; 162: 1737–45.

11 Fagan TC, Sowers J. Type 2 diabetes mellitus: Greater cardiovascular risks and greater benefits of therapy. *Arch Intern Med* 1999; 159: 1033–4.

12 Leiter LA, Lewanczuk RZ. Of the renin-angiotensin system and reactive oxygen species Type 2 diabetes and angiotensin II inhibition. *Am J Hypertens* 2005; 18: 121–8.

13 Sharma AM, Engeli S. The role of renin-angiotensin system blockade in the management of hypertension associated with the cardiometabolic syndrome. *J Cardiometab Syndr* 2006; 1: 29–35.

14 Shoelson SE, Lee J, Goldfine AB. Inflammation and insulin resistance. *J Clin Invest* 2006; 116: 1793–801.

15 Sarwar N, Gao P, Seshasai SR et al. Diabetes mellitus, fasting blood glucose concentration, and risk of vascular disease: A collaborative meta-analysis of 102 prospective studies. *Lancet* 2010; 375: 2215–22.

16 Stratton IM, Adler AI, Neil HA et al. Association of glycaemia with macrovascular and microvascular complications of type 2 diabetes (UKPDS 35): Prospective observational study. *Brit Med J* 2000; 321: 405–12.

17 Stamler J, Vaccaro O, Neaton JD, Wentworth D. Diabetes, other risk factors, and 12-yr cardiovascular mortality for men screened in the Multiple Risk Factor Intervention Trial. *Diabetes Care* 1993; 16: 434–44.

18 Gerstein HC, Miller ME, Byington RP et al. Effects of intensive glucose lowering in type 2 diabetes. *N Engl J Med* 2008; 358: 2545–59.

19 Mancia G, Laurent S, Agabiti-Rosei E et al. Reappraisal of European guidelines on hypertension management: A European Society of Hypertension Task Force document. *J Hypertens* 2009; 27(11): 2121–58.

20 Braunwald E et al. Angiotensin-converting-enzyme inhibition in stable coronary artery disease. *N. Engl J Med* 2004; 351: 2058–68.

21 Heart Protection Study Collaborative Group. MRC/BHF Heart Protection Study of cholesterol lowering with simvastatin in 20,536 high-risk individuals: A randomised placebo-controlled trial. *Lancet* 2002; 360: 7–22.

22 UK Prospective Diabetes Study Group. Tight blood pressure control and risk of macrovascular and microvascular complications in type 2 diabetes: UKPDS 28. *Brit Med J* 1998; 317: 703–13.

23 UK Prospective Diabetes Study Group. Efficacy of atenolol and captopril in reducing risk of macrovascular and microvascular complications in type 2 diabetes: UKPDS 39. *Brit Med J* 1998; 317: 713–20.

24 Hansson L, Lindholm LH, Niskanen L et al. Effect of angiotensin-converting-enzyme inhibition compared with conventional therapy on cardiovascular morbidity and mortality in hypertension: The Captopril Prevention Project (CAPPP) randomised trial. *Lancet* 1999; 353: 611–16.

25 Niskanen L, Hedner T, Hansson L et al; CAPPP Study Group. Reduced cardiovascular mobidity and mortality in hypertensive diabetic patients on first-line therapy with an ACE inhibitor compared with a diuretic/beta-blocker-based treatment regimen: A subanalysis of the Captopril Prevention Project. *Diabetes Care* 2001; 24: 2091–6.

26 Yusuf S, Sleight P, Pogue J et al. Effects of and angiotensin-converting-enzyme inhibitor, ramipril, on cardiovascular events in high-risk patients. The Heart Outcomes Prevention Evaluation Study Investigators. *N Engl J Med* 2000; 342: 145–53.

27 Heart Outcomes Prevention Evaluation Study Investigators. Effects of ramipril on cardiovascular and microvascular outcomes in people with diabetes mellitus: Results of the HOPE study and MICRO-HOPE substudy. Heart Outcomes Prevention Evaluation Study Investigators. *Lancet* 2000; 355: 253–9.

28 Mann JF, Gerstein HC, Pogue J et al; HOPE Investigators. Renal insufficiency as a predictor of cardiovascular outcomes and the impact of ramipril: The HOPE randomized trial. *Ann Intern Med* 2001; 134: 629–36.

29 PROGRESS Collaborative Group. Randomised trial of a perindopril-based blood-pressure-lowering regimen among 6105 individuals with previous stroke or transient ischaemic attack. *Lancet* 2001; 358: 1033–41.

30 Berthet K, Neal BC, Chalmers JP; Perindopril Protection Against Recurrent Stroke Study Collaborative Group. Reductions in the risks of recurrent stroke in patients with and without diabetes: The PROGRESS Trial. *Blood Press* 2004; 13: 7–13.

31 Hansson L, Zanchetti A, Carruthers SG et al. Effects of intensive blood-pressure lowering and low-dose aspirin in patients with hypertension: Principal results of the Hypertension Optimal Treatment (HOT) randomised trial. HOT Study Group. *Lancet* 1998; 351: 1755–62.

32 Schrier RW, Estacio RO, Jeffers B. Appropriate Blood Pressure Control in NIDDM (ABCD) Trial. *Diabetologia* 1996; 39: 1646–54.

33 Estacio RO, Jeffers BW, Hiatt WR et al. The effect of nisoldipine as compared with enalapril on cardiovascular outcomes in patients with non-insulin-dependent diabetes and hypertension. *N Engl J Med* 1998; 338: 645–52.

34 Schrier RW, Estacio RO, Esler A, Mehler P. Effects of aggressive blood pressure control in normotensive type 2 diabetic patients on albuminuria, retinopathy and strokes. *Kidney Int* 2002; 61: 1086–97.

35 Cushman WC, Evans GW, Byington RP et al.; ACCORD Study Group. Effects of intensive blood-pressure control in type 2 diabetes mellitus. *N Engl J Med* 2010; 362: 1575–85.

36 Cushman WC, Grimm RH Jr,, Cutler JA et al.' ACCORD Study Group. Rationale and design for the blood pressure intervention of the Action to Control Cardiovascular Risk in Diabetes (ACCORD) trial. *Am J Cardiol* 2007; 99: 44i–55i.

37 Lewis EJ, Hunsicker LG, Clarke WR et al. Renoprotective effect of the angiotensin-receptor antagonist irbesartan in patients with nephropathy due to type 2 diabetes. *N Engl J Med* 2001; 345: 851–60.

38 Berl T, Hunsicker LG, Lewis JB et al. Impact of achieved blood pressure on cardiovascular outcomes in the Irbesartan Diabetic Nephropathy Trial. *J Am Soc Nephrol* 2005; 16: 2170–79.

39 Pepine CJ, Handberg EM, Cooper-DeHoff RM et al. A calcium antagonist vs a non-calcium antagonist hypertension treatment strategy for patients with coronary artery disease. The International verapamil-Trandolapril Study (INVEST): A randomized controlled trial. *JAMA* 2003; 290: 2805–16.

40 Tuomilehto J, Rastenyte D, Birkenhäger WH et al. Effects of calcium-channel blockade in older patients with diabetes and systolic hypertension. Systolic Hypertension in Europe Trial Investigators. *N Engl J Med* 1999; 340: 677–84.

41 Patel A, MacMahon S, Chalmers J et al. Effects of a fixed combination of perindopril and indapamide on macrovascular and microvascular outcomes in patients with type 2 diabetes mellitus (the ADVANCE trial): A randomised controlled trial. *Lancet* 2007; 370: 829–40.

42 Holman RR, Paul SK, Bethel MA et al. Long-term follow-up after tight control of blood pressure in type 2 diabetes. *N Engl J Med* 2008; 359: 1565–76.

43 Chew EY, Ambrosius WT, Davis MD et al. Effects of medical therapies on retinopathy progression in type 2 diabetes. *N Engl J Med* 2010; 363: 233–44.

44 Perneger TV, Brancati FL, Whelton PK, Klag MJ. End-stage renal disease attributable to diabetes mellitus. *Ann Intern Med* 1994; 121: 912–18.

45 Bakris GL, Ritz E; World Kidney Day Steering Committee. The message for World Kidney Day 2009: Hypertension and kidney disease – a marriage that should be prevented. *J Hypertens* 2009; 27: 666–9.

46 Adler AI, Stevens RJ, Manley SE et al.; UKPDS Group. Development and progression of nephropathy in type 2 diabetes: The United Kingdom Prospective Diabetes Study (UKPDS 64). *Kidney Int* 2003; 63: 225–32.

47 McCullough PA, Verrill TA. Cardiorenal interaction: Appropriate treatment of cardiovascular risk factors to improve outcomes in chronic kidney disease. *Postgrad Med* 2010; 122: 25–34.

48 Strippoli GF, Craig M, Schena FP, Craig JC. Role of blood pressure targets and specific antihypertensive agents used to prevent diabetic nephropathy and delay its progression. *J Am Soc Nephrol* 2006; 17(4 Suppl 2): S153–S155.

49 Brenner BM, Cooper ME, de Zeeuw D et al.; RENAAL Study Investigators. Effects of losartan on renal and cardiovascular outcomes in patients with type 2 diabetes and nephropathy. *N Engl J Med* 2001; 345: 861–9.

50 Berl T, Hunsicker LG, Lewis JB et al.; Irbesartan Diabetic Nephropathy Trial Collaborative Study Group. Cardiovascular outcomes in the Irbesartan Diabetic Nephropathy Trial of patients with type 2 diabetes and overt nephropathy. *Ann Intern Med* 2003; 138: 542–9.

51 Parving HH, Lehnert H, Bröchner-Mortensen J et al.; Irbesartan in Patients with Type 2 Diabetes and Microalbuminuria Study Group. The effect of irbesartan on the development of diabetic nephropathy in patients with type 2 diabetes. *N Engl J Med* 2001; 345: 870–78.

52 Bakris GL, Sarafidis PA, Weir MR et al.; ACCOMPLISH Trial Investigators. Renal outcomes with different fixed-dose combination therapies in patients with hypertension at high risk for cardiovascular events (ACCOMPLISH): A prespecified secondary analysis of a randomised controlled trial. *Lancet* 2010; 375: 1173–81.

53 Weber MA, Bakris GL, Jamerson K et al.; ACCOMPLISH Investigators. Cardiovascular events during differing hypertension therapies in patients with diabetes. *J Am Coll Cardiol* 2010; 56, 77–85.

54 Mann JF, Schmieder RE, Dyal L et al.; Telmisartan Randomised Assessment Study in ACE Intolerant Subjects with Cardiovascular Disease (TRANSCEND) Investigators. Effect of telmisartan on renal outcomes: A randomised trial. *Ann Intern Med* 2009; 151: 1–10.

55 Yusuf S, Teo K, Anderson C et al.; Telmisartan Randomised Assessment Study in ACE Intolerant Subjects with Cardiovascular Disease (TRANSCEND) Investigators. Effects of the angiotensin-receptor blocker telmisartan on cardiovascular events in high-risk patients intolerant to angiotensin-converting enzyme inhibitors: A randomised controlled trial. *Lancet* 2008; 372: 1174–83.

56 Sjølie AK, Klein R, Porta M et al.; DIRECT Programme Study Group. Effect of candesartan on regression of retinopathy in type 2 diabetes (DIRECT-Protect 2): A randomised placebo-controlled trial. *Lancet* 2008; 372: 1385–93.

57 Bilous R, Chaturvedi N, Sjølie AK et al. Effect of candesartan on microalbuminuria and albumin excretion rate in diabetes: Three randomized trials. *Ann Intern Med* 2009; 151: 11–20.

58 Chaturvedi N, Porta M, Klein R et al.; DIRECT Programme Study Group. Effect of candesartan on prevention (DIRECT-Prevent 1) and progression (DIRECT-Protect 1) of retinopathy in type 1 diabetes: Randomised, placebo-controlled trials. *Lancet* 2008; 372: 1394–402.

59 Bertrand ME, Mourad JJ. Reduction in mortality with antihypertensive agents: Evidence from clinical trials in at-risk hypertensive patients. *Eur Heart J* 2010; 31(Abstr Suppl): 321–2.

60 Dahlöf B, Sever PS, Poulter NR et al.; ASCOT Investigators. Prevention of cardiovascular events with an antihypertensive regimen of amlodipine adding perindopril as required versus atenolol adding bendroflumethiazide as required, in the Anglo-Scandinavian Cardiac Outcomes Trial-Blood Pressure Lowering Arm (ASCOT-BPLA): A multicentre randomised controlled trial. *Lancet* 2005; 366: 895–906.

61 Beckett NS, Peters NS, Fletcher AE et al.; HYVET Study Group. Treatment of hypertension in patients 80 years of age or older. *N Engl J Med* 2008; 358: 1887–98.

62 Blood Pressure Lowering Treatment Trialists' Collaboration. Effects of different blood pressure lowering regimens on major cardiovascular events: Results of prospectively designed overviews of randomised trials. *Lancet* 2003; 362: 1527–35.

63 Prospective Studies Collaboration. Age-specific relevance of usual blood pressure to vascular mortality: A meta-analysis of individual data for one million adults in 61 prospective studies. *Lancet* 2002; 360: 1903–13.

64 Jackson R, Lawes CM, Bennett DA et al. Treatment with drugs to lower blood pressure and blood cholesterol based on an individual's absolute cardiovascular risk. *Lancet* 2005; 365: 434–41.

65 The INDANA Project Collaborators. Effect of antihypertensive treatment in patients having already suffered from stroke. *Stroke* 1997; 28: 2557–62.

66 Rothwell PM, Howard SC, Spence D. Relationship between blood pressure and stroke risk in patients with symptomatic carotid occlusive disease. *Stroke* 2003; 34: 2583–90.

67 Bosch J, Yusuf S, Pogue J et al. on behalf of the HOPE Investigators. Use of ramipril in preventing stroke: Double blind randomised trial. *Brit Med J* 2002; 324: 1–5.

68 McAlister FA; Renin Angiotension System Modulator Meta-Analysis Investigators. Angiotensin-converting enzyme inhibitors or angiotensin receptor blockers are beneficial in normotensive atherosclerotic patients: A collaborative meta-analysis of randomized trials. *Eur Heart J* 2012; 33: 505–14.

69 Mann JF, Schmeider RE, McQueen M et al.; ONTARGET Investigators. Renal outcomes with telmisartan, ramipril, or both, in people at high vascular risk (the ONTARGET study): A multicentre, randomised, double-blind, controlled trial. *Lancet* 2008; 372: 547–53.

70 de Galan BE, Perkovic V, Ninomiya T et al.; ADVANCE Collaborative Group. Lowering blood pressure reduces renal events in type 2 diabetes. *J Am Soc Nephrol* 2009; 20: 883–92.

71 Lambers Heerspink HJ, Ninomiya T, Perkovic V et al.; for the ADVANCE Collaborative Group. Effects of a fixed combination of perindopril and indapamide in patients with type 2 diabetes and chronic kidney disease. *Eur Heart J* 2010; 31: 2888–96.

72 Su DC, Kim CM, Choi IS et al. Trends in blood pressure control and treatment among type 2 diabetes with comorbid hypertension in the United States: 1988–2004. *J Hypertens* 2009; 27: 1908–18.

73 Jamerson K, Weber MA, Bakris GL et al.; ACCOMPLISH Trial Investigators. Benazepril plus amlodipine or hydrochlorothiazide for hypertension in high-risk patients. *N Engl J Med* 2008; 359: 2417–28.

Answers to Multiple-Choice Questions for Case Study 1

1 A

2 B

3 B

4 B

5 A

CHAPTER 7

Dyslipidemia and Its Management in Type 2 Diabetes

D. John Betteridge
University College London Hospital, London, UK

Key Points

- Dyslipidemia is an integral component of metabolic syndrome and type 2 diabetes.

- Dyslipidemia involves both quantitative and qualitative lipid and lipoprotein abnormalities: moderate hypertriglyceridemia, low HDL-cholesterol, small dense LDL particles, and accumulation of cholesterol-rich remnant particles.

- Dyslipidemia is a major independent risk predictor for atherosclerosis-related disease.

- Increasing LDL-cholesterol concentrations and decreasing HDL-cholesterol concentrations were the strongest risk predictors for myocardial infarction observed in UKPDS.

- Patients with type 2 diabetes are at high risk of CVD events and the majority will fulfill criteria for pharmacotherapy to lower LDL-cholesterol.

- Statins are the cornerstone of therapy and their use is based on a wealth of data from well-conducted robust RCT.

- Some patients are statin intolerant and other drug classes such as ezetimibe, fibrates, nicotinic acid, and colesevalam may be required.

- New LDL-cholesterol-lowering strategies are in development that should ensure, if proved to be effective and safe, that more patients achieve LDL-cholesterol goals.

- Low HDL-cholesterol remains a significant risk predictor even when low LDL-cholesterol levels are achieved in the statin trials.

- To date no evidence is available from RCT to support measures to increase HDL-cholesterol to lower CVD events.

- Intensive management of dyslipidemia should be part of a global approach to CVD risk reduction in the diabetic population.

Introduction

Atherosclerosis-related disease, coronary heart disease (CHD), peripheral vascular disease (PVD), and thrombotic stroke are major complications in

---

Managing Cardiovascular Complications in Diabetes, First Edition.
Edited by D. John Betteridge and Stephen Nicholls.
© 2014 John Wiley & Sons, Ltd. Published 2014 by John Wiley & Sons, Ltd.

people with type 2 diabetes mellitus [1]. A recent meta-analysis of 102 prospective studies demonstrated a hazard ratio of 2 for coronary death and non-fatal myocardial infarction (MI) and 2.5 for ischemic stroke [2]. In the United Kingdom Prospective Diabetes Study (UKPDS), for each 1% increase in HbA1c there was a 28% inc rease in PVD [3].

The main focus for CVD risk management relates to patients with type 2 diabetes, but the increased lifetime risk for those with type 1 diabetes should be remembered when considering lipid lowering, particularly those with albuminuria, hypertension, and chronic kidney disease [4].

The pathogenesis of atherosclerosis in diabetes is multifactorial and the task for the physician is to manage all modifiable risk factors to prevent CVD events. However, it is clear from prospective studies that plasma cholesterol and low-density lipoprotein (LDL)-cholesterol in particular are major independent risk factors. In the United Kingdom Prospective Diabetes Study (UKPDS) of newly presenting patients with type 2 diabetes, LDL-cholesterol was the strongest predictor of MI. The second strongest predictor of MI was low levels of high-density lipoprotein (HDL)-cholesterol ahead of glycated hemoglobin, systolic blood pressure, and cigarette smoking [5].

Diabetic Dyslipidemia

The dyslipidemia of metabolic syndrome, insulin resistance, and type 2 diabetes consists of both quantitative and qualitative lipid and lipoprotein abnormalities [6]. Moderate hypertriglyceridemia is accompanied by low levels of HDL-cholesterol and an increase in cholesterol-rich remnant particles of chylomicrons and very low-density lipoprotein (VLDL) metabolism. LDL-cholesterol concentrations reflect those of the background population. However, important qualitative changes are present in the LDL particle distribution, with the accumulation of smaller, denser particles that are thought to be more atherogenic [7].

This complex phenotype is present at the time of diabetes diagnosis as it is part of the metabolic syndrome and prediabetes. In an individual patient it will be influenced by gender and lifestyle factors, particularly central obesity, the degree of physical activity, poor glycemic control, cigarette smoking, and alcohol intake. In addition, other secondary causes including renal and hepatic dysfunction, hypothyroidism, and concurrent medication may have a significant effect. Concurrent primary dyslipidemias such as familial hypercholesterolemia, familial combined hyperlipidemia, and type III dyslipidemia should be identified and managed appropriately.

Although understanding of the impact of insulin resistance on lipid and lipoprotein metabolism has increased enormously, much remains to be learned. A basic abnormality is the overproduction of large VLDL from the liver, partly as a result of an increased flux of fatty acids from adipose tissue combined with lack of inhibition of VLDL assembly [8]. In the postprandial state, hepatic VLDL production is not suppressed and this, together with exogenous fat absorbed in the form of chylomicrons, saturates activity of the enzyme lipoprotein lipase (LPL). LPL activity itself can also be reduced by increased levels of apoprotein C-III, apoprotein A-V, excess levels of fatty acids, low adiponectin levels, and insulin resistance.

Prolongation of the postprandial phase of lipid metabolism is associated with increased cholesterol and triglyceride exchange through the activity of cholesterol ester transport protein (CETP). CETP facilitates a mole-for-mole transfer of cholesterol esters from HDL to VLDL, IDL and chylomicron remnants, and LDL in exchange for triglycerides. As a result, LDL and HDL are triglyceride enriched and become substrates for the enzyme hepatic lipase, the activity of which is increased in diabetes. As a result of the triglyceride hydrolysis by this enzyme, LDL and HDL become smaller and denser. Smaller, denser HDL particles are cleared more rapidly, contributing to the low plasma levels observed [7, 9].

Dyslipidemia and CVD Risk

It is those patients with diabetes and concomitant metabolic syndrome including dyslipidemia that are at highest risk. In the National Health and Nutrition Examination (NHANES III) performed in the USA, the prevalence of metabolic syndrome in diabetes was 86%. The prevalence of CHD in this group was 19.2%. In those with diabetes and no evidence of metabolic syndrome, CHD prevalence was 7.5%, which is comparable to those without diabetes or metabolic syndrome [10].

Many studies in different populations have confirmed that dyslipidemia is a common finding in type 2 diabetes. The prevalence of low HDL-cholesterol (<0.9 mmol/l in men; <1.0 mmol/l in women) and/or raised triglycerides (>1.7 mmo/l) was increased about threefold compared to the background population in the Botnia study from Finland [11]. In a Canadian study, the prevalence of dyslipidemia ranged from 55% to 66% depending on the duration of disease: the longer the diabetes duration, the higher the prevalence of dyslipidemia [12].

LDL-cholesterol concentrations are generally similar to those of the background population. However, LDL-cholesterol remains a major risk factor and was indeed the best predictor of risk of MI in the UKPDS [5]. Qualitative changes in LDL particles increase their atherogenicity. The particles are smaller and denser with less lipid core. Parts of the apoprotein B molecule are exposed which have increased affinity to glycosaminoglycans. As a result, the particles are more likely to be retained in the subintimal space of the artery. Small, dense LDL are also more susceptible to oxidation, and it is oxidized LDL that is central to the development of atherosclerosis. Glycation of apoprotein B may also contribute to the increased atherogenicity [6].

HDL-cholesterol concentrations are inversely related to the risk of CVD events. In UKPDS, low HDL was the second best predictor of MI risk [5]. Baseline HDL concentrations remain a significant risk predictor in the major CVD outcome trials with statins, even in those subjects who achieved LDL-cholesterol concentrations <1.8 mmol/l [13]. The mechanism(s) by which HDL protects remains to be fully understood, although its role in reverse cholesterol transport has received considerable attention. Other potential mechanisms include antioxidant, anti-inflammatory, and antithrombotic effects [14].

The relationship of plasma triglycerides to CVD risk remains unresolved. Present in univariate analyses, the relationship is not maintained after other factors are adjusted for, particularly non-HDL-cholesterol [15]. Remnants of triglyceride-rich lipoproteins, enriched in cholesterol through lipid exchange mediated by CETP in prolonged postprandial lipemia, are atherogenic, as they are rapidly taken up by arterial wall macrophages to form foam cells. In several studies including the more recent FIELD and ACCORD studies, subjects with raised triglyceride (>2.3 mmol/l) and low HDL-cholesterol (<0.9 mmol/l) have been shown to be at higher CVD risk. Clearly, these parameters are intimately linked through postprandial lipemia [16, 17]. In the Copenhagen General Population Study, which included over 2,000 subjects with diabetes, nonfasting triglyceride concentrations were highly predictive of CVD events independent of other factors [18]. This relationship probably reflects the link between nonfasting triglycerides and remnant lipoprotein cholesterol.

Management of Diabetic Dyslipidemia

Management of dyslipidemia should be part of overall CVD risk prevention, with attention to all modifiable risk factors. A lipid profile including total cholesterol and triglycerides, HDL-cholesterol with calculation of LDL-cholesterol by the Friedwald formula generally provides sufficient information for clinical management. Non-HDL-cholesterol is an important measure readily calculated by subtracting HDL-cholesterol from total cholesterol; this value is closely correlated with measurements of apoprotein B and therefore the number of atherogenic particles. It is often inconvenient for patients to fast for these measurements and this is not crucial, as apart from triglycerides, nonfasting concentrations do not differ significantly. Furthermore, as has been discussed, nonfasting triglycerides appear to be a strong CVD predictor.

As already discussed, the lipid phenotype may be influenced by other primary and secondary dyslipidemias [19].These other conditions should be diagnosed and treated appropriately. In the individual patient poor glycemic control, central obesity, excess alcohol intake, suboptimal diet and lack of physical activity are common and open to lifestyle intervention. It cannot be overemphasized that lifestyle measures should be the cornerstone of therapy in the management of vascular risk. The reader is referred to a comprehensive review of the topic [20].

Are all patients with type 2 diabetes at sufficient CVD risk (20% 10-year CVD risk) to receive pharmacotherapy for dyslipidemia? In the author's opinion, risk calculation is not necessary, as most patients above the age of 40 years will fulfill this risk criterion. However, risk engines such as the one based on the UKPDS epidemiology data are available [21]. In the recent European Society of Cardiology/European Atherosclerosis Society guidelines for the management of dyslipidaemias [19], in patients with type 2 diabetes and CVD or chronic kidney disease (CKD), and those without CVD who are over the age of 40 years with one or more other CVD risk factors or markers of target organ damage, the recommended goal for LDL-cholesterol is <1.8 mmo/l and the secondary goal for non-HDL-cholesterol is <2.6 mmo/l. These guidelines also give a target for apoprotein B of less than <0.8 g/L. This, in the author's opinion, is forward thinking and particularly helpful (if available) in diabetic dyslipidemia, as potentially atherogenic cholesterol is carried on lipoproteins other than LDL. There is one molecule of apoprotein B per particle of the VLDL, IDL, LDL cascade and its concentration therefore gives important information on particle numbers. For all other people with type 2 diabetes, an LDL-cholesterol <2.5 mmol/l is the primary target. The non-HDL-cholesterol target is below 3.3 mmol/l and apoprotein B <1.0 g/L. In this and other guidelines, different targets are set depending on the risk. The author fails to see the rationale for this and in his practice, once the decision to introduce pharmacotherapy has been taken, the more intensive target is applied to all.

Secondary Prevention

Statins are first-line pharmacotherapy for diabetic dyslipidemia. Their use is based on a wealth of data from robust, randomized trials for both primary and secondary prevention of CVD events. First discovered in the 1970s by the Japanese scientist Dr. Akiro Endo, the introduction of these drugs into clinical practice in the 1980s enabled the first definitive CVD end-point trials of cholesterol lowering to be performed. They act by decreasing hepatic cholesterol synthesis (by about 40%) by specific competitive inhibition of the rate-determining enzyme, HMG-CoA reductase, which catalyzes the first committed step in cholesterol synthesis. As a result, the expression of hepatic LDL receptors is increased, which bind and take up more plasma LDL, thereby decreasing plasma LDL. The Scandinavian Simvastatin Survival Study (4S) was the first landmark statin trial [22] performed in patients with established CHD ($n = 4,444$, 827 females). The primary endpoint was overall mortality. Simvastatin reduced LDL-cholesterol concentration by 35% and, after a mean follow-up of 5.4 years, there were 182 deaths in the treated group compared to 256 in the placebo group (HR 0.7; 95% CI 0.59–0.85; $p < 0.0003$). In addition, there were highly significant reductions in all coronary events.

In 4S 202 known diabetic patients (age 60 years, 78% male) were included and approximately half of those on placebo suffered a major coronary event during the study period [23]. In the simvastatin group, CVD events were reduced by 55% ($p = 0.002$). Numbers were too small to assess the effect on overall mortality, although there was a 47%, nonsignificant reduction. In a further analysis, additional diabetic patients ($n = 483$) were identified on the basis of a baseline fasting glucose >7.0 mmol/l [24]. In addition, 678 patients were identified with impaired fasting glucose (IFT) with glucose levels between 6.1 and 6.9 mmol/l. Major CHD events were reduced by simvastatin (HR 0.58; 95% CI 0.42–0.81, $p < 0.001$). The 28% reduction in overall mortality did not reach significance. In the IFT group there was a significant reduction in overall mortality (HR 0.57; 95% CI 0.31–0.91, $p < 0.02$) [24].

The results of 4S have been confirmed in further subgroup analyses from several large RCT (Table 7.1), including The Heart Protection Study (HPS), which incorporated a large diabetes subgroup and its analysis was prespecified [25]. It is clear that patients with diabetes and CHD respond in a similar way to the nondiabetic population. However, a substantial residual vascular risk persists, as demonstrated by the HPS study. The residual risk of suffering a major CVD event in diabetic patients with CHD receiving 40 mg/day simvastatin remained higher than in nondiabetic patients with CHD on placebo (Figure 7.1).

The question arose as to whether more intensive statin therapy would result in further risk reduction. This has been tested in formal RCT in both acute coronary syndromes and stable coronary disease. In the Treat to New Targets (TNT) trial, more intensive therapy with atorvastatin 80 mg/day was compared to atorvastatin 10 mg/day in 10,001 patients with stable CHD [26]. In the diabetic subgroup ($n = 1,501$), LDL-cholesterol was 2.0 mmol/l compared to 2.55 mmol/l in the standard treatment group,

Table 7.1 Impact of statin therapy in subgroups of diabetic patients in the major statin trials. Diabetic patients show the same benefit in terms of CVD reduction to those without diabetes.

Variables / Trial	Type of event	Treatment	Proportion of events (%) Diabetes		Relative risk reduction (%) Patient group	
			No	Yes	All	Diabetes
4S Diabetes n = 202	CHD death or non-fatal MI	Simvastatin	19	23	32	55
		Placebo	27	45		
4S Reanalysis Diabetes n = 483	CHD death or non-fatal MI	Simvastatin	19	24	32	42
		Placebo	26	38		
HPS Diabetes n = 3050	Major coronary event, stroke, or revascularization	Simvastatin	20	31	24	18
		Placebo	25	36		
CARE Diabetes n = 586	CHD death, non-fatal MI	Pravastatin	12	19	23	25
		Placebo	15	23		
LIPID Diabetes n = 782	CHD death, non-fatal MI, revascularization	Pravastatin	19	29	24	19
		Placebo	25	37		
LIPS Diabetes n = 202	CHD death, non-fatal MI, revascularization	Fluvastatin	21	22	22	47
		Placebo	25	38		
GREACE Diabetes n = 313	CHD, death, non-fatal MI, UAP, CHF, revascularization, stroke	Atorvastatin	12	12	51	58
		Standard care	25	30	–	–

4S, Scandinavian Simvastatin Survival Study; HPS, Heart Protection Study; CARE, Cholesterol and Recurrent Events Trial; LIPID, Long-Term Intervention with Pravastatin in Ischaemic Disease Study; LIPS, Lescol Intervention Prevention Study; GREACE, Greek Atorvastatin and CHD Evaluation Study. CHD, coronary heart disease; CHF, congestive heart failure; MI, myocardial infarction; revasc, revascularization; UAP, unstable angina pectoris.

(Source: Rydén L et al. Guidelines on diabetes, pre-diabetes, and cardiovascular diseases: executive summary. The Task Force on Diabetes and Cardiovascular Diseases of the European Society of Cardiology (ESC) and of the European Association for the Study of Diabetes (EASD). *Eur Heart J.* 2007 Jan;28(1):88–136. Reproduced with permission of Oxford University Press.)

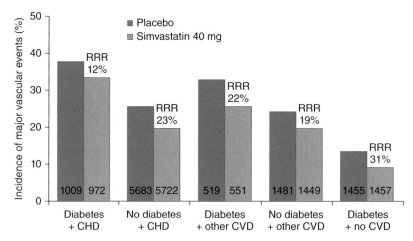

Figure 7.1 Residual CVD risk in nondiabetes with CVD. Those patients in the 4S study with diabetes and established CVD on statin therapy remained at higher risk than those nondiabeteic patients with CVD on placebo. RRR, relative risk reduction. (Source: HPS Collaborative Group 2003 [25]. Reproduced with permission of Elsevier.)

and this was associated with a significant reduction in major CVD events (HR 0.75, 95% CI 0.58–0.97, p = 0.026). 5584 patients (56%) were identified with metabolic syndrome; in this subgroup intensive therapy was associated with a 29% risk reduction in the primary endpoint (HR 0.71, 95% CI 0.61–0.84, $p < 0.0001$) [27].

A meta-analysis has examined data from four trials of intensive versus conventional statin therapy in 27,584 patients with acute coronary syndromes or with stable coronary disease involving [28]. Intensive statin therapy (higher dose or more potent drug) was associated with a further 16% reduction in coronary death and MI (HR 0.84; 955CI 0.77–0.91; $p < 0.0001$; Figure 7.2). This large database supports results from individual trials showing the benefit from more intensive therapy. This finding has been confirmed by an analysis from the Cholesterol Treatment Trialists' Collaboration [29, 30]. Given the high risk in the diabetic patient with established CVD disease, intensive LDL-lowering therapy should become part of routine clinical practice.

The only trial to recruit a specific population of stroke or transient ischemic attack survivors (n = 4,731) with time to subsequent stroke as the primary endpoint was SPARCL [31]. High-intensity statin therapy with atorvastatin 80 mg/day was associated with a reduction in subsequent stroke of 16% (HR 0.84 95% CI 0.71–0.99, $p < 0.03$). As might be predicted, secondary endpoints of major coronary events showed highly significant reductions. In the diabetes subgroup of 794 patients, there was a 30% reduction in stroke and a 51% reduction in major coronary events.

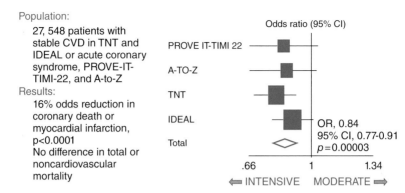

Population:
27, 548 patients with stable CVD in TNT and IDEAL or acute coronary syndrome, PROVE-IT-TIMI-22, and A-to-Z

Results:
16% odds reduction in coronary death or myocardial infarction, p<0.0001 No difference in total or noncardiovascular mortality

Figure 7.2 The impact of more intensive stain therapy compared with conventional therapy in a meta-analysis of four major trials in patients with stable coronary disease and patients post acute coronary syndrome. More intensive therapy produced a further 16% reduction in coronary events. (Source: Cannon et al. 2006 [28]. Reproduced with permission of Elsevier.)

Primary Prevention

Higher case fatality in diabetes with the first CVD event points to the importance of primary CVD prevention. A large number of diabetic patients (n = 2,912) was included in HPS. Simvastatin, which reduced LDL-cholesterol by 0.9 mmol/l, was associated with a 33% relative risk reduction in major CVD events (p = 0.0003). This benefit was independent of baseline lipids, diabetes duration, glycemic control, and age. The authors calculated that simvastatin therapy over five years should prevent a first major cardiovascular event in about 45 people per 1,000 treated [25]. Support for the HPS findings came from the Collaborative Atorvastatin Diabetes Study (CARDS): 2,838 type 2 diabetic patients, aged 40–75 years, without clinical CVD but with one other risk factor (hypertension, current cigarette smoking, retinopathy, or albuminuria), received atorvastatin 10 mg/day or matching placebo [32]. Patients were excluded if baseline LDL-cholesterol was >4.14 mmol/l, the treatment threshold at the time, and baseline triglyceride levels up to 6.78 mmol/l were permitted. The trial was terminated two years earlier than expected because the prespecified early stopping rule for efficacy had been met. Atorvastatin reduced LDL-cholesterol by 40% compared to placebo, representing an absolute reduction of 1.2 mmol/l; this reduction was associated with a 37% (95% CI −52 to −17, p = 0.001) relative risk reduction in major CVD events (Figure 7.3). CARDs was not powered for overall mortality; however, there was a 27% reduction of borderline statistical significance (p = 0.059). Stroke was reduced by 48%. There was no heterogeneity of effect in relation to baseline lipids, age, diabetes duration, glycemic control,

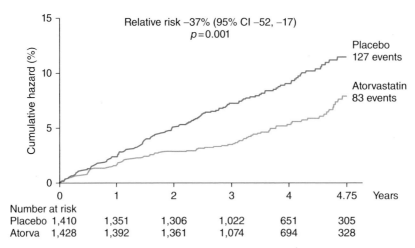

Figure 7.3 Main results from the Collaborative Atorvastatin Diabetes study (CARDS), which demonstrated that atorvastatin 10 mg/day reduced first major CVD events by 37% in patients with type 2 diabetes. (Source: Colhoun et al. 2004 [32]. Reproduced with permission of Elsevier.)

systolic blood pressure, smoking, or albuminuria. The authors concluded that atorvastatin was safe and effective in reducing the risk of first CVD events in patients without high LDL-cholesterol levels, mean baseline 3 mmol/l [32]. On the basis of this trial together with HPS, there seems to be no justification for a particular threshold level of LDL to determine which patients should receive statin therapy; rather, their absolute CVD risk should be the primary determinant.

The diabetes subgroup ($n = 2,532$) from the Anglo Scandinavian Cardiac Outcomes Trial Lipid-Lowering Arm (ASCOT-LLA) showed a similar trend (test for heterogeneity not significant) to reduction of CVD events as seen in those without diabetes. This trial is of particular interest because the benefits of statin therapy with atorvastatin 10 mg/day were seen in well-treated hypertensive patients [33].

Cholesterol Goal Achievement in Practice

The availability of the highly effective and well-tolerated statin class of drugs for LDL-cholesterol lowering should ensure that most patients with diabetes achieve their therapeutic goals. However, much still needs to be done to translate the findings from well-conducted RCT to the benefit of the individual patient. The EUROASPIRE epidemiology surveys performed across many European countries have certainly demonstrated improvement in risk-factor management in those with symptomatic coronary disease over recent years. However, in the most recent survey from 2009, over 40% of patients remained with cholesterol >4.5 mmol/l. Of interest is that the number of patients with diabetes among the sample of CHD patients is about 35% [34].

A contributory factor to the failure to achieve therapeutic goals is statin intolerance. Meta-analysis of the RCT of statin trials involving over 100,000 participants has confirmed the safety of this drug class [35]. However, in practice there is a significant minority of patients who cannot tolerate statins at all, or can only tolerate a small dose, insufficient to achieve the LDL goal. The main reported side effects are muscle aches and pains, often with a normal creatine phosphokinase level [36]. In addition, concurrent medication with drugs that can increase statin concentrations because they interfere with their metabolism may preclude an effective dose.

In patients who complain of perceived statin side effects, it is important to reiterate the benefits of the statins and to exclude other problems. In the patient with myalgia, the author measures vitamin D levels and corrects low levels, often with benefit. It is of course also important to exclude hypothyroidism. Some patients have reported benefit by taking Co-Enzyme Q 10 supplements, although the evidence base for this is not robust. In the author's clinic, the fallback position is to give a long-acting statin such as atorvastatin or rosuvastatin in low dose once or twice weekly, plus the specific cholesterol absorption inhibitor ezetimibe.

Recently, an analysis of a large database of ezetimibe studies has been reported [37]. Notably, people with diabetes appeared to respond better to a statin/ezetimibe combination than those without diabetes (Figure 7.4). Is this likely to be a true finding and if so, what is the explanation? When ezetimibe was first introduced, its mechanism of action was not understood. However, subsequently it became clear that its action is to block Niemann-Pick C1-Like 1 (NPC1L1), which is a transmembrane receptor found at the apical membranes of enterocytes that mediates cholesterol absorption [38]. Subsequently, experiments in NPC1L1 knockout and ezetimibe-fed experimental animals have shown that NPC1L1 deficiency prevents diet-induced hepatic fatty liver and obesity development [39]. Ezetimibe has also been shown to reduce hepatic fat in humans [40, 41]. The mechanism(s) of these effects remains to be fully explained. As hepatic fat is a central feature of metabolic syndrome and type 2 diabetes, it is possible that modulation of this by ezetimibe may have an impact on hepatic insulin resistance and lipoprotein output.

The combination of simvastatin and ezetimibe was the treatment arm of a large study of patients with chronic end-stage kidney disease, which included a significant number of patients with diabetes. This trial showed significant reductions in CVD events with the combination therapy, which correlated with the degree of LDL-cholesterol reduction [42].

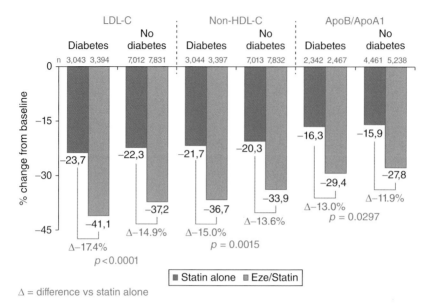

Figure 7.4 The impact of statin/ezetimibe combination compared to statin therapy alone in patients with and without diabetes. A meta-analysis of 27 controlled trials. Patients with diabetes appear to respond better to combination therapy compared to those without diabetes. (Source: Leiter et al. 2011 [37]. Reproduced with permission of John Wiley & Sons, Ltd.)

A not uncommon situation when managing diabetic dyslipidemia relates to the persistence of modest hypertriglyceridemia, despite achievement of the LDL-cholesterol goal. The author's approach here is to look at the important secondary goal of non-HDL-cholesterol, which is set 0.8 mmol/l above the LDL goal. This measures potentially atherogenic cholesterol carried on lipoproteins (remnant particles and IDL) other than LDL. Another possibility is to add a fibrate such as fenofibrate or bezafibrate. Although recent RCT of fenofibrate, FIELD, and ACCORD [43, 17] in diabetic patients have disappointed in terms of the primary endpoint, a consistent finding from these and other fibrate trials has been the apparent CVD benefit in those patients with hypertriglyceridemia and low HDL [44]. In addition, in both FIELD and ACCORD significant reductions in development of retinopathy were reported [45, 46].

Severe Hypertriglyceridemia

Diabetic patients may develop severe hypertriglyceridemia, with fasting serum triglyceride concentrations over 11 mmol/l and sometimes in the 20–60 mmol/l range or higher. Increased hepatic output of VLDL from the liver, together with postprandial absorption of chylomicrons, swamps the clearance pathway through the enzyme lipoprotein lipase. Diabetes alone does not result in such high triglyceride levels and there is usually an underlying lipid disorder such as familial combined hyperlipidemia. Other secondary causes – for example, hypothyroidism, high alcohol intake, central obesity and renal disease – should be excluded.

Severe hypertriglyceridemia (fasting levels >11 mmol/l) may be associated with recurrent attacks of abdominal pain and sometimes pancreatitis. Hepatosplenomegaly due to accumulation of lipid-laden macrophages may occur. Rarely, there may be memory disturbances and lack of concentration. Some patients develop spectacular skin eruptions, eruptive xanthomata, which appear as crops of raised pinkish, yellow spots over elbows, knees, and buttocks.

Massive hypertriglyceridemia may interfere with the measurement of other analytes such as hemoglobin, bilirubin, and liver transaminases and, by decreasing water volume in plasma, can lead to artificially low sodium measurement.

Treatment is of some urgency given the risk of pancreatitis. It is important that the patient is counseled to follow a low total fat diet together with reductions in alcohol and refined carbohydrate. In addition, high doses of omega 3 fish oils are beneficial, combined with a fibrate or nicotinic acid. As diet and lifestyle measures progress, it is often possible to stop the fish oils. If significant mixed lipemia persists, a statin is indicated with the possible addition of a fibrate.

A Look to the Future

It was the study of cultured cells from a rare inborn error of metabolism, homozygous familial hypercholesterolemia (FH), by the Nobel laureates Brown and Goldstein that led to the discovery of the LDL receptor and ultimately drugs to target its expression [47]. It is the activity of hepatic LDL receptors that is the major determinant of plasma LDL concentration. Subsequently, the study of other families with a severe FH phenotype has identified a previously unknown cellular process important for LDL receptor activity [48, 49]. Proprotein convertase subtilisin/kexin type 9 (PCSK9), a serine protease synthesized in the liver, reduces the number of LDL receptors. The circulating enzyme binds to the receptor on the hepatic cell surface, is internalized with it, and promotes its lysosomal degradation; so as a result of the action of PCSK9, LDL receptor numbers are reduced and plasma LDL increases. Mutations in the PCSK9 gene resulting in overactivity produce a severe FH phenotype. Monoclonal antibodies have been developed that bind to and inactivate PCSK9, leading to increased LDL receptor activity and reduction of plasma LDL. The monoclonal antibodies, which need to be administered subcutaneously every two or four weeks, produce plasma LDL reductions of around 60% on top of statin therapy [50, 51]. If this new approach proves to be effective and safe in the long term, it will facilitate LDL goal attainment in the majority of patients.

Increasing HDL-cholesterol is an attractive lipoprotein target following the reduction of LDL. HDL-cholesterol concentrations remain predictors of risk in the statin trials, even when intensive LDL reduction has been achieved. However, as yet there is no evidence from definitive RCT of the benefit of increasing HDL for CVD reduction. Nicotinic acid will increase HDL-cholesterol by around 20%, but the AIM HIGH study, which was designed to test the benefit of statin/nicotinic acid combination compared to statin alone, was terminated prematurely for futility [52]. The design, conduct, and power of this trial have been subject to much criticism; however, at the end of 2012 it was announced that HPS2Thrive, a much larger trial involving over 25,000 subjects and a high number of people with diabetes, comparing the nicotinic acid/laropiprant combination product and statin therapy to intensive LDL-cholesterol lowering with statin (± ezetimibe) alone, did not show added benefit (www.ctsu.ox.ac .uk/research/megatrials/hps-thrive). Following the results of HPS3Thrive, the nicotinic acid/laropiprant combination is to be withdrawn.

Inhibitors of cholesterol ester transfer protein (CETP) can increase HDL-cholesterol much more than nicotinic acid, but initial experience has been profoundly disappointing, either because of off-target toxic effects with torceptrapib or futility with dalcetrapib [53, 54]. However anacetrapib [55] and evacetrapib [56] are in ongoing CVD outcome trials. These drugs lead to large increases in HDL-cholesterol (>100%), but also lower LDL-cholesterol and apoprotein B. If positive, these trials will not answer the HDL hypothesis, however, as benefit may accrue from their other lipid effects.

The PPAR gamma agonist pioglitazone, in use as an oral hypoglycemia agent, consistently increases HDL-cholesterol by approximately 10%. Of interest is its apparent benefit in delaying the progression of coronary atheroma, as demonstrated by intravascular ultrasound in the PERISCOPE study, and carotid artery intima-media thickness, as demonstrated by high-resolution ultrasound in the CHICAGO study and clinical events in the PROACTIVE study; this appears to relate to its increase in HDL-cholesterol rather than the reduction in HbA1c [57, 58, 59]. The author uses this agent extensively, but is mindful of potential adverse effects, including fluid retention, the possibility of increased fracture incidence, and bladder cancer, although the latter is by no means certain.

Conclusions

Dyslipidemia is an important component of metabolic syndrome, insulin resistance, and type 2 diabetes. It is a major risk factor for CVD, the most important cause of premature morbidity and mortality in this high-risk population. It is open to therapeutic intervention principally with statins, which have been subject to well-conducted RCT in both primary and secondary CVD prevention. It is important that the benefits demonstrated in these RCT are transferred to everyday clinical practice for the benefit of individual patients. Survey data suggest that much still needs to be done to ensure that all patients at high risk receive effective lipid-lowering therapy.

Case Study 1

A 58-year-old businessman attends the clinic for annual review of diabetes. He was diagnosed with type 2 diabetes at the age of 49 years. His sister and mother also have type 2 diabetes. His mother had a myocardial infarction at 65 years. He is a nonsmoker and does not drink excess alcohol. He has no relevant past medical history apart from hypertension diagnosed at the age of 53 years. He is asymptomatic. His current medication consists of metformin modified release 500 mg twice daily, sitagliptin 100 mg daily, simvastatin 40 mg daily, losartan 100 mg daily, amlodipine 5 mg daily, and indapamide 1.25 mg daily. Concordance with therapy was excellent. His BMI was 27. There were no abnormal findings on examination, BP 133/83. His HbA1c was 7.1%, estimated GFR 78, liver function normal apart from alanine transferase of 57 (<50), thyroid function normal, urine albumin/creatinine ratio slightly raised at 3.6, cholesterol 5.3 mmol/l, triglycerides 3.9 mmol/l, HDL-cholesterol 0.9mol/l, calculated LDL-cholesterol 2.56 mmol/l.

His glycemic control is pretty good and there would be general agreement that an HbA1c of 7% is a reasonable goal for him. His oral agents are unlikely to precipitate hypoglycemia. Rather than adding additional medication, he was advised to tighten up on his diet and lifestyle measures, which had been somewhat relaxed over the holiday period.

His hypertension appears reasonable in the clinic and his home-monitored readings show an average systolic pressure of around 126 mmHg. However, he does have microalbuminuria, although this is less than on previous visits when his antihypertensive regimen was increased.

His lipid profile is reasonable, but not optimal. His non-HDL-cholesterol of 4.4 mmol/l indicates a significant residual cholesterol burden despite the calculated LDL. This patient should be treated more intensively given his age and additional risk factors of hypertension and microalbuminuria. In addition, his mother developed symptomatic ischemic heart disease at 65 years. The target is LDL-cholesterol <1.8 mmol/l and non-HDL-cholesterol <2.6 mmol/l.

There are several options, but my preferred one would be to switch to atorvastatin 40 mg daily in the first instance. His alanine transferase is slightly raised. This probably represents a degree of fatty liver (this was confirmed with abdominal ultrasound), which is not a contraindication to statin therapy. It is likely that the more effective statin together with his improved diet and lifestyle efforts will produce a significant improvement, although they may not fully achieve the intensive goal. In that case, I would add ezetimibe 10 mg/day, which has a more than additive effect in lowering cholesterol when added to statin therapy.

Multiple-Choice Questions

1 Are the following statements true or false?
    A Statins lower LDL-cholesterol by reducing hepatic lipoprotein output
    B Ezetimibe reduces the absorption of bile salt in the terminal ileum.
    C Fibrates are effective if reducing plasma triglyceride concentrations.
    D Statins should not be combined with other lipid-lowering drugs.
    E Triglyceride concentrations are the best independent predictor of cardiovascular events in type 2 diabetes.

2 Are the following statements true or false?
    A Non-HDL-cholesterol concentrations correlate well with apoprotein B levels.
    B Consistent evidence from randomized controlled clinical trials demonstrates that raising HDL-cholesterol by pharmacotherapy is associated with a significant reduction in CVD events.
    C Statin therapy is contradicted in patients with fatty liver.
    D The addition of ezetimibe to statin therapy leads to a more than an additive effect in reducing plasma LDL-cholesterol concentrations.
    E Fenofibrate has been shown to reduce the progression of retinopathy in type 2 diabetes.

3 Are the following statements true or false?
    A Insulin resistance is associated with increased activity of the enzyme lipoprotein lipase.
    B LDL receptor activity is directly related to hepatic cholesterol concentrations.
    C Low-density lipoprotein particles are smaller, denser, and potentially more atherogenic in type 2 diabetes.
    D Remnant lipoprotein particles are important carriers of potentially atherogenic cholesterol.
    E The flux of free fatty acids from visceral fat to the liver is decreased in type 2 diabetes.

Answers provided after the References

References

1 Bloomgarden ZT. Cardiovascular disease in diabetes. *Diabetes Care* 2008; 31: 1260–66.

2 Fletcher AE, Sarwar N, Gao P et al. Diabetes mellitus: Fasting blood glucose concentration and risk of vascular disease, a collaborative meta-analysis of 102 prospective studies. *Lancet* 2010; 375: 2215–22.

3 Adler AI, Stevens RJ, Neil A et al. UKPDS 59 Hyperglycaemia and other potentially modifiable risk factors for peripheral vascular disease in type 2 diabetes. *Diabetes Care* 2002; 25: 894–9.

4 Soedamah-Muthu SS, Fuller JH, Mulnier HE et al. High risk of cardiovascular disease in patients with type 1 diabetes in the UK: A cohort study using the general practice research data base. *Diabetes Care* 2006; 29: 798–804.

5 Turner RC, Millns H, Neil HAW et al.; for the United Kingdom Prospective Diabetes Study Group. Risk factors for coronary artery disease in non-insulin dependent diabetes mellitus: United Kingdom Prospective Diabetes Study (UKPDS:23). *Brit Med J* 1998; 316: 823–8.

6 Mazzone T, Chait A, Plutzky J. Cardiovascular disease risk in type 2 diabetes mellitus: Insights from mechanistic studies. *Lancet* 2008; 371: 1800–9.

7 Taskinen M-R. Diabetic dyslipidaemia: From basic research to clinical practice. *Diabetologia* 2003; 46: 733–49.

8 Adiels M, Olofsson S-O, Taskinen M-R et al. Overproduction of very low density lipoproteins is the hallmark of the dyslipidaemia in the metabolic syndrome. *Arterioscler Thromb Vasc Biol* 2008; 28: 1225–36.

9 Chahil TJ, Ginsberg HN. Diabetic dyslipidaemia. *Endocrinol Metab Clin North Am* 2006; 35: 491–510.

10 Alexander CM, Landsman PB, Teutsch SM et al. Third National Health and Nutrition Examination Survey (NHANES III) National Cholesterol Education Program (NCEP). NECP-defined metabolic syndrome, diabetes and prevalence of coronary heart disease among NHANES III participants aged 50 years and older. *Diabetes* 2003; 52: 1210–14.

11 Isomaa B, Almgren P, Tuomi T et al. Cardiovascular morbidity and mortality associated with the metabolic syndrome. *Diabetes Care* 2001; 24: 683–9.

12 Harris SB, Ekoe J-M, Zdanowicz Y et al. Glycaemic control and morbidity in the Canadian primary care setting (results of the diabetes in Canada evaluation study). *Diabetes Res Clin Pract* 2005; 70: 90–97.

13 Barter P, Gotto AM, LaRosa JC et al.; for the Treating to New Targets Investigators. HDL cholesterol, very low levels of LDL cholesterol and cardiovascular events. *N Engl J Med* 2007; 357: 1301–10.

14 deGoma EM, deGoma RL, Rader DJ. Beyond high density lipoprotein cholesterol levels: Evaluating high-density lipoprotein function as influenced by novel therapeutic approaches. *J Am Coll Cardiol* 2008; 51: 2199–211.

15 Di Angelantonio E, Sarwar N, Perry P et al. Major lipids, apolipoproteins and risk of vascular disease. *JAMA* 2009; 302: 1993–2000.

16 Scott R, O'Brien R, Fulcher G et al. Effects of fenofibrate treatment on cardiovascular disease risk in 9795 individuals with type 2 diabetes and various components of the metabolic syndrome: The Fenofibrate Intervention and Event Lowering in Diabetes (FIELD) study. *Diabetes Care* 2009; 32: 493–8.

17 Ginsberg HN, Elam MB, Lovato LC et al. Effects of combination lipid therapy in type 2 diabetes mellitus. *N Engl J Med* 2010; 362: 1563–74.

18 Nordestgaard BG, Benn M, Schnohr P, Tybjaerg-Hansen A. Non fasting triglycerides and risk of myocardial infarction, ischaemic heart disease and death in men and women. *JAMA* 2007; 298: 299–308.

19 The Task Force for the Management of Dyslipidaemias of the European Society of Cardiology (ESC) and the European Atherosclerosis Society (EAS).

ESC/EAS Guidelines for the management of dyslipidaemias. *Eur Heart J* 2011; 32: 1769–818.

20 American Diabetes Association. Nutritional recommendations and interventions for diabetes: A position statement of the American Diabetes Association. *Diabetes Care* 2008; 31(Suppl 1): s61–s78.

21 Stevens RJ, Kothari V, Adler AI, Stratton IM. The UKPDS risk engine: A model for the risk of coronary heart disease in type 2 diabetes (UKPDS 56). *Clin Sci (London)* 2001; 101: 671–9.

22 The Scandinavian Simvastatin Survival Study Group. Randomised trial of cholesterol lowering in 4444 people with coronary heart disease: The Scandinavian Simvastatin Survival Study (4S). *Lancet* 1994; 344: 1383–9.

23 Pyorala K, Pedersen TR, Kjekshus J et al. Cholesterol lowering with simvastatin improves prognosis of diabetic patients with coronary heart disease: A subgroup analysis of the Scandinavian Simvastatin Survival Study (4S). *Diabetes Care* 1997; 20: 614–20.

24 Haffner SM, Alexander CM, Cook TJ et al. Reduced coronary events in simvastatin-treated patients with coronary heart disease and diabetes or impaired fasting glucose levels. Subgroup analysis in the Scandinavian Simvastatin Survival Study. *Arch Int Med* 1999; 159: 2661–7.

25 Heart Protection Study Collaborative Group. MRC/BHF Heart Protection Study of cholesterol lowering with simvastatin in 5963 people with diabetes: A randomized placebo-controlled trial. *Lancet* 2003; 361: 2005–16.

26 La Rosa JC, Grundy SG, Waters DD et al. Intensive lipid lowering with atorvastatin in patients with stable coronary disease. *N Engl J Med* 2005; 352: 1425–35.

27 Shepherd J, Barter P, Carmena R et al. Effect of lowering LDL cholesterol substantially below recommended levels in patients with diabetes and coronary heart disease: The Treating to New Targets (TNT) Study. *Diabetes Care* 2006; 29: 1220–26.

28 Cannon CP, Steinberg BA, Murphy SA et al. Meta-analysis of cardiovascular outcomes trials comparing intensive versus moderate statin therapy. *J Am Coll Cardiol* 2006; 48: 438–45.

29 Cholesterol Treatment Trialists' (CTT) Collaboration. Efficacy of cholesterol lowering in 18,686 people with diabetes in 14 randomised trials of statins: A meta-analysis. *Lancet* 2008; 371: 117–25.

30 Cholesterol Treatment Trialists' (CTT) Collaboration. Efficacy and safety of more intensive lowering of LDL cholesterol: A meta-analysis of data from 170,000 participants in 26 randomised trials. *Lancet* 376: 1670–81.

31 The Statin Prevention by Aggressive Reduction in Cholesterol Levels (SPARCL) Investigators. High dose atorvastatin after stroke or transient ischaemic attack. *N Engl J Med* 2006; 355: 549–59.

32 Colhoun HM, Betteridge DJ, Durrington PN et al.; on behalf of the CARDS investigators. Primary prevention of cardiovascular disease in type 2 diabetes in the Collaborative Atorvastatin Diabetes Study (CARDS): Multicentre randomized placebo-controlled trial. *Lancet* 2004; 364: 685–96.

33 Sever PS, Poulter NR, Dahlof B et al.; for the ASCOT Investigators. Reduction in cardiovascular events with atorvastatin in 2532 patients with type 2 diabetes. *Diabetes Care* 2005; 28: 1151–7.

34 Kotseva K, Wood D, De Backer G et al.; for the Euroaspire Study Group. Cardiovascular prevention guidelines in daily practice: A comparison of Euroaspire I, II and III surveys in eight European countries. *Lancet* 2009; 373: 929–40.

35 Armitage J. The safety of statins in clinical practice. *Lancet* 2007; 370: 1782–90.

36 Rosenbaum D, Dallongeville J, Sabouret P, Bruckert E. Discontinuation of statin therapy due to muscular side effects: A survey in real life. *Nutr Metab Cardiovasc Dis* 2013; 23(9): 871–5.

37 Leiter LA, Betteridge DJ, Farnier M et al. Lipid-altering efficacy and safety profile of combination therapy with ezetimibe/statin vs staatin monotherapy in patients with and without diabetes: An analysis of pooled data from 27 clinical trials. *Diabetes Obes Metab* 2011; 13: 615–28.

38 Garcia-Calvo M, Lisnock JM, Bull HG et al. The target of ezetimibe is Niemann-Pick C1-Like 1 (NPC1L1). *Proc Nat Acad Sci USA* 2005; 102: 8132–7.

39 Jia L, Betters JL, Yu L. Niemann-Pick C1-Like 1 (NPC1L1) in intestinal and hepatic cholesterol transport. *Annu Rev Physiol* 2011; 73: 239–59.

40 Chan DC, Watts GF, Gan SK et al. Effects of ezetimibe on hepatic fat, inflammatory markers and apolipoprotein B-100 kinetics in insulin resistant obese subjects on a weight loss diet. *Diabetes Care* 2010; 33: 1134–9.

41 Park H, Shima T, Yamaguchi K, Mitsuyoshi H. Efficacy of long-term ezetimibe therapy in patients with non alcoholic fatty liver disease. *J Gastroenterol* 2011; 46: 101–7.

42 Baigent C, Landray MJ, Reith C et al. The effects of lowering LDL-cholesterol with simvastatin plus ezetimibe in patients with chronic kidney disease (Study of Heart and Renal Protection): A randomised placebo-controlled trial. *Lancet* 2011; 377: 2181–92.

43 FIELD study investigators. Effects of long-term fenofibrate therapy on cardiovascular events in 9795 people with type 2 diabetes mellitus (the FIELD study): A randomised controlled trial. *Lancet* 2005; 366: 1849–61.

44 Chapman MJ, Ginsberg HN, Amarenco P et al. Triglyceride-risk lipoproteins and high density lipoprotein cholesterol in patients at high risk of cardiovascular disease: Evidence and guidance for management. *Eur Heart J* 2011; 32: 1345–61.

45 Keech AC, Mitchell P, Summanen PA et al. Effect of fenofibrate on the need for laser treatment for diabetic retinopathy (FIELD study): A randomised controlled trial. *Lancet* 2007; 370: 1687–97.

46 The ACCORD Study Group and ACCORD Eye Study Group. Effects of medical therapies on retinopathy progression in type 2 diabetes. *N Engl J Med* 2010; 363: 233–44.

47 Goldstein JL, Brown MS. The LDL receptor. *Arterioscler Thromb Vasc Biol* 2009; 29: 431–8.

48 Abifadel M, Varret M, Rabee JD et al. Mutations in PCSK9 cause autosomal dominant hypercholesterolaemia. *Nat Genet* 2003; 34: 154–6.

49 Lambert G, Sjouke B, Choque B, Kastelein JJP, Kees Hovingh G. The PCSK9 decade. *J Lipid Res* 2012; 53: 2515–24.

50 McKenny JM, Koren MJ, Kereiakis DJ, Hanotin C, Ferrand AC, Stein EA. Safety and efficacy of a monoclonal antibody to proprotein convertase subtilisin/kexin type 9 serine protease, SAR 236553/REGN 727 in patients with primary hypercholesterolaemia receiving ongoing stable atorvastatin therapy. *J Am Coll Cardiol* 2012; 59: 2344–53.

51 Sullivan D, Olsson AG, Scott R et al. Effect of a monoclonal antibody to PCSK9 on low density lipoprotein cholesterol levels in statin-intolerant patients: The GAUSS randomised trial. *JAMA* 2012; 308. Epub Nov 5.

52 The AIM HIGH Investigators. Niacin in patients with low HDL-cholesterol levels receiving statin therapy. *N Engl J Med* 2011; 365: 2255–67.

53 Barter PJ, Caulfield M, Eriksson M et al.; for the ILLUMINATE Investigators. Effects of torcetrapib in patients at high risk for coronary events. *N Engl J Med* 2007; 357: 2109–22.

54 Schwartz GG, Olsson AG, Abt M et al. Effects of dalcetrapib in patients with a recent acute coronary syndrome. *N Engl J Med* 2012; 367: 2089–99.

55 Cannon CP, Shah S, Dansky HM et al. Safety of anacetrapib in patients with or at high risk of coronary heart disease. *N Engl J Med* 2010; 363: 2406–15.

56 Nicholls SJ, Brewer B, Kastelein JJP et al. Effects of the CETP inhibitor evacetrapib administered as monotherapy or in combination with statins on HDL and LDL cholesterol: A randomised controlled trial. *JAMA* 2011; 306: 2099–109.

57 Nicholls SJ, Tuzcu M, Wolski K et al. Lowering the triglyceride/high density lipoprotein cholesterol ratio is associated with the beneficial impact of pioglitazone on progression of coronary atherosclerosis in diabetic patients. *J Am Coll Cardiol* 2011; 57: 153–9.

58 Davidson M, Meyer PM, Haffner S et al. Increased high-density lipoprotein cholesterol predicts the piogltazone-mediated reduction of carotid intima-media thickness progression in patients with type 2 diabetes mellitus. *Circulation* 2008; 117: 2123–30.

59 Ferrannini E, Betteridge DJ, Dormandy JA et al. High density lipoprotein-cholesterol and not HbA1c was directly related to cardiovascular outcome in PROactive. *Diabetes Obes Metab* 2011; 13: 759–64.

Answers to Multiple-Choice Questions for Case Study 1

1 A, B, D, E – False
   C – True

2 A, D, E – True
   B, C – False

3 A, B, E – False
   C, D – True

CHAPTER 8

Thrombosis in Diabetes and Its Clinical Management

R.A. Ajjan and Peter J. Grant
University of Leeds, Leeds, UK

Key Points

- Longstanding diabetes is frequently accompanied by the development of a prothrombotic state.

- Thrombotic changes include an increase in some clotting factors, inhibition of fibrinolysis, posttranslational modifications to fibrin(ogen), and platelet activation.

- Therapeutics have been developed that inhibit platelet activation (aspirin, P2Y12 inhibitors) and coagulation processes (heparins, bivalirudin).

- In the primary prevention of cardiovascular disease in low-risk diabetes, the use of aspirin is not recommended as the risk of side effects outweighs any potential beneficial effects.

- In high-risk diabetes (those with end-organ damage) aspirin is recommended for primary prevention.

- In the acute setting, combinations of aspirin, P2Y12 inhibitors, and anticoagulants are used to protect the myocardium against the effects of occlusive arterial thrombosis.

- Post-ACS, a combination of aspirin and a P2Y12 inhibitor is recommended for 12 months after the acute event.

- Cessation of P2Y12 inhibitors earlier than 12 months post-ACS is not recommended as there is a higher incidence of recurrent events in this group.

- Aspirin is effective in secondary prevention of ACS in subjects with diabetes and should be continued after cessation of P2Y12 inhibition at 12 months post-ACS.

Introduction

The development of occlusive thrombotic vascular disease has become one of the major causes of morbidity and mortality in the modern world. Subjects with both type 1 and type 2 diabetes are at increased risk of developing cardiovascular disease, with approximately three-quarters

---

Managing Cardiovascular Complications in Diabetes, First Edition.
Edited by D. John Betteridge and Stephen Nicholls.
© 2014 John Wiley & Sons, Ltd. Published 2014 by John Wiley & Sons, Ltd.

of patients with diabetes ultimately dying from vascular causes. In the arterial system, subjects with diabetes have an increased prevalence of stroke, acute coronary syndromes, and peripheral vascular disease, while in the venous system a small increase in venous thrombotic disease has been observed, much of which may be related to associated comorbidities. Arterial disease is a chronic process characterized by the early development of endothelial dysfunction and fatty streaks followed by plaque formation, plaque instability, and occlusive thrombus formation on a ruptured plaque. Diabetes can affect all aspects of these processes, and clinical studies indicate that coronary artery plaques from subjects with diabetes have increased plaque thrombus and monocyte/macrophage infiltration compared to nondiabetes controls [1]. This, together with more extensive disease affecting both the proximal and distal coronary vasculature, describes a situation in which the circulation supplying the heart has more lesions, with a greater propensity to rupture and to produce more thrombus. The arterial clot is characterized by the development of a platelet-rich fibrin mesh, the fibrin being generated by activation of the fluid phase of coagulation, while venous thrombosis is characterized by a fibrin-rich, platelet-poor thrombus. Type 2 diabetes is associated with increased platelet activation [2], and with a range of abnormalities in coagulation and fibrinolysis related to the metabolic abnormalities associated with insulin resistance and hyperglycemia [3]. These prothrombotic changes contribute to the increased prevalence of acute coronary syndromes and other arterial disorders; increased platelet reactivity in particular has been reported to prospectively predict risk of major adverse cardiovascular events in type 2 diabetes patients with stable coronary artery disease [4]. Most evidence seems to indicate that thrombotic disorders start to appear with the development of insulin resistance and in the presence of advanced complications such as chronic kidney disease. Glycemia has an additional effect on many of these processes, which tend to deteriorate as the chronic nature of diabetes unfolds. Clinical studies suggest that as a consequence, uncomplicated type 1 diabetes has relatively minor alterations in thrombotic profile, while nondiabetes insulin-resistant relatives of subjects with diabetes have clustering of inflammatory thrombotic risk prior to the appearance of frank hyperglycemia [5, 6, 7]; and in both groups further changes occur as the disorder progresses.

The recognition that myocardial infarction usually results from thrombus formation on a ruptured plaque led to a revolution in therapeutic approaches that has improved primary and secondary prevention of cardiovascular disease as well as the management of acute coronary syndromes. Among these, the development of increasingly sophisticated inhibitors of platelet activation, direct thrombin inhibitors, and heparin-like molecules have transformed care of both diabetes and nondiabetes subjects with coronary artery disease. In this chapter we will describe the mechanisms that underpin abnormalities in platelet function and the fluid phases of coagulation and fibrinolysis in subjects with diabetes, the way in which these changes relate to cardiovascular disease, and how antiplatelet agents and anticoagulants ameliorate cardiovascular outcomes in subjects with diabetes.

Mechanisms of Thrombosis

The hemostatic system consists of a fluid phase of activators and inhibitors of coagulation and fibrinolysis that regulate the formation and breakdown of fibrin and a cellular, platelet phase that interacts with sites of vascular damage and fibrin to release a range of procoagulant and inflammatory mediators. Thrombin is the pivotal enzyme in the coagulation pathway, having a crucial role in both fibrin formation and platelet activation. Thrombin is generated by the cleavage of prothrombin by a Factor Xase complex, which occurs as the result of interactions between tissue factor-activated Factor VII and Factor X secondary to vascular damage. Thrombin, while having major procoagulant and pro-inflammatory effects, can express an anticoagulant effect when thrombin binds to the cell-associated receptor thrombomodulin to change thrombin's substrate [8].

Fibrinogen Cleavage

Fibrinogen is a large protein produced by the liver that consists of two sets of three α, β, and γ chains linked by disulfide bonds [9]. Thrombin cleaves fibrinogen by cutting small fibrinopeptides from each of the fibrinogen α chains, allowing the α chains to open out and interact with other cleaved fibrinogen molecules, leading to the formation of double-stranded fibrils that branch out to create a complex fibrin network. Cleavage of fibrinopeptide B allows lateral aggregation of the developing fibrin structure.

Factor XIII Activation and Fibrin Cross-linking

Coagulation FXIII is a transglutaminase that circulates in plasma in a heterodimeric structure consisting of two A and two B subunits. Thrombin activates Factor XIII by cleaving a 37 amino acid peptide from the A subunit, which promotes separation of the A and B subunits and permits exposure of the active site on FXIIIA. Activated Factor XIIIA covalently cross-links fibrin fibrils, which creates a fibrin structure that is insoluble, with altered mechanical properties and increased resistance to fibrinolytic activity [10].

Fibrinolysis

Analogous to thrombin, plasmin is the pivotal enzyme in the fibrinolytic cascade. Plasmin is generated by the cleavage of plasminogen by tissue plasminogen activator (tPA), and this reaction occurs 1,000-fold faster in the presence of fibrin. A lysine binding site on plasmin binds plasmin to fibrin, which facilitates fibrin breakdown and also protects plasmin from local inhibition by antiplasmin. Plasmin cleaves arginine and lysine sites on a range of molecules and its activity is tightly controlled by antiplasmin to prevent systemic proteolysis [11]. Cleavage of fibrin by plasmin leads to the generation of fibrin degradation products, which can be measured in plasma, and one of which, D-dimer, is used as an indicator of the presence of venous thrombotic disease. In addition to antiplasmin, other inhibitors of this pathway include plasminogen activator inhibitor-1 (PAI-1) and thrombin activatable fibrinolysis inhibitor (TAFI). PAI-1 is the fast-acting inhibitor of tPA that binds to and inhibits tPA activity. PAI-1 is produced by endothelial cells and platelets and circulates in plasma in excess over tPA, and is also found in fairly high concentrations in thrombus. TAFI is found in large quantities in platelets and plasma, and is activated by thrombin, a cleavage event that is much enhanced when thrombin is bound to thrombomodulin. Activated TAFI cleaves the N-terminal lysine residues from degrading fibrin to prevent binding of plasminogen and tPA to fibrin, which results in inhibition of plasmin generation and clot lysis [12].

Platelet Activation

Damage to the vascular wall leads to two key events in platelet associated clot formation: 1) receptor-mediated platelet adherence and aggregation; and 2) thrombin-mediated platelet activation. Adherence to the subendothelial matrix is facilitated by a range of glycoprotein receptors (GP Ib/IX, GPVI, and GPIa), which interact with von Willebrand factor to promote platelet adhesion. This interaction leads to activation of platelet GPIIb/IIIa, which binds fibrinogen and promotes platelet aggregation. Thrombin is the most potent platelet activator, which exerts its effects through binding to protease-activated receptor 1 (PAR-1) on the platelet surface. This leads to a cascade of signaling processes, culminating in the release of a range of inflammatory and thrombotic mediators, which further promote clot formation. In addition to thrombin, a range of other mediators, including ADP, collagen, and thromboxane, can activate the platelet through a receptor-binding event. These receptors provide some of the novel targets for therapeutic approaches described later and are discussed in a number of excellent reviews [13, 14, 15]. The main steps in clot formation and lysis are summarized in Figure 8.1.

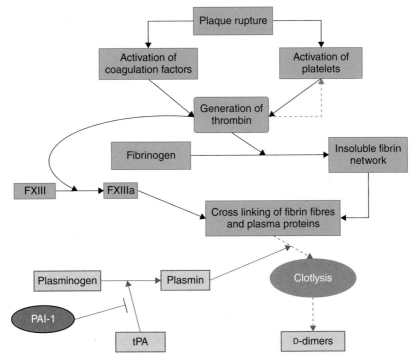

Figure 8.1 Clot formation and fibrinolysis. Rupture of an atherosclerotic plaque exposes a prothrombotic core, resulting in activation of platelets and coagulation proteins. Thrombin is formed with subsequent conversion of soluble fibrinogen to insoluble fibrin, which is further strengthened by thrombin-activated FXIII. Thrombin further activates platelets, enhancing the thrombotic process. Tissue plasminogen activator mediates conversion of plasminogen to plasmin, which lyzes the clot, generating D-dimers. Fibrinolysis is inhibited by a number of proteins, including plasminogen activator inhibitor (PAI)-1.

Summary of the Mechanisms of Thrombosis

In describing the individual components of these processes, it is easy to lose sight of the exquisite control that is exerted at all levels of clot formation. In addition to platelets, thrombosis involves binding events on endothelium, subendothelial layers, macrophages, and leukocytes, with the balance between thrombosis and clot lysis and the localization of clot formation depending on these interactions. Emerging evidence demonstrates the importance of thrombotic inflammatory interactions, both at the cellular level where platelet/macrophage binding initiates the release of a range of soluble procoagulant and inflammatory molecules, and in the fluid phase where, for example, complement C3 binds fibrin to inhibit fibrinolysis [16]. As these events cycle toward fibrin formation and fibrin/platelet interactions, further levels of control are exerted by the interaction of activators and inhibitors of lysis on fibrin itself. All of these levels of control direct and limit thrombus formation and fibrinolysis to the site of need to prevent systemic thrombus formation and proteolysis.

Mechanisms of Thrombosis in Diabetes

Coagulation and Fibrinolysis

The major consistent hemostatic abnormality observed in insulin-resistant type 2 diabetes is marked suppression of fibrinolysis associated with increased levels of both PAI-1 and tPA [17]. Studies of euglycemic first-degree relatives of subjects with type 2 diabetes indicate that such individuals tend to be insulin resistant and have raised triglyceride, tPA, and PAI-1 before a diagnosis of diabetes is made; there is little evidence to suggest that glycemia influences this pattern. Several studies have reported strong associations between insulin resistance, triglyceride, and PAI-1 levels, and it appears that the severity of suppression of fibrinolysis clusters with an increasing number of conventional risk factors. The PAI-1 gene has a 4G/5G polymorphism 675 bp from the start site, and the 4G allele has been associated with both higher PAI-1 levels and increased risk of acute coronary syndrome [18]. Additionally, there are indications that interactions between the 4G/5G genotype and features of the metabolic syndrome regulate circulating PAI-1 levels, providing a path for increasing cardiovascular risk [19]. TAFI levels seem to be unaffected by insulin resistance or hyperglycemia, although there are indications that levels are increased in type 2 diabetes with microalbuminuria [20]. Coagulation Factor VII levels show a similar association with insulin resistance and type 2 diabetes is also associated with elevated fibrinogen and Factor XII levels [17]. The importance of insulin resistance in these early manifestations of thrombotic risk is emphasized by studies of insulin-sensitizing agents, which consistently demonstrate that metformin and thiazolidinedione use is associated with reductions in PAI-1 and tPA, while metformin has additionally been reported to lower levels of Factors VII and XIIIA [17].

Clot Structure

Jörneskog reported changes in clot structure in type 1 diabetes subjects showing reduced permeability to indicate a more compact structure [21]. Other studies have made similar observations using plasma-purified fibrinogen from type 2 diabetes patients [22]. The evidence indicates that posttranslational modifications to fibrin(ogen) are promoting structural alterations to fibrin [23]. However, such changes facilitate decreased plasmin generation on the clot surface and increased antiplasmin binding, with an overall effect on fibrinolysis rather than clot formation [24]. Compact structures have been associated with increased cardiovascular risk and poorer cardiovascular outcome in nondiabetes populations, and it is likely that a range of metabolic influences affect this phenotype.

Platelet Activation

The circulating platelet is sensitive to a wide range of metabolic changes associated with diabetes, of which hyperglycemia is the most clinically apparent. Short-term exposure to hyperglycemia increases platelet reactivity and improvements in glycemic control ameliorate these effects. It has been proposed that hyperglycemia may have osmotic effects on the platelet, alter protein kinase C expression, and/or have indirect effects through exposure to glycated proteins. In this respect, recent evidence indicates that AGE proteins induce a prothrombotic state through interactions with the platelet CD36 receptor mediated by a JNK2 pathway [25]. Oxidized LDL is reported to activate platelets in insulin-resistant subjects [26], and CD36 is involved in platelet activation through interactions with dyslipidemia and oxidative stress, effects that are absent in CD36 null mice [27]. It is interesting to note that the macrophage CD36 receptor is well established as having a role in the formation of early fatty streaks through interactions with oxidized LDL leading to increased foam cell formation. This response in macrophages is accentuated in insulin-resistant states and is ameliorated by thiazolidinediones. Thiazolidinediones are reported to possess antiplatelet effects, although it is not known whether this effect on platelets is mediated to any extent through effects on CD36. Other potential influences include effects of insulin resistance. Insulin has anti-aggregatory effects in platelets from insulin-sensitive subjects and emerging data indicate that IGF-1 may have prothrombotic effects on the platelet through interaction with the hetrodimerized insulin/IGF-1 receptor in insulin-resistant states. In a population of 208 type 2 diabetes patients with stable coronary artery disease followed up for 24 months, carriers of a particular insulin receptor substrate-1 (IRS-1) genotype exhibited both increased platelet reactivity and a significantly higher risk of major adverse cardiovascular events [28]. These findings both implicate the insulin-signaling pathway in cardiovascular outcomes and provide a potential mechanism for inter-individual differences between subjects with diabetes.

Overall, the available data indicate that diabetes is associated with a range of metabolic abnormalities that adversely influence platelet function. Management of the platelet aspect of this prothrombotic state should involve normalization of the metabolic changes seen in diabetes and the appropriate use of antiplatelet therapy, as discussed below.

Management and Prevention of Thrombotic Events in Diabetes

Individuals with diabetes are at increased risk of cardiovascular events and their prognosis following vascular ischemia is worse than the nondiabetes population. This increase in mortality is related to a combination of more extensive vascular pathology associated with increased thrombotic milieu, secondary to enhanced platelet activation and quantitative/qualitative changes in procoagulant and antifibrinolytic factors. The detailed discussion of the management of vascular ischemic events is covered elsewhere in this book; we will concentrate on highlighting diabetes-specific antithrombotic therapy.

Antiplatelet Agents

There are a number of antiplatelet agents in use for the treatment and prevention of cardiovascular disease in diabetes, which mainly affect three pathways of platelet activation, although agents are under development that target additional pathways. In this section the various antiplatelet agents used in the treatment and prevention of cardiovascular disease are discussed, with an emphasis on the role of these agents in diabetes.

Aspirin

Aspirin acetylates serine residue 529 in cyclo-oxygenase (COX)-1, irreversibly inhibiting enzyme activity and blocking the production of thromboxane A2, resulting in diminished platelet aggregation. Another mode of action that we and others have shown is that aspirin acetylates fibrinogen, altering fibrin network characteristics, making the clot easier to lyze [29, 30, 31, 32]. Also, aspirin may influence clot lysis indirectly through a nitric oxide-dependent mechanism [33, 34]. These platelet-independent fibrinolytic properties of aspirin are potentially important clinically, and may explain the enhanced fibrinolytic effects of streptokinase when used with aspirin in the ISIS-2 study [35].

Aspirin is regularly used in the setting of acute coronary syndrome (ACS), the benefit of which has been repeatedly demonstrated in individuals with or without diabetes [35, 36, 37]. Aspirin should be given as early as possible in ACS, regardless of whether the diagnosis is unstable angina/NSTEMI (non-ST-elevation myocardial infarction) or STEMI (ST-elevation myocardial infarction), at an initial dose of 162–325 mg (300 mg is used in the UK) with a combination of other anti-thrombotic agents (detailed below). This is followed by a maintenance dose of 75–162 mg/day (75 mg/day in the UK) in those with proven vascular pathology. In the longer term, aspirin is used for secondary cardiovascular protection in diabetes [38, 39], a practice supported by two large meta-analyses [40, 41]. The percentage reduction in vascular ischemia with the use of aspirin for secondary prevention is 17% (from 22.3 to 18.5%; $p < 0.01$) and 22% (from 16.4 to 12.8%; $p < 0.00001$) in subjects with and without diabetes respectively. These data indicate that aspirin may be less effective in secondary cardiovascular protection in diabetes, a concept supported by a relatively recent observational study failing to show a benefit for aspirin in secondary prevention [42].

The use of aspirin for primary cardiovascular protection in diabetes is more controversial. Until recently, aspirin has been regularly used in these circumstances, although the evidence supporting such practice was surprisingly scarce. Indeed, several pieces of evidence suggest that aspirin should not be used in all diabetes subjects for primary prevention. In the Primary Prevention Project (PPP) trial, aspirin treatment failed to offer significant cardiovascular protection in diabetes patients, in contrast to individuals with no diabetes [43]. A meta-analysis of more than 140,000 subjects has shown that the use of antiplatelet agents (mainly aspirin) resulted in a 22% reduction in cardiovascular events, but in a subgroup of around 5,000 diabetic subjects the risk reduction was only 7%, which was not statistically significant [41]. Moreover, two recent primary prevention studies, JPAD and POPADAD, failed to show an impact of aspirin on cardiovascular events in individuals with diabetes [44, 45]. However, JPAD demonstrated an overall benefit in the older population, suggesting that a subgroup of patients may benefit from this therapy. A longitudinal observational study of 651 diabetes individuals over 11.6 years' follow-up period (7,537 patient-years) has shown a reduction in CV events in aspirin-treated subjects after adjustment for significant CV variables (HR 0.30 CI 0.09–0.95), indicating that aspirin may be beneficial in some patients with diabetes [46]. In contrast, an increase in cardiovascular events was reported in aspirin-treated Chinese diabetes subjects with no history of ischemic heart disease [47]. Similar results were documented in the Swedish record linkage study, although again, a beneficial effect was observed in the older population [48]. A meta-analysis of seven studies, including 11,618 diabetes individuals, reported a 9% reduction in overall major adverse cardiovascular events (MACE) without an effect on mortality, which may be due to the relatively short period of follow-up [49].

Data indicate that the efficacy of aspirin in primary prevention in diabetes is compromised and should not be used in all patients. However, it appears that some individuals with diabetes, perhaps those at high cardiovascular risk, benefit from aspirin therapy for primary prevention. Given this situation, current national and international guidelines limit the use of aspirin for primary prevention in diabetes to individuals at "high cardiovascular risk" without clearly categorizing this group and leaving the decision at the discretion of the attending physician. There are two ongoing outcome studies investigating the appropriate use of aspirin for primary cardiovascular protection in diabetes (ASCEND and ACCEPT-D, clinical trial registration number NCT00135226 and IS-RCTN48110081 respectively), which are expected to report in the next three to four years.

In summary, 1) aspirin continues to be used in ACS (inclusive of unstable angina, NSTEMI, and STEMI), in combination with other antiplatelet agents in both diabetes and nondiabetes subjects; 2) aspirin is used as monotherapy for secondary cardiovascular protection, but may be less efficacious in subjects with diabetes; 3) there is no convincing evidence for the use of aspirin monotherapy for primary cardiovascular protection in diabetes, although some guidelines recommend its use in high-risk subjects.

Clopidogrel

Clopidogrel, a thienopyridine agent, is an irreversible antagonist of the platelet P2Y12 receptor. Clopidogrel is a pro-drug and is converted to the active metabolite by the P450 system in the liver; the onset of action may be delayed by CYP genetic polymorphisms. Clopidogrel is used in combination with aspirin in subjects with acute coronary syndrome and as monotherapy in those intolerant to aspirin or in patients with symptomatic cerebrovascular disease despite aspirin therapy [50, 51].

The combination of aspirin and clopidogrel in the setting of ACS (usually 300–600 mg loading dose of clopidogrel followed by maintenance of 75 mg/day) has been established through a number of large-scale clinical trials, with benefits shown in diabetes and nondiabetes subjects [52, 53, 54, 55]. However, newer agents have recently shown superior efficacy (detailed below), and dual therapy with clopidogrel is now used less frequently in some centers, where the cost of the newer agents can be absorbed. Combination aspirin and clopidogrel is usually given for a year following ACS (clopidogrel at 75 mg/day) and aspirin monotherapy continued beyond this period. However, routine combination therapy in high-risk diabetes individuals with no recent ACS is not recommended due to the absence of clinical benefit, supported by data from the CHARISMA trial [56].

There is evidence to suggest that clopidogrel monotherapy is superior to aspirin when used for secondary cardiovascular prevention in diabetes. The CAPRIE study enrolled 19,185 subjects with established cardiovascular disease and randomized to aspirin 325 mg/day or clopidogrel 75 mg/day. In the post hoc analysis of the diabetes group, a 12% reduction in vascular ischemia was documented comparing aspirin with clopidogrel users (from 17.7% to 15.6%, respectively; $p = 0.04$); the difference was even more pronounced in insulin users [57]. However, as this was an unspecified post hoc analysis, it has largely gone unnoticed and the data failed to find their way into clinical practice.

It should be noted that variability in the biochemical efficacy of clopidogrel is largely due to variability in drug metabolism. The prevalence of clopidogrel low responsiveness varies widely between studies (5–40%), related to the test used, definition of resistance, and population studied [58]. Diabetes is one factor accounting for the reduced response to clopidogrel, particularly in the presence of poor diabetes control, microvascular complications, or in those having insulin treatment [59]. Some of the suggested mechanisms for the reduced efficacy of clopidogrel in diabetes include insulin resistance resulting in diminished platelet response to insulin, upregulation of P2Y12 receptor signaling, and higher platelet turnover.

In summary, 1) clopidogrel is used in combination with aspirin for diabetes subjects with ACS, although it is gradually being replaced in some centers by newer P2Y12 antagonists; 2) clopidogrel monotherapy is used for secondary cardiovascular prevention in diabetes in individuals intolerant to aspirin and in those with symptomatic cerebroavascular disease despite aspirin therapy; 3) there is no evidence to suggest that use of clopidogrel monotherapy for primary prevention in diabetes is beneficial. It is worth noting that some clinicians use clopidogrel instead of aspirin therapy for secondary cardiovascular protection in very high-risk diabetes subjects, although the evidence supporting such practice is limited.

Prasugrel

Prasugrel, a third-generation thienopyridine, is a pro-drug requiring metabolism to the active compound that irreversibly blocks the P2Y12 receptor. A key difference between clopidogrel and prasugrel is related to the quicker metabolism of prasugrel to the active compound, resulting in faster action. This translated clinically in the TRITON-TIMI 38 trial into an 18% reduction in primary endpoint (cardiovascular death or vascular events) when prasugrel (60 mg loading followed by 10 mg/day maintenance) was used instead of clopidogrel (300 mg loading followed by 75 mg/day maintenance) in combination with aspirin in 13,608 ACS subjects undergoing PCI (9.9% and 12.1%, respectively; $p < 0.001$), over a 15-month follow-up [60]. This clinical benefit was canceled out by a significant increase in bleeding in the prasugrel group (2.4% vs. 1.8% respectively, $p = 0.03$), and the use of prasugrel over clopidogrel could not be recommended in all ACS patients. Interestingly, subgroup analysis of the diabetes group yielded somewhat different results. There was an impressive 30% reduction in the primary endpoint comparing the prasugrel with the clopidogrel group (12.2% and 17.0%, respectively; $p < 0.001$), an effect that was particularly pronounced in insulin users (a 37% reduction). In contrast to the nondiabetic population, the reduction in primary endpoint was not associated with an increased risk of bleeding (2.6%

and 2.5% for the prasugrel and clopidogrel groups, respectively; $p > 0.1$). Although the results for the diabetes subgroup are impressive, this study has attracted a number of criticisms mainly related to the "modest" loading dose of clopidogrel. However, OPTIMUS-3 has shown that prasugrel 60 mg loading and 10 mg/day maintenance achieved better inhibition of platelet function than clopidogrel 600 mg loading and 150 mg/day maintenance dose in subjects with diabetes who were on long-term aspirin treatment, suggesting superior efficacy to clopidogrel when used in combination with aspirin [61]. Further trials are currently ongoing investigating prasugrel in unstable angina and NSTEMI [62].

Prasugrel is not licensed as monotherapy and there are no large-scale clinical trials investigating its use in this context. It remains unclear whether prasugrel is superior to clopidogrel when used as monotherapy for primary or secondary cardiovascular protection.

Therefore, current evidence suggests that 1) prasugrel in combination with aspirin is superior to clopidogrel and aspirin in diabetes individuals with ACS, a finding that has led some centers to use prasugrel instead of clopidogrel in this group of patients; 2) prasugrel is not licensed or recommended for monotherapy either in secondary or primary cardiovascular protection in diabetes.

Ticagrelol

Ticagrelol, an agent of the cyclopentyltriazolopyrimidine class, blocks the platelet P2Y12 receptor; however, it differs from the thienopyridines by being an active drug (no metabolism necessary), with reversibility of action and a shorter half-life, necessitating twice-daily administration. The PLATO trial showed the superior efficacy of ticagrelol compared with clopidogrel when used in combination with aspirin in 18,642 ACS patients treated medically or following PCI [63]. The primary endpoint of vascular event or cardiovascular death was reduced at 12 months in the ticagrelol group by 16% (10.2% and 12.3% in ticagrelol and clopidogrel groups, respectively; $p < 0.0001$), with no associated increase in the study's predefined bleeding rate (11.6% and 11.2%, respectively; $p = 0.43$). In a predefined subgroup analysis of diabetes patients, a similar pattern emerged (risk reduction of 12%), although this failed to reach statistical significance, probably due to the relatively limited number of diabetes subjects.

Results of the PLATO study are certainly impressive given that patients were aggressively treated for cardiovascular risk factors, and some centers adopted the use of this agent instead of clopidogrel without differentiating between diabetes and nondiabetes subjects. It is worth noting that ticagrelol is not without drawbacks, as it has to be administered twice daily and can be associated with shortness of breath and cardiac rhythm disturbances.

Clinical use of this agent outside the randomized controlled trial setting will clarify whether compliance is an issue and whether the additional side effects have clinical consequences.

There are no studies on the use of ticagrelol monotherapy for primary or secondary cardiovascular protection, and to our knowledge no studies are planned in this area.

In summary, ticagrelol is an interesting alternative to clopidogrel with superior efficacy when used in combination with aspirin in the ACS setting, in both diabetes and nondiabetes subjects.

Dipyridamol and Cilostazol

These agents modulate the phosphodiesterase pathway to reduce platelet activation. On their own, these are very weak agents and are always used in combination with other antiplatelets. Dipyridamol has no role in coronary artery disease, but has been recommended in combination with aspirin in individuals with recurrent cerebrovascular ischemia [64, 65]. However, others have demonstrated that this combination is not superior to monotherapy with clopidogrel [50]. Given the absence of an indication for dipyridamol in coronary artery disease and the questionable efficacy in cerebrovascular disease, this agent is not used frequently in clinical practice.

In contrast to dipyridamol, the use of cilostazol appears to be gaining momentum in diabetes. This agent is primarily indicated for the treatment of symptomatic peripheral vascular disease, but recent work suggests that this agent has additional benefits in diabetes, which may be partly related to enhanced P2Y12 inhibition [66]. Triple therapy with cilostazol has been shown to reduce coronary artery restenosis following PCI in diabetes subjects [67, 68], and long-term outcome studies are needed to assess further the clinical efficacy of cilostazol in diabetes. One limitation of cilostazol use may prove to be the side-effect profile and increased mortality in those with heart failure.

Inhibitors of Platelet–Fibrinogen Interaction

Platelets interact with fibrinogen through the GPIIb/IIIa receptor, with the protein forming a bridge between platelets, resulting in platelet aggregation. There are three inhibitors of the receptor currently in use, including abciximab, eptifibatide, and tirofiban. These agents are used intravenously and are only suitable in acute clinical settings. Evidence from studies conducted more than a decade ago suggests that GPIIb/IIIa inhibitors have superior efficacy in subjects with diabetes with a reduction in 30-day mortality following ACS, particularly in those undergoing PCI [69].

However, these data were derived during an era when antiplatelet therapy was less effective; indeed, a more recent trial (ISAR-SWEET) showed that use of abciximab and high-loading-dose clopidogrel (600 mg), compared with clopidogrel alone, was not associated with a reduction of one-year mortality in 701 diabetes subjects with ACS undergoing PCI [70]. In contrast, ISAR-REACT2, which had a similar design except that patients with NSTEMI were enrolled, showed a reduction in vascular events/death in abciximab-treated individuals, and this applied to both diabetes and nondiabetes subjects. Studies using eptifibatide and tirofiban showed mixed results in the populations studied and did not demonstrate superior efficacy in subjects with diabetes [71]. Furthermore, recent evidence suggests that bivalirudin is superior to abciximab and enoxaparin in diabetes, with reduced bleeding rate, limiting GPIIb/IIIa inhibitor use in diabetes. Overall, however, there is still a role for these agents in diabetes patients with ACS, depending on the individual needs of the patient and the clinical decision of the attending physician.

Agents Affecting the Coagulation Pathway

The main agents currently in use include thrombin and Factor X (FX) inhibitors. Their use in diabetes is briefly discussed below.

Heparin

Agents in this family are indirect inhibitors of FX and prothrombin, through modulation of antithrombin III activity. Fractionated heparin is regularly used in individuals with ACS, including those with diabetes. These agents are indirect thrombin inhibitors and enoxaparin is the main low molecular weight heparin (LMWH) used due to its predictive anticoagulation effect, ease of injections, and lower risk of thrombocytopenia. A recent meta-analysis showed that enoxaparin is superior to unfractionated heparin at reducing mortality and bleeding complications, particularly when used in subjects with STEMI undergoing primary PCI [72]. Therefore, enoxaparin remains a cornerstone in the management of subjects with ACS, regardless of whether the diagnosis is STEMI or NSTEMI and irrespective of planned conservative therapy or invasive coronary intervention.

Bivalirudin

This agent is a direct thrombin inhibitor. Compared with the combination of GPIIa/bIII and heparin, bivalirudin showed similar protection from vascular ischemia following ACS, but with fewer bleeding complications [73]. In the Acute Catheterization and Urgent Intervention Triage

Strategy (ACUITY) trial, subgroup analysis of diabetes subjects showed that bivalirudin use was associated with similar ischemic events compared with the combination of GPIIb/IIIa inhibitors (GPI) plus heparin (7.9% and 8.9% respectively; $p = 0.40$), but with far less major bleeding (3.7% and 7.1%, respectively; $p < 0.001$), resulting in a clear net clinical benefit [74]. Similar data were obtained from Harmonizing Outcomes with Revascularization and Stents in Acute Myocardial Infarction (HORIZONS-AMI), which enrolled 3,602 patients, 593 of whom had diabetes. This study showed that diabetes subjects treated with bivalirudin had reduced mortality at 30 days compared with the combination of GPIIb/IIIa inhibitors and unfractionated heparin (2.1% and 5.5%, respectively; $p = 0.04$), and this benefit was also evident in insulin-treated patients. Bleeding complications were lower in bivalirudin compared with the GPI/heparin combination group (2.5% and 7.1%, respectively; $p = 0.01$), although no difference in mortality was demonstrated at 12 months (14.2% and 16.2%, respectively, $p = 0.4$) [75].

Therefore, bivalirudin is recommended for clinical use in diabetes subjects with ACS in whom coronary intervention is planned, particularly in those who have a high bleeding risk; individuals on insulin therapy equally benefit from this treatment. Given the heterogeneity of patients with diabetes, more work is needed to clarify the type of individuals who would benefit the most from this therapy.

Fondaparinux

This agent binds reversibly to antithrombin III, indirectly inhibiting FX activity. Oasis 5 enrolled 20,078 patients with unstable angina and NSTEMI and confirmed the noninferiority of fondaparinux compared with LMWH in the composite efficacy endpoint of death, myocardial infarction, or refractory ischemia. However, mortality was lower in fondaparinux-treated individuals compared with LMWH at 30 days (2.9% and 3.5%, respectively; $p = 0.02$) and 6 months (5.8% and 6.5%, respectively; $p = 0.05$), and was associated with a lower bleeding rate after nine days' treatment (2.2% and 4.1%, respectively; $p < 0.01$) [76]. OASIS 6 investigated 12,092 patients with STEMI, who underwent thrombolysis or PCI. The study had a complex design, but data indicated that fondaparinux was superior to LMWH in those who had thrombolysis or conservative management, whereas the opposite was true in individuals undergoing PCI [77]. Therefore, fondaparinux is not recommended in STEMI patients undergoing PCI. Although diabetes patients constituted 25% in OASIS 5 and 18% in OASIS 6, no data were provided for this subgroup of patients and it is unclear whether diabetes has an effect on response to fondaparinux therapy.

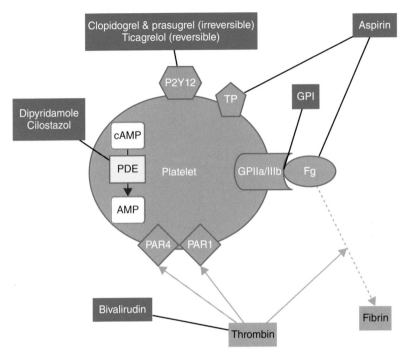

Figure 8.2 Mode of action of various antiplatelet agents. Aspirin acetylates and inhibits cyclo-oxygenase 1, resulting in reduced thromboxane production, and it also acetylates fibrinogen, thereby modulating the fibrin network structure and efficiency of fibrinolysis. Clopidogrel and prasugrel are irreversible inhibitors of the P2Y12 pathway, whereas ticagrelol is a reversible inhibitor. Dipyridamole and cilostazol affect phosphphodiesterase, thereby modulating cAMP coversion to AMP. GPIIa/IIIb inhibitors interfere with platelet fibrinogen interactions, whereas bivalirudin is a direct thrombin inhibitor.

Figure 8.2 illustrates the mode of action of the main antithrombotic agents used in ACS, whereas Table 8.1 summarizes the role of antiplatelet and anticoagulant therapy in atherothrombotic disease in diabetes.

Hypoglycemic Agents and Thrombosis Risk

There is evidence to suggest that the type of hypoglycemic agent used may modulate predisposition to future ischemic events. Metformin is normally used as first-line therapy in subjects with type 2 diabetes. The UK Prospective Diabetes Study (UKPDS) has demonstrated reduced ischemic heart disease (IHD) risk in overweight patients using metformin compared with subjects not on this therapy, and the concept of cardiovascular protection by metformin emerged [78]. Further observational work supported

Table 8.1 Summary of the clinical use of various antiplatelet therapies in diabetes.

Agent	Mode of action	Use in ACS	Secondary prevention (monotherapy)	Primary prevention (monotherapy)
Aspirin	Cox-1 inhibitor	Yes	Yes	Only in high risk subjects
Clopidogrel	Irreversible P2Y12 inhibitor	Yes	Yes	High risk aspirin intolerant individuals (possibly superior to aspirin)
Prasugrel	Irreversible P2Y12 inhibitor	Yes (probably better than clopidogrel in DM)	No	No
Ticagrelol	Reversible P2Y12 inhibitor	Yes (superior toclopidogrel regardless of diabetes status)	No	No
Cilostazol	Phosphodiesterase inhibitor	Yes (possible future role as triple therapy in DM)	No	No
GPIIb/IIIa inhibitors	Modulators of platelet fibrinogen interactions	Yes (possible advantage in DM)	No	No
Bivalirudin	Direct thrombin inhibitor	Yes (possibly superior to combination GPI&LMWH in DM)	No	No

this concept, including data from the REACH registry including 19,691 patients [79]. The mechanisms for reduced cardiovascular events in metformin users may be related, at least in part, to the antithrombotic actions of this agent, reviewed elsewhere [80].

Thiazolidinediones (TZD) are peroxisome proliferator-activated receptor (PPAR)-γ stimulators and directly affect insulin resistance, the key pathogenic mechanism in diabetes. TZD can lower fibrinogen and PAI-1 levels, which reduces thrombosis potential and improves fibrinolysis [81, 82, 83, 84]. Furthermore, these agents can delay intra-arterial thrombus formation and modulate the progression of atherothrombotic lesions [85, 86, 87]. In the PROactive trial, pioglitazone failed to show a benefit for a complex primary endpoint, but was associated with a reduction in the prespecified secondary endpoint (all-cause mortality, nonfatal MI, and stroke) [88]. This latter analysis created a debate in the scientific community, as some commentators argued that the negative findings in relation to the primary endpoint invalidate analysis of the secondary endpoint. Overall, this study indicates that pioglitazone is at worst cardioneutral and certainly does not cause an increase in cardiovascular events or death. In contrast, a much-debated meta-analysis suggested that rosiglitazone increases the risk of cardiovascular events in diabetes [89], which subsequently resulted in the withdrawal of this agent from the market.

Gliptins and glucagon-like peptide (GLP)-1 analogs are relatively new hypoglycemic agents, which may modulate thrombosis potential. Retrospective analysis of various studies suggest that these agents reduce vascular ischemic events and clinical outcome studies are currently underway to clarify their role in CVD prevention further [90].

Insulin is mainly used in type 2 diabetes after the failure of other hypoglycemic agents. Insulin-treated type 2 diabetes subjects are at a greater risk of cardiovascular events compared with noninsulin-treated subjects, which may simply be a reflection of longer disease duration, with a consequent increase in the risk of complications [91]. In healthy individuals, insulin has antithrombotic effects, but it has the opposite effects in the presence of insulin resistance, secondary to enhanced platelet activation and increased plasma levels of fibrinogen and PAI-1.

Management of Venous Thromboembolism in Diabetes

Diabetes is associated with an increased risk of venous thromboembolism, which appears to be related to diabetic complications rather than hyperglycemia per se [92.93]. Treatment of diabetes subjects with venous thromboembolic disease is similar to that of the nondiabetic population, and relies on the administration of LMWH until vitamin K antagonists take effect (the latter agents require a few days to exert full therapeutic activity).

Fondaparinux has also been used for prophylaxis and treatment, whereas thrombin inhibitors are emerging as future therapeutic agents.

Management Guidelines

There are no clear guidelines for the treatment of diabetes with ACS and there is a great variability between countries and even centers in the same country, which is largely dependent on local resources and

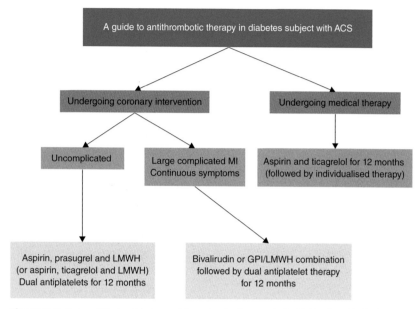

Figure 8.3 A simplified guide to antithrombotic therapy in individuals with diabetes.

data interpretation of different trials. Given the current evidence, we attempt to draw up a simplistic guide to the treatment of ACS patient with diabetes, which is summarized in Figure 8.3. The large number of agents in development and the ongoing clinical trials make this an ever-changing clinical area and the proposed guide will need to be continually updated.

Conclusions

Despite major advances in therapy, atherothrombotic complications remain the main cause of morbidity and mortality in individuals with diabetes. Formation of an obstructive thrombus, the final step in the atherothrombotic process, occurs secondary to a complex interaction between the cellular and fluid phases of coagulation, often resulting in irreversible end-organ damage.

Antithrombotic treatment for diabetes can be divided into primary and secondary prevention, as well as treatment of the acute vascular event. Aspirin used to be the main agent used for primary cardiovascular prevention in diabetes, but recent studies failed to show a beneficial role for this agent, and therefore it is reserved for individuals with high cardiovascular risk, and at the discretion of the attending physician. Large clinical studies are currently underway to clarify further the role of aspirin in primary prevention in individuals in diabetes, which are expected to report in the next three years. In contrast to primary prevention, the role of aspirin in secondary cardiovascular protection in diabetes is well established, although it remains less effective in this population compared to individuals with no diabetes.

Antithrombotic therapy following ACS has been through major changes over the past decade. Diabetes individuals are treated largely similarly to the nondiabetic population, using dual antiplatelet inhibition with LMWH, and coronary artery intervention as appropriate. However, recent evidence has demonstrated differences in response to antithrombotic therapy in those with deranged glucose metabolism. For example, prasugrel is thought to have a superior efficacy to clopidogrel in diabetes subjects when combined with aspirin following ACS. Bivalirudin has also shown promising outcomes in diabetes subjects with complicated ACS, indicating that different treatment strategies will be needed for individuals with diabetes following vascular ischemia.

Several difficulties are encountered when trying to assess the efficacy of antithrombotic therapy in diabetes. First, studies investigating novel antithrombotic therapy are not usually powered to analyze diabetes subjects separately, and therefore results are often inconclusive. Second, the diagnosis of diabetes does not always follow strict criteria and therefore a significant number of diabetes patients are missed, which may bias the results. Third, diabetes is a heterogeneous condition and not a single clinical entity, and therefore cardiovascular risk can vary a great deal between diabetes individuals, dependent on diabetes duration and the presence of various complications; studies have rarely taken this point into account, making data interpretation problematic.

Considered together, current evidence indicates that diabetes subjects have a differential response to antiplatelet and anticoagulant drug therapy compared to subjects with normal glucose metabolism. Further studies are still needed to clarify the optimal antithrombotic strategy in this high-risk population.

Case Study 1

A 62-year-old man with type 2 diabetes is seen in clinic for routine review. His diabetes was diagnosed seven years earlier and he developed background retinopathy and microalbuminuria five years following the diagnosis of diabetes. There is no family history of diabetes, but his father died aged 64 years of myocardial infarction, as did his uncle at the age of 58 years. He used to smoke 20 cigarettes a day for 30 years and stopped at the age of 51 years, whereas his alcohol intake is minimal (around 2 units/month). His current treatment includes metformin 850 mg tds; gliclazide 160 mg bd; sitagliptin 100 mg od; simvastatin 40 mg od; ramipril 10 mg od.

His weight was 102 kg with a BMI of 34 kg/m², his blood pressure 128/71 mmHg, and he had no significant proteinuria. He had palpable peripheral pulses but signs of early neuropathy as assessed by the monofilament test. His blood tests showed HbA1c 63 mmol/mol; creatinine 103 umol/l; eGFR 51 ml/min/m²; total cholesterol 5.2 mmol/l; LDL 3.6 mmol/l; triglycerides 2.1 mmol/l.

Questions

1 Is this patient a candidate for aspirin therapy?
   He leaves the clinic, but contacts the diabetes nurse by phone two hours later to say he has been feeling slightly breathless since leaving the clinic and he thinks this is due to a "cold running in the family." The diabetes nurse reassures him and plans to ring him the next day. She checks with the doctor to make sure this is the right course of action.

2 Do you agree with the diabetes nurse that this is the safest and easiest course of action?
   The patient is brought back to the clinic and on further questioning he denies chest pain, but says the breathlessness is getting worse.

3 What is your next step?
   His ECG is shown in Figure 8.4.

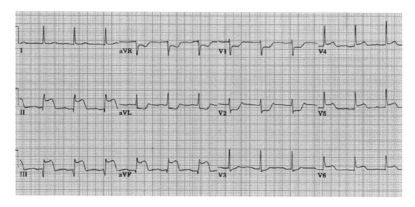

Figure 8.4 ECG.

4 What is your next step?
   He is immediately admitted under the cardiologists and given a loading dose of aspirin 300 mg and prasugrel 60 mg.

5 Do you agree with this approach? If not, what is the alternative?
   Almost immediately after aspirin and clopidogrel, his breathlessness worsens and he starts to complain of chest pain. Cardiologists have

already made arrangements for coronary PCI, but are awaiting the arrival of support staff. The nurse is about to inject the patient with LMWH, but the cardiologist has other ideas.

6 What are the options at this stage?

The patient undergoes an uneventful PCI and a stent is placed in the LAD. He is symptom free after the procedure and an echocardiogram shows normal left ventricular function. His glucose levels are running between 14 and 20 mmol/l.

7 Should this be treated or would you rather wait for 72 hours before deciding on hypoglycemic therapy?

The patient is discharged from hospital after four days and he is completely symptom free.

8 What is the best antithrombotic strategy in this patient in the medium and long term (in the first 12 months following the event and longer term)?

Answers provided after the References

Multiple-Choice Questions

1 Which of the following is/are true in relation to bivalirudin?

 A The main side effect of bivalirudin is shortness of breath, which limits the use of this agent.

 B Bivalirudin is a direct inhibitor of FX.

 C In diabetes patients with ACS, the combination of abciximab and heparin has similar efficacy to bivalirudin monotherapy, but the risk of bleeding is lower with the latter therapy.

 D Recent work suggests that the combination of bivalirudin with insulin is particularly effective at reducing future cardiovascular events following ACS in subjects with diabetes.

 E Bivalirudin should never be used with metformin due to the higher risk of heart failure with this combination.

2 Which of the following is *not* true in relation to aspirin?

 A Aspirin should not be used routinely for primary cardiovascular protection in diabetes.

 B Aspirin affects both platelet function and fibrin network structure.

 C Aspirin is effective in secondary cardiovascular protection in diabetes.

 D Limited evidence suggests that clopidogrel monotherapy is superior to aspirin when used for secondary cardiovascular protection in diabetes.

 E Recent evidence suggests that prasugrel is superior to aspirin when used in diabetes subjects in the setting of acute coronary syndrome.

3 Which of the following statements is/are not true? (There can be more than one option.)

  A The inhibition of fibrinolysis by TAFI is related to the modulation of thrombin production.

  B FXIII stabilizes the clot by cross-linking fibrin fibres and plasma proteins into the fibrin network.

  C Fibrinogen plasma levels are increased in diabetes and predict future cardiovascular events.

  D The generation of plasmin from plasminogen occurs 1,000-fold faster in the presence of fibrin.

  E Thrombin and ADP both directly activate platelets and cleave fibrinogen to form the fibrin network.

Answers provided after the References

Guidelines and Web Links

http://www.ncbi.nlm.nih.gov/pubmed/23996285
ESC Guidelines on diabetes, pre-diabetes, and cardiovascular diseases developed in collaboration with the EASD: The Task Force on diabetes, pre-diabetes, and cardiovascular diseases of the European Society of Cardiology (ESC) and developed in collaboration with the European Association for the Study of Diabetes (EASD).

References

1 Moreno PR, Murcia AM, Palacios IF et al. Coronary composition and macrophage infiltration in atherectomy specimens from patients with diabetes mellitus. *Circulation* 2000; 102: 2180–84.

2 Ferreiro JL, Angiolillo DJ. Diabetes and antiplatelet therapy in acute coronary syndrome. *Circulation* 2011; 123: 798–813.

3 Hess K, Grant PJ. Inflammation and thrombosis in diabetes. *Thromb Haemost* 2011; 105(Suppl 1): S43–S54.

4 Angiolillo DJ, Bernardo E, Sabate M et al. Impact of platelet reactivity on cardiovascular outcomes in patients with type 2 diabetes mellitus and coronary artery disease. *J Am Coll Cardiol* 2007; 50: 1541–7.

5 Mansfield MW, Heywood DM, Grant PJ. Circulating levels of factor VII, fibrinogen, and von Willebrand factor and features of insulin resistance in first-degree relatives of patients with NIDDM. *Circulation* 1996; 94: 2171–6.

6 Mansfield MW, Stickland MH, Grant PJ. PAI-1 concentrations in first-degree relatives of patients with non-insulin-dependent diabetes: Metabolic and genetic associations. *Thromb Haemost* 1997; 77: 357–61.

7 Schroeder V, Carter AM, Dunne J, Mansfield MW, Grant PJ. Proinflammatory and hypofibrinolytic phenotype in healthy first-degree relatives of patients with Type 2 diabetes. *J Thromb Haemost* 2010; 8: 2080–82.

8 Siller-Matula JM, Schwameis M, Blann A, Mannhalter C, Jilma B. Thrombin as a multi-functional enzyme: Focus on in vitro and in vivo effects. *Thromb Haemost* 2011; 106: 1020–33.

9 La Corte AL, Philippou H, Ariens RA. Role of fibrin structure in thrombosis and vascular disease. *Adv Protein Chem Struct Biol* 2011; 83: 75–127.

10 Ariens RA, Lai TS, Weisel JW, Greenberg CS, Grant PJ. Role of factor XIII in fibrin clot formation and effects of genetic polymorphisms. *Blood* 2002; 100: 743–54.

11 Weisel JW, Litvinov RI. The biochemical and physical process of fibrinolysis and effects of clot structure and stability on the lysis rate. *Cardiovasc Hematol Agents Med Chem* 2008; 6: 161–80.

12 Antovic JP. Thrombin activatable fibrinolysis inhibitor (TAFI): A link between coagulation and fibrinolysis. *Clin Lab* 2003; 49: 475–86.

13 Storey RF. Biology and pharmacology of the platelet P2Y12 receptor. *Curr Pharm Des* 2006; 12: 1255–9.

14 Kleiman NS, Freedman JE, Tracy PB et al. Platelets: Developmental biology, physiology, and translatable platforms for preclinical investigation and drug development. *Platelets* 2008; 19: 239–51.

15 Angiolillo DJ, Ueno M, Goto S. Basic principles of platelet biology and clinical implications. *Circ J* 2010; 74: 597–607.

16 Hess K, Alzahrani SH, Mathai M et al. A novel mechanism for hypofibrinolysis in diabetes: The role of complement C3. *Diabetologia* 2012; 55: 1103–13.

17 Alzahrani SH, Ajjan RA. Coagulation and fibrinolysis in diabetes. *Diab Vasc Dis Res* 2010; 7: 260–73.

18 Hoekstra T, Geleijnse JM, Schouten EG, Kluft C. Plasminogen activator inhibitor-type 1: Its plasma determinants and relation with cardiovascular risk. *Thromb Haemost* 2004; 91: 861–72.

19 Zorio E, Gilabert-Estelles J, Espana F et al. Fibrinolysis: The key to new pathogenetic mechanisms. *Curr Med Chem* 2008; 15: 923–9.

20 Chudy P, Kotulicova D, Stasko J, Kubisz P. The relationship among TAFI, t-PA, PAI-1 and F1 + 2 in type 2 diabetic patients with normoalbuminuria and microalbuminuria. *Blood Coagul Fibrinolysis* 2011; 22: 493–8.

21 Jorneskog G, Egberg N, Fagrell B et al. Altered properties of the fibrin gel structure in patients with IDDM. *Diabetologia* 1996; 39: 1519–23.

22 Dunn EJ, Ariens RA, Grant PJ. The influence of type 2 diabetes on fibrin structure and function. *Diabetologia* 2005; 48: 1198–206.

23 Henschen-Edman AH. Fibrinogen non-inherited heterogeneity and its relationship to function in health and disease. *Ann NY Acad Sci* 2001; 936: 580–93.

24 Dunn EJ, Philippou H, Ariens RA, Grant PJ. Molecular mechanisms involved in the resistance of fibrin to clot lysis by plasmin in subjects with type 2 diabetes mellitus. *Diabetologia* 2006; 49: 1071–80.

25 Zhu W, Li W, Silverstein RL. Advanced glycation end products induce a prothrombotic phenotype in mice via interaction with platelet CD36. *Blood* 2012; 119(25): 6136–44.

26 Colas R, Sassolas A, Guichardant M et al. LDL from obese patients with the metabolic syndrome show increased lipid peroxidation and activate platelets. *Diabetologia* 2011; 54: 2931–40.

27 Podrez EA, Byzova TV, Febbraio M et al. Platelet CD36 links hyperlipidemia, oxidant stress and a prothrombotic phenotype. *Nat Med* 2007; 13: 1086–95.

28 Angiolillo DJ, Bernardo E, Zanoni M et al. Impact of insulin receptor substrate-1 genotypes on platelet reactivity and cardiovascular outcomes in patients with type 2 diabetes mellitus and coronary artery disease. *J Am Coll Cardiol* 2011; 58: 30–39.

29 Fatah K, Beving H, Albage A, Ivert T, Blomback M. Acetylsalicylic acid may protect the patient by increasing fibrin gel porosity: Is withdrawing of treatment harmful to the patient? *Eur Heart J* 1996; 17: 1362–6.

30 He S, Blomback M, Yoo G, Sinha R, Henschen-Edman AH. Modified clotting proper-
    ties of fibrinogen in the presence of acetylsalicylic acid in a purified system. *Ann NY
    Acad Sci* 2001; 936: 531–5.

31 Undas A, Brummel-Ziedins KE, Mann KG. Antithrombotic properties of aspirin
    and resistance to aspirin: Beyond strictly antiplatelet actions. *Blood* 2007; 109:
    2285–92.

32 Ajjan RA, Standeven KF, Khanbhai M et al. Effects of aspirin on clot structure and
    fibrinolysis using a novel in vitro cellular system. *Arterioscler Thromb Vasc Biol* 2009;
    29: 712–17.

33 Karmohapatra SK, Chakraborty K, Kahn NN, Sinha AK. The role of nitric oxide in
    aspirin induced thrombolysis in vitro and the purification of aspirin activated nitric
    oxide synthase from human blood platelets. *Am J Hematol* 2007; 82: 986–95.

34 Karmohapatra SK, Kahn NN, Sinha AK. The thrombolytic effect of aspirin in animal
    model. *J Thromb Thrombolysis* 2007; 24: 123–9.

35 Randomised trial of intravenous streptokinase, oral aspirin, both, or neither
    among 17,187 cases of suspected acute myocardial infarction: ISIS-2. ISIS-2 (Sec-
    ond International Study of Infarct Survival) Collaborative Group. *Lancet* 1988; 2:
    349–60.

36 Lewis HD, Jr., Davis JW, Archibald DG et al. Protective effects of aspirin against acute
    myocardial infarction and death in men with unstable angina. Results of a Veterans
    Administration Cooperative Study. *N Engl J Med* 1983; 309: 396–403.

37 Theroux P, Ouimet H, McCans J et al. Aspirin, heparin, or both to treat acute unstable
    angina. *N Engl J Med* 1988; 319: 1105–11.

38 Patrono C, Garcia Rodriguez LA, Landolfi R, Baigent C. Low-dose aspirin for the
    prevention of atherothrombosis. *N Engl J Med* 2005; 353: 2373–83.

39 Colwell JA. Aspirin therapy in diabetes. *Diabetes Care* 2004; 27(Suppl 1): S72–S73.

40 Collaborative overview of randomised trials of antiplatelet therapy – I: Prevention
    of death, myocardial infarction, and stroke by prolonged antiplatelet therapy in var-
    ious categories of patients. Antiplatelet Trialists' Collaboration. *Brit Med J* 1994; 308:
    81–106.

41 Collaborative meta-analysis of randomised trials of antiplatelet therapy for preven-
    tion of death, myocardial infarction, and stroke in high risk patients. *Brit Med J* 2002;
    324: 71–86.

42 Cubbon RM, Gale CP, Rajwani A et al. Aspirin and mortality in patients with diabetes
    sustaining acute coronary syndrome. *Diabetes Care* 2008; 31: 363–5.

43 Sacco M, Pellegrini F, Roncaglioni MC et al. Primary prevention of cardiovascular
    events with low-dose aspirin and vitamin E in type 2 diabetic patients: Results of the
    Primary Prevention Project (PPP) trial. *Diabetes Care* 2003; 26: 3264–72.

44 Belch J, MacCuish A, Campbell I et al. The prevention of progression of arterial dis-
    ease and diabetes (POPADAD) trial: Factorial randomised placebo controlled trial of
    aspirin and antioxidants in patients with diabetes and asymptomatic peripheral arte-
    rial disease. *Brit Med J* 2008; 337: a1840.

45 Ogawa H, Nakayama M, Morimoto T et al. Low-dose aspirin for primary prevention
    of atherosclerotic events in patients with type 2 diabetes: A randomized controlled
    trial. *JAMA* 2008; 300: 2134–41.

46 Ong G, Davis TM, Davis WA. Aspirin is associated with reduced cardiovascular and
    all-cause mortality in type 2 diabetes in a primary prevention setting: The Fremantle
    Diabetes study. *Diabetes Care* 2010; 33: 317–21.

47 Leung WY, So WY, Stewart D et al. Lack of benefits for prevention of cardiovascular
    disease with aspirin therapy in type 2 diabetic patients: A longitudinal observational
    study. *Cardiovasc Diabetol* 2009; 8: 57.

48 Welin L, Wilhelmsen L, Bjornberg A, Oden A. Aspirin increases mortality in diabetic patients without cardiovascular disease: A Swedish record linkage study. *Pharmacoepidemiol Drug Saf* 2009; 18: 1143–9.

49 Butalia S, Leung AA, Ghali WA, Rabi DM. Aspirin effect on the incidence of major adverse cardiovascular events in patients with diabetes mellitus: A systematic review and meta-analysis. *Cardiovasc Diabetol* 2011; 10: 25.

50 Sacco RL, Diener HC, Yusuf S et al. Aspirin and extended-release dipyridamole versus clopidogrel for recurrent stroke. *N Engl J Med* 2008; 359: 1238–51.

51 Diener HC, Bogousslavsky J, Brass LM et al. Aspirin and clopidogrel compared with clopidogrel alone after recent ischaemic stroke or transient ischaemic attack in high-risk patients (MATCH): Randomised, double-blind, placebo-controlled trial. *Lancet* 2004; 364: 331–7.

52 Mehta SR, Yusuf S, Peters RJ et al. Effects of pretreatment with clopidogrel and aspirin followed by long-term therapy in patients undergoing percutaneous coronary intervention: The PCI-CURE study. *Lancet* 2001; 358: 527–33.

53 Steinhubl SR, Berger PB, Mann JT, III, et al. Early and sustained dual oral antiplatelet therapy following percutaneous coronary intervention: A randomized controlled trial. *JAMA* 2002; 288: 2411–20.

54 Chen ZM, Jiang LX, Chen YP et al. Addition of clopidogrel to aspirin in 45,852 patients with acute myocardial infarction: Randomised placebo-controlled trial. *Lancet* 2005; 366: 1607–21.

55 Sabatine MS, Cannon CP, Gibson CM et al. Addition of clopidogrel to aspirin and fibrinolytic therapy for myocardial infarction with ST-segment elevation. *N Engl J Med* 2005; 352: 1179–89.

56 Bhatt DL, Fox KA, Hacke W et al. Clopidogrel and aspirin versus aspirin alone for the prevention of atherothrombotic events. *N Engl J Med* 2006; 354: 1706–17.

57 Bhatt DL, Marso SP, Hirsch AT et al. Amplified benefit of clopidogrel versus aspirin in patients with diabetes mellitus. *Am J Cardiol* 2002; 90: 625–8.

58 Ferreiro JL, Angiolillo DJ. Clopidogrel response variability: Current status and future directions. *Thromb Haemost* 2009; 102: 7–14.

59 Ferreiro JL, Cequier AR, Angiolillo DJ. Antithrombotic therapy in patients with diabetes mellitus and coronary artery disease. *Diab Vasc Dis Res* 2010; 7: 274–88.

60 Wiviott SD, Braunwald E, McCabe CH et al. Prasugrel versus clopidogrel in patients with acute coronary syndromes. *New Engl J Med* 2007; 357: 2001–15.

61 Angiolillo DJ, Badimon JJ, Saucedo JF et al. A pharmacodynamic comparison of prasugrel vs. high-dose clopidogrel in patients with type 2 diabetes mellitus and coronary artery disease: Results of the Optimizing anti-Platelet Therapy In diabetes MellitUS (OPTIMUS)-3 Trial. *Eur Heart J* 2011; 32: 838–46.

62 Chin CT, Roe MT, Fox KA et al. Study design and rationale of a comparison of prasugrel and clopidogrel in medically managed patients with unstable angina/non-ST-segment elevation myocardial infarction: The TaRgeted platelet Inhibition to cLarify the Optimal strateGy to medicallY manage Acute Coronary Syndromes (TRILOGY ACS) trial. *Am Heart J* 2010; 160: 16–22.

63 James S, Angiolillo DJ, Cornel JH et al. Ticagrelor vs. clopidogrel in patients with acute coronary syndromes and diabetes: A substudy from the PLATelet inhibition and patient Outcomes (PLATO) trial. *Eur Heart J* 2010; 31: 3006–16.

64 Leonardi-Bee J, Bath PM, Bousser MG et al. Dipyridamole for preventing recurrent ischemic stroke and other vascular events: A meta-analysis of individual patient data from randomized controlled trials. *Stroke* 2005; 36: 162–8.

65 Halkes PH, van GJ, Kappelle LJ, Koudstaal PJ, Algra A. Aspirin plus dipyridamole versus aspirin alone after cerebral ischaemia of arterial origin (ESPRIT): Randomised controlled trial. *Lancet* 2006; 367: 1665–73.

66 Angiolillo DJ, Capranzano P, Goto S et al. A randomized study assessing the impact of cilostazol on platelet function profiles in patients with diabetes mellitus and coronary artery disease on dual antiplatelet therapy: Results of the OPTIMUS-2 study. *Eur Heart J* 2008; 29: 2202–11.

67 Lee SW, Chun KJ, Park SW et al. Comparison of triple antiplatelet therapy and dual antiplatelet therapy in patients at high risk of restenosis after drug-eluting stent implantation (from the DECLARE-DIABETES and -LONG Trials). *Am J Cardiol* 2010; 105: 168–73.

68 Jennings DL, Kalus JS. Addition of cilostazol to aspirin and a thienopyridine for prevention of restenosis after coronary artery stenting: A meta-analysis. *J Clin Pharmacol* 2010; 50: 415–21.

69 Roffi M, Chew DP, Mukherjee D et al. Platelet glycoprotein IIb/IIIa inhibitors reduce mortality in diabetic patients with non-ST-segment-elevation acute coronary syndromes. *Circulation* 2001; 104: 2767–71.

70 Mehilli J, Kastrati A, Schuhlen H et al. Randomized clinical trial of abciximab in diabetic patients undergoing elective percutaneous coronary interventions after treatment with a high loading dose of clopidogrel. *Circulation* 2004; 110: 3627–35.

71 Schneider DJ. Anti-platelet therapy: Glycoprotein IIb-IIIa antagonists. *Brit J Clin Pharmacol* 2011; 72: 672–82.

72 Silvain J, Beygui F, Barthelemy O et al. Efficacy and safety of enoxaparin versus unfractionated heparin during percutaneous coronary intervention: Systematic review and meta-analysis. *Brit Med J* 2012; 344: e553.

73 Stone GW, McLaurin BT, Cox DA et al. Bivalirudin for patients with acute coronary syndromes. *N Engl J Med* 2006; 355: 2203–16.

74 Feit F, Manoukian SV, Ebrahimi R et al. Safety and efficacy of bivalirudin monotherapy in patients with diabetes mellitus and acute coronary syndromes: A report from the ACUITY (Acute Catheterization and Urgent Intervention Triage Strategy) trial. *J Am Coll Cardiol* 2008; 51: 1645–52.

75 Witzenbichler B, Mehran R, Guagliumi G et al. Impact of diabetes mellitus on the safety and effectiveness of bivalirudin in patients with acute myocardial infarction undergoing primary angioplasty: Analysis from the HORIZONS-AMI (Harmonizing Outcomes with RevasculariZatiON and Stents in Acute Myocardial Infarction) trial. *JACC Cardiovasc Interv* 2011; 4: 760–68.

76 Yusuf S, Mehta SR, Chrolavicius S et al. Comparison of fondaparinux and enoxaparin in acute coronary syndromes. *N Engl J Med* 2006; 354: 1464–76.

77 Yusuf S, Mehta SR, Chrolavicius S et al. Effects of fondaparinux on mortality and reinfarction in patients with acute ST-segment elevation myocardial infarction: The OASIS-6 randomized trial. *JAMA* 2006; 295: 1519–30.

78 UK Prospective Diabetes Study (UKPDS) Group. Effect of intensive blood-glucose control with metformin on complications in overweight patients with type 2 diabetes (UKPDS 34). *Lancet* 1998; 352: 854–65.

79 Roussel R, Travert F, Pasquet B et al. Metformin use and mortality among patients with diabetes and atherothrombosis. *Arch Intern Med* 2010; 170: 1892–9.

80 Alzahrani SH, Ajjan RA. Coagulation and fibrinolysis in diabetes. *Diabetes Vasc Dis Res* 2010; 7: 4260–73.

81 Haffner SM, Greenberg AS, Weston WM et al. Effect of rosiglitazone treatment on nontraditional markers of cardiovascular disease in patients with type 2 diabetes mellitus. *Circulation* 2002; 106: 679–84.

82 Buckingham RE. Thiazolidinediones: Pleiotropic drugs with potent anti-inflammatory properties for tissue protection. *Hepatol Res* 2005; 33: 167–70.

83 Chen IC, Chao TH, Tsai WC, Li YH. Rosiglitazone reduces plasma levels of inflammatory and hemostatic biomarkers and improves global endothelial function in habitual heavy smokers without diabetes mellitus or metabolic syndrome. *J Formos Med Assoc* 2010; 109: 113–19.

84 Perriello G, Pampanelli S, Brunetti P, di Pietro C, Mariz S. Long-term effects of pioglitazone versus gliclazide on hepatic and humoral coagulation factors in patients with type 2 diabetes. *Diab Vasc Dis Res* 2007; 4: 226–30.

85 Li D, Chen K, Sinha N et al. The effects of PPAR-gamma ligand pioglitazone on platelet aggregation and arterial thrombus formation. *Cardiovasc Res* 2005; 65: 907–12.

86 Mieszczanska H, Kaba NK, Francis CW et al. Effects of pioglitazone on fasting and postprandial levels of lipid and hemostatic variables in overweight non-diabetic patients with coronary artery disease. *J Thromb Haemost* 2007; 5: 942–9.

87 Marx N, Wohrle J, Nusser T et al. Pioglitazone reduces neointima volume after coronary stent implantation: A randomized, placebo-controlled, double-blind trial in nondiabetic patients. *Circulation* 2005; 112: 2792–8.

88 The PROactive Study Executive Committee and Data and Safety Monitoring Committee.PROactive study. *Lancet* 2006; 367: 982.

89 Nissen SE, Wolski K. Effect of rosiglitazone on the risk of myocardial infarction and death from cardiovascular causes. *N Engl J Med* 2007; 356: 2457–71.

90 De Caterina R, Madonna R, Sourij H, Wascher T. Glycaemic control in acute coronary syndromes: Prognostic value and therapeutic options. *Eur Heart J* 2010; 31: 1557–64.

91 Margolis DJ, Hoffstad O, Strom BL. Association between serious ischemic cardiac outcomes and medications used to treat diabetes. *Pharmacoepidemiol Drug Saf* 2008; 17: 753–9.

92 Stein PD, Goldman J, Matta F, Yaekoub AY. Diabetes mellitus and risk of venous thromboembolism. *Am J Med Sci* 2009; 337: 259–64.

93 Heit JA, Leibson CL, Ashrani AA et al. Is diabetes mellitus an independent risk factor for venous thromboembolism? A population-based case-control study. *Arterioscler Thromb Vasc Biol* 2009; 29: 1399–405.

Answers to Case Study 1 Questions

1 There is a general lack of evidence supporting the use of aspirin for primary prevention in individuals with diabetes. Recent primary prevention studies have failed to show an effect of aspirin therapy on future cardiovascular events, although some subgroups of diabetes patients showed a benefit. Unfortunately, studies to date have not been adequately powered to give a clear answer. Therefore, current guidelines recommend the use of aspirin for primary prevention in high-risk diabetes subjects. Our patient is overweight, has a strong family history of cardiovascular disease, has signs of microvascular complications, and he used to be a heavy smoker. Therefore, there is

an argument for starting him on aspirin treatment, with the acknowledgment that no concrete evidence exists at present for such a practice. This should be discussed with the patient, including the side effects of aspirin (gastrointestinal and intra-cerebral bleeding), before making a final decision.

2 Silent myocardial infarction (i.e., myocardial infarction without chest pain) is not uncommon in diabetes, particularly in those with microvascular complications. Therefore, sudden onset breathlessness in a diabetes subject should be taken seriously and the possibility of a cardiac event should be ruled out.

3 He will need an ECG and cardiac enzymes requested to rule out a cardiac cause for his sudden-onset shortness of breath.

4 His ECG shows ST elevation in II, III, AVF, V5, and V6 consistent with inferior infarction and lateral extension. Cardiologists should be contacted immediately and the patient should be given antiplatelet agents.

5 Given the evidence for the superior efficacy of prasugrel in diabetes, this approach is not unreasonable. Alternatively, the patient could have been given ticagrelol with aspirin.

6 LMWH has been shown to be effective in patients with and without diabetes. This treatment is sometimes given in association with GPIIb/IIIa inhibitors in subjects with continuing symptoms before PCI. An alternative to combined LMWH and GPIIb/IIIa inhibitors is bivalirudin, which has shown overall a better clinical profile in subjects with diabetes (reduced risk of bleeding).

7 It is advisable to treat hyperglycemia early, supported by data from the DIGAMI1 trial. However, care should be taken to avoid hypoglycemia in these subjects and therefore frequent monitoring of glucose levels and early input from the diabetes team is required.

8 The patient will require dual antiplatelet therapy for at least a year. Given that the patient has diabetes, his risk of mortality and/or recurrent ischemic event within the first year is high (two- to threefold that of an individual with no diabetes). Patients are usually treated with clopidgrel and aspirin for a year following MI, but in our patient the combination of prasugrel and aspirin or ticagrelol and aspirin should be considered. There is no clear evidence for the benefit of dual therapy past one year following MI and therefore patients are usually maintained on aspirin alone in the longer term (for secondary cardiovascular protection).

Answers to Multiple-Choice Questions for Case Study 1

1 C

2 E

3 A, E

CHAPTER 9

Diet and Lifestyle in CVD Prevention and Treatment

Alice H. Lichtenstein
Tufts University, Boston, MA, USA

Key Points

- Modifications to dietary patterns and lifestyle behaviors (physical activity and tobacco use) can decrease an individual's risk of developing cardiovascular disease.

- Moderate fat intake (25% to 35% of energy) is associated with lower triglyceride concentrations than a low-fat diet.

- In most individuals, a reduction in saturated fat (animal fats – meat and dairy) and *trans* fat (partially hydrogenated fat) intake will result in a decrease in LDL-cholesterol concentrations.

- Whole grain products should be substituted for refined grain products to reduce cardiovascular disease risk.

- Energy-containing beverage intake should be monitored to avoid overconsumption of excess calories and nutrient dilution.

- Nutrient supplements are not associated with reduced risk of cardiovascular disease.

Introduction

Cardiovascular disease (CVD) is the leading cause of morbidity and mortality in developed countries and more recently in developing countries. Modifications to habitual dietary patterns and lifestyle behaviors (physical activity and tobacco use) can strongly influence the risk of developing CVD. This relationship is multifactorial, and can be influenced through effects on body weight, body composition, plasma lipid and lipoprotein concentrations, cardiorespiratory fitness, glucose homeostasis, blood pressure, and inflammatory status. The goals for any diet and lifestyle intervention with the intent of reducing CVD risk should include achieving and maintaining a healthy body weight, systolic and diastolic blood pressure values within the normal range, and plasma lipoprotein profiles and glucose concentrations associated with optimal health outcomes. This chapter will focus on diet, physical activity, and tobacco use.

Managing Cardiovascular Complications in Diabetes, First Edition.
Edited by D. John Betteridge and Stephen Nicholls.
© 2014 John Wiley & Sons, Ltd. Published 2014 by John Wiley & Sons, Ltd.

Diet

There is a wide range of dietary variables that have been associated with CVD risk. Some were first identified early in the early twentieth century (e.g., dietary cholesterol), while others have been recognized more recently (e.g., *trans* fatty acids). Many have been the topic of controversy and as new data emerge our relative assessment of each evolves. For example, the importance of dietary cholesterol has diminished relative to the importance of saturated fat.

It is difficult, if not impossible, to assess directly the efficacy of individual dietary components on CVD risk because of the challenges, both practical and financial, in modifying the diets of a large group of people for long periods of time, as well as the difficulty that arises in studying individual dietary components within the context of habitual dietary patterns. Therefore, most dietary factors with the intent of reducing CVD risk are evaluated on the basis of short-term interventions (weeks or months) using biomarkers (e.g., plasma cholesterol concentrations, inflammatory factors) rather than hard endpoints. By combining data from different types of studies, dietary patterns have emerged that are associated with a lower risk of CVD [1, 2].

Total Dietary Fat

Dietary fat serves as a major energy source in the human diet. One gram of fat has the equivalent of 9 calories, whereas one gram of protein and carbohydrate has the equivalent of 4 calories, and alcohol has the equivalent of 7 calories per gram. The two major issues to consider with regard to total amount of dietary fat and CVD risk are body weight and plasma lipoprotein profiles. The range of total fat intake is relatively wide, from 15% of energy (%E) to 45%E. Current recommendations are to consume a diet containing 25%E to 35%E as total fat [3, 4]. For individuals with diabetes, the recommendation is to consume diets toward the higher end of this range [5, 6].

Body weight

Long-term data indicated that reducing total fat intake by 10%E resulted in only modest reductions in body weight over a 12-month period, approximately 1 kg in normal-weight individuals, and 3 kg in overweight or obese individuals [7, 8, 9]. More recent data indicate that total fat intake is not significantly related to annual body weight changes [8, 10] and only weakly related to annual changes in waist circumference [8]. One mitigating factor may be the fiber content of the diet [7, 8, 9]. Higher fiber intakes have been associated with lower body weights and waist circumferences [8]. These data suggest that consuming fruits, vegetables, and whole grains rather

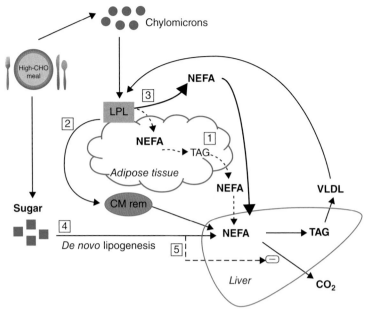

Figure 9.1 Mechanisms of carbohydrate (CHO)-induced hypertriacylglycerolemia. (1) Impaired ability of insulin to suppress lipolysis, leading to increase NEFA flux (┄►); (2) accumulation of chylomicron remnants (CM rem; ►); (3) down-regulation of adipose tissue lipoprotein lipase (LPL) activity (►; (4) *de novo* lipogenesis (►); (5) less hepatic fatty acid oxidation, possibly inhibited through malonyl-CoA produced in *de novo* lipogenesis (┄►). (Source: Chong et al. 2007 [17]. Reproduced with permission of Cambridge University Press.)

than fat-free cookies, cakes, and fat-free savory snacks may be preferential in preventing weight gain or promoting weight loss.

Lipoprotein Profiles

Low-fat diets are associated with elevated triglyceride concentrations and depressed high-density lipoprotein (HDL)-cholesterol concentrations resulting from what is commonly referred to as carbohydrate-induced hypertriglyceridemia [11, 12, 13]. Carbohydrate-induced hypertriglyceridemia, resulting in elevated triglyceride concentrations, is caused by an enhanced rate of hepatic fatty acid synthesis and is precipitated by an excess flow of glucose from the gut to the liver [14, 15] and subsequent production of hepatic triglyceride-rich particles, termed very low-density lipoprotein (VLDL) [16, 17, 18] (Figure 9.1). In some cases delayed triglyceride clearance associated with low-fat diets has also been observed, contributing to the elevated triglyceride concentrations [19].

The metabolic response to a low-fat diet can vary depending on the experimental design or characteristics of the study subjects. Within the context of a stable body weight, replacement of dietary fat with carbohydrate results in higher triglyceride and VLDL-cholesterol concentrations, lower HDL-cholesterol concentrations, and a higher (less favorable) total cholesterol to HDL-cholesterol ratio [20, 21, 22, 23, 24, 25]. This effect is blunted when an individual is in negative energy balance, engages in regular physical activity, or consumes a fiber-rich source of carbohydrate [11, 23, 24]. Sedentary individuals with visceral adiposity are at particularly high risk for carbohydrate-induced hypertrygliceridemia [13]. The associated elevated insulin concentrations (insulin resistance) may enhance VLDL synthesis or delay clearance.

The extent to which the fat to carbohydrate ratio of the diet is altered predicts the change in triglyceride and HDL-cholesterol concentrations [26, 27] or CVD outcomes [28]. Moderate carbohydrate restriction and weight loss have been reported to provide equivalent but nonadditive improvements in the atherogenic dyslipidemic pattern, characterized by an elevated triglyceride concentration and total cholesterol to HDL-cholesterol ratio [29].

Type of Dietary Fat

Studies performed in the mid-1960s demonstrated that changes in dietary fatty acid profiles altered plasma total cholesterol concentrations in most individuals [30, 31]. In using a variety of different experimental designs, more recent work has confirmed these early findings [25, 32, 33, 34]. When carbohydrate is displaced by saturated fatty acids, low-density lipoprotein (LDL)-cholesterol concentrations increase, whereas when carbohydrate is displaced by unsaturated fatty acids, LDL-cholesterol concentrations decrease. The effect of polyunsaturated fatty acids is greater than that of monounsaturated fatty acids [25, 35]. When carbohydrate is displaced by saturated, monounsaturated, or polyunsaturated fatty acids, HDL-cholesterol concentrations are increased, with saturated fatty acids having the greatest effect and polyunsaturated fatty acids having the least effect. With respect to dietary fat and total cholesterol to HDL-cholesterol ratios, there is little effect when carbohydrate is displaced by saturated fatty acids, whereas monounsaturated and polyunsaturated fatty acids decrease the ratio (more favorable) to a similar magnitude. Relative to carbohydrate, all types of dietary fat decrease triglyceride concentrations. Changes in LDL-cholesterol concentrations induced by changes in the fatty acid profile of the diet are primarily attributed to differences in the fractional catabolic rate of LDL rather than production rate [36, 37]. Differences in HDL-cholesterol concentrations induced by changes in the fatty acid profile of the diet are primarily attributed to differences in the production rate rather than the fractional catabolic rate [38, 39].

The major sources of saturated fatty acids in the diet are meat and dairy fats. The major sources of monounsaturated fatty acids in the diet are canola and olive oils. The major sources of polyunsaturated fatty acids (PUFA) in the diet are soybean, corn, safflower, and sunflower oils. The common dietary fatty acids are listed in Table 9.1.

Unique Fatty Acid Classes
Omega-3 (n-3) PUFA

A difference in the prevalence of CVD between Greenland Inuits and genetically similar Scandinavians was first reported in the early 1980s [40, 41]. The lower rate of CVD in the Greenland Inuits was attributed to higher HDL-cholesterol concentrations, resulting from higher intakes of marine foods, particularly the n-3 PUFA.

Since that time, a number of studies have reported an inverse association between dietary n-3 PUFA and CVD and stroke risk [42]. Intervention studies have demonstrated that eicosapentaenoic acid (EPA, 20:5n-3) and docosahexaenoic acid (DHA,22:6n-3), but not alpha-linolenic acid (ALA, 18:3n-3), positively affect CVD outcomes in both primary and secondary prevention settings [43]. The effect of EPA and DHA on CVD has been attributed to antiarrhythmic properties and effects on lowering plasma triglyceride concentrations, platelet reactivity, and blood pressure [44, 45, 46]. A meta-analysis suggested that for beneficial effects on CVD outcomes to be achieved, the minimum intake should be 250 mg EPA+DHA per day [47]. This intake can be achieved by adhering to the recommendation to consume at least two fish meals per week, particularly oily fish for the general population [3, 4, 48].

The three major dietary n-3 PUFA are ALA, EPA, and DHA. ALA is found in plants and plant oils. Of oils commonly used in food preparation, soybean oil and canola oil have the highest levels of ALA. EPA and DHA, sometimes referred to as very long chain n-3 PUFA, are found in marine foods, predominantly fatty fish. Humans can convert ALA to EPA and DHA. However, this conversion capacity is low [49, 50, 51]. For this reason, the recommendation, with respect to CVD risk reduction, is made on the basis of fish meals per week [3, 4, 48]. For individuals with established disease, the current recommendation is to consume the equivalent of 1 g EPA+DHA per day. Due to their hypotriglyceridemic effect, 3–5 g EPA+DHA is recommended for individuals with chronically elevated triglyceride concentrations and use should be monitored by a physician [48, 52]. A new source of DHA, algal oil, has also been shown to decrease triglyceride concentrations significantly [53].

Trans Fatty Acids

The double bonds in fatty acids occur in the *cis* or *trans* configuration. The *cis* configuration is the predominant form, representing the majority of double bonds in plant oils and animal fats.

Table 9.1 Common dietary fatty acids.

Code	Common Name	Formula
SATURATED		
12:0	lauric acid	$CH_3(CH_2)_{10}COOH$
14:0	myristic acid	$CH_3(CH_2)_{12}COOH$
16:0	palmitic acid	$CH_3(CH_2)_{14}COOH$
18:0	stearic acid	$CH_3(CH_2)_{16}COOH$
MONOUNSATURATED		
16:1n-7 cis	palmitoleic acidCH_3	$(CH_2)_5CH=(c)CH(CH_2)_7COOH$
18:1n-9 cis	oleic acid	$CH_3(CH_2)_7CH=(c)CH(CH_2)_7COOH$
18:1n-9 trans	elaidic acid	$CH_3(CH_2)_7CH=(t)CH(CH_2)_7COOH$
POLYUNSATURATED		
18:2n-6,9 all cis	linoleic acid	$CH_3(CH_2)_4CH=(c)CHCH_2CH=(c)CH(CH_2)_7COOH$
18:3n-3,6,9 all cis	α-linolenic acid	$CH_3CH_2CH=(c)CHCH_2CH=(c)CHCH_2CH=(c)CH(CH_2)_7COOH$
18:3n-6,9,12 all cis	γ-linolenic acid	$CH_3(CH_2)_4CH=(c)CHCH_2CH=(c)CHCH_2CH=(c)CH(CH_2)_4COOH$
20:4n-6,9,12,15 all cis	arachidonic acid	$CH_3(CH_2)_4CH=(c)CHCH_2CH=(c)CHCH_2CH=(c)CHCH_2CH=(c)CH(CH_2)_3COOH$
20:5n-3,6,9,12,15 all cis	eicosapentaenoic acid	$CH_3(CH_2CH=(c)CH)_5(CH_2)_3COOH$
22:6n-3,6,9,12,15,18 all cis	docosahexaenoic acid	$CH_3(CH_2CH=(c)CH)_6(CH_2)_2COOH$

Since the 1990s attention has focused on the effect of *trans* fatty acids on CVD and other health outcomes [54, 55]. Similar to saturated fatty acids, *trans* fatty acids increase LDL-cholesterol concentrations. In contrast to saturated fatty acids, *trans* fatty acids do not increase HDL-cholesterol concentrations. Taken together, these changes result in a less favorable LDL-cholesterol/HDL cholesterol ratio with respect to CVD risk [25, 56]. A trend toward increased triglyceride concentrations is frequently reported. Some research has also suggested that *trans* fatty acids may increase lipoprotein (a) and high-sensitivity C-reactive protein concentrations, insulin resistance, metabolic syndrome, and diabetes [57, 58].

There are two main sources of dietary *trans* fatty acids: those that occur naturally in meat and dairy products as a result of anerobic bacteria fermentation in ruminant animals, and those formed during partial hydrogenation of vegetable or fish oils. Traditionally, oils have been partially hydrogenated to increase their viscosity (changing liquid oil into a semi-liquid or solid) and extend their shelf life (decreasing susceptibility to oxidation). In recent decades the major source of dietary *trans* fatty acids has been from partially hydrogenated fat, primarily from commercially prepared fried foods and baked goods [57].

The *trans* fat intake has declined in recent years in the USA. In 2003 the Food and Drug Administration mandated that by 2006 the *trans* fat content of packaged food should be listed on the Nutrient Facts panel [59]. As a result, between 2005 and 2010 the US Department of Agriculture documented a decline in the *trans* fat content of newly introduced foods and a rise in the use of "no *trans* fat" claims on food packages [60]. Around that same time some US cities restricted the use of partially hydrogenated fats by chain restaurants. In one such city, New York, between 2006 and 2008 the proportion of restaurants using partially hydrogenated fat declined from 51% to 2% [61]. Between the years 2000 and 2009, plasma *trans* fatty acid levels in non-Hispanic white adults living in the USA decreased by 50% [62]. Similar trends have been seen in other counties [63, 64].

Dietary Cholesterol

The observation that dietary cholesterol increased blood cholesterol concentrations and is associated with the development of CVD was first made early in the twentieth century in rabbits [65]. In humans, a positive association between dietary cholesterol and both plasma cholesterol concentrations and CVD risk has been repeatedly observed [66, 67, 68]. However, within the range currently consumed in the USA, 250–350 mg per day, the impact of further decreasing dietary cholesterol on plasma cholesterol concentrations, in most people, is modest [69].

The effect of dietary cholesterol on plasma lipoprotein concentrations is less than that of saturated and *trans* fatty acids, and as such receives less emphasis with respect to dietary recommendations [3, 70]. Of note is that there is a relatively high degree of variability in response to dietary cholesterol among individuals, and this hypo- and hyper-responsiveness has been attributed to genotype differences [71].

With few exceptions, dietary cholesterol is present in foods of animal origin. Eggs provide a particularly rich source of dietary cholesterol. Other sources include milk and meat fat. With regard to the latter source, restricting saturated fat intake is likely to result in a decrease in dietary cholesterol intake.

Dietary Carbohydrate

The area of dietary carbohydrate and CVD risk is less defined than dietary fat and CVD risk, notwithstanding the relationship, as it pertains to low-fat/high-carbohydrate diets and both body weight and lipoprotein profiles.

A positive association has been reported between diet patterns high in simple carbohydrate (primarily sucrose and high-fructose corn syrup) and CVD outcomes, and a negative association between diet patterns high in unrefined carbohydrate (whole grains) and CVD risk factors [72–84]. The intervention data have been heterogeneous and limited in scope [79, 80, 81, 82, 85, 86, 87, 88].

A negative association has been reported between diets high in unrefined carbohydrate and diabetes risk [76, 87, 89, 90, 91]. Studies directly comparing the effect of refined carbohydrate (products made with white flour) and simple carbohydrate on plasma glucose and insulin concentrations have yielded mixed results [92, 93, 94]. Likewise, study results directly comparing the effect of unrefined carbohydrate and refined carbohydrate on plasma glucose and insulin concentrations have been mixed [95, 96, 97].

This discordance between the observational and interventional data is likely attributable to experimental difficulties in distinguishing among the differences associated with substituting foods high in simple carbohydrate and whole grains in the diet. However, on the basis of the totality of the data, dietary recommendations consistent with emphasizing the intake of products made with whole grains is prudent and consistent with overall dietary pattern guidance to minimize CVD risk.

Fiber

An inverse association between fiber and CVD risk has been reported for whole-grain intake and CVD [98]. Studies that have estimated the independent effect of dietary fiber on CVD risk have ranged from concluding a modest [99–103] to a more substantial (20% to 40%) [98] effect for those who eat whole grain foods regularly relative to those who eat them rarely. To avoid increased energy intake, recommendations to increase dietary fiber should be focused on substituting foods made with refined carbohydrate with those made with whole grains rather than adding whole-grain foods to the diet.

Most evidence suggests that soluble fiber exerts its hypocholesterolemic effect by binding bile acids and cholesterol in the intestine, resulting in increased fecal loss and altered colonic metabolism of bile acids [104]. The fermentation of fiber polysaccharides in the colon yields short-chain fatty acids. Some evidence suggests that these compounds may have hypo-cholesterolemic effects via alterations in hepatic metabolism. Interestingly, observational data has consistently associated dietary insoluble fiber from cereals, but not vegetables and fruits, with lower CVD risk and slower progression of atherosclerotic lesions [105, 106, 107]. Current recommendations for adults are the consumption of 25–28 g dietary fiber daily.

Fructose

In adults, higher intakes of sugar-sweetened beverages, frequently made from high-fructose corn syrup, have been associated with weight gain over time and increased risk for developing type 2 diabetes. In children, higher intakes of sugar-sweetened beverages have been associated with higher body weights [108, 109, 110]. Due to these relationships, concern was raised about the potential relationship between fructose and high-fructose corn syrup and both body weight and CVD risk factors [111].

Intervention data have suggested that at least in the short term, an increase in fructose intake, either alone or as high-fructose corn syrup, relative to glucose or sucrose, resulted in similar effects on insulin sensitiv-ity or secretion, glucose kinetics, lipolysis, and glucose, insulin, C-peptide, triglycerides, HDL-cholesterol, and LDL-cholesterol concentrations [112, 113, 114]. Recent attention has now shifted from the type of carbohydrate per se to the form carbohydrate – liquid (beverage) verses solid (food) [115, 116]. This is an active area of investigation at this time.

Protein
Type of Protein

Target dietary recommendations for protein as a percentage of energy have changed little over the years [3, 70, 117, 118, 119, 120]. Dietary protein can be divided into two categories as defined by origin: animal, primarily meat, fish and dairy; and vegetable, primarily grains and legumes. For the most part, the former source of protein contributes the majority of dietary saturated fatty acids and much of the monounsaturated fatty acids to the diet, while the latter, with the exception of tropical oils (palm, palm kernel, and coconut), contributes the majority of the polyunsaturated and some of the monounsaturated fatty acids to the diet. Fish contributes the majority of the very long-chain n-3 fatty acids to the diet, whereas soybean and canola oils contribute the majority of the ALA to the diet. The implications of fatty acids accompanying the sources of protein has already been discussed.

Soy Protein

The potential relationship between soy protein and the risk of developing CVD has a long history dating back to the 1940s [121]. Despite this relatively protracted lead time, attempts at more precisely defining this relationship were slow in coming and somewhat inconsistent [122]. Reinvigorated interest developed about the relationship between soy protein and lipoprotein concentrations in the mid-1990s [123, 124]. At that time it was unclear whether the effect of soy protein on lipoprotein concentrations was attributable to the soy protein per se, or to other soybean-derived factor(s) such as isoflavones. The most recent data suggest either a null or a small LDL-cholesterol-lowering effect of relativity large amounts of soy protein (25–50 grams) [125, 126, 127]. Soy-derived isoflavones do not appear to have an independent effect on lipoprotein concentrations [127, 128, 129]. Nevertheless, consumption of soy protein–rich foods may indirectly reduce CVD risk if they displace animal and full-fat dairy foods that contain saturated fat and cholesterol from the diet.

Dietary Supplements
Phytosterols (Plant Sterols/Stanols)

Plant sterols (phytosterols) are a group of alcoholic derivatives of cyclopentanoperhydrophenanthrene. They are structurally similar to cholesterol, differing only in the aliphatic side chain. Plant sterols occur naturally in plants, and their function is analogous to cholesterol in humans. The most common forms are sitosterol, campesterol, and stigmasterol. In the gut, plant sterols have a higher affinity for micelles than cholesterol, causing them to displace cholesterol from the micelles. This displacement causes about a 50% decrease in the bioavailability of intestinal cholesterol [130, 131, 132, 133, 134]. The decrease in plasma LDL-cholesterol concentrations may be mediated by an increase in the expression of LDL receptors on peripheral cells [130].

Two forms of plant sterols have been used to lower LDL-cholesterol concentrations, plant sterols in their natural state, and a saturated form of plant sterols, termed plant stanols. Some plant sterol/stanol preparations are esterified to a fatty acid prior to incorporation into foods [135]. This extra step increases the miscibility of the plant sterols/stanols with the food components. More recently, additional modifications to increase the miscibility of the plant sterols/stanols with the food components have been developed such as microencapsulation. As a group, these forms of plant stanols/sterols or stanol/sterol esters lower LDL-cholesterol concentrations, on average, by 10% [136, 137, 138]. Maximal effects have been observed at about 2 g per day. It was generally concluded that intakes above that level do not confer additional benefit, although this has recently been questioned [134]. By comparison, the mean intake of naturally occurring plant sterols in the diet ranges from 150–350 mg per day and plant stanols 15–50 mg per day. Controversy remains as to whether the efficacy of plant sterols and stanols is similar [134, 137, 139].

Habitual consumption of plant sterols results in a small increase in plasma sterol concentrations, an increase that is greater for the sterol than the stanol form. This has led to concern about the potential adverse effects of higher plasma plant sterol concentrations on CVD outcomes [140, 141]. The data, in both mice models and humans, are inconsistent [142, 143]. This issue is of particular concern because statin therapy increases the rate of plant sterol absorption [140]. The area remains under active investigation.

Plant stanols/sterols are currently available in a wide variety of foods, drinks, and soft gel capsules. The choice of vehicle should be determined by availability and by other considerations, including the energy content of the products. To sustain LDL-cholesterol reductions from plant sterols/stanols, individuals need to consume them daily, just as they would a lipid-lowering medication.

Policosanols

Policosanols are a mixture of higher primary aliphatic alcohols that can be isolated from sugar cane wax, wheatgerm, rice, beeswax, and other plants [144, 145, 146]. Early work suggested that policosanols were highly efficacious as a cholesterol-lowering agent, decreasing LDL-cholesterol concentrations up to 31% and increasing HDL-cholesterol concentrations up to 29% [146, 147, 148]. The vast majority of studies demonstrating the efficacy of policosanols on plasma lipoprotein profiles were conducted using a preparation of policosanols isolated from sugar cane wax [148]. More recent work conducted under controlled conditions in individuals with hypercholesterolemia [145, 149, 150, 151] and heterozygous familial hypercholesterolemia [152, 153] have consistently failed to supported these earlier findings. At this time the evidence does not support the use of policosanols, regardless of source, to treat elevated LDL-cholesterol concentrations or optimize lipoprotein profiles.

Red yeast rice

Red yeast rice is used as an alternative therapy for hyperlipidemia, particularly in place of drugs that inhibit cholesterol biosynthesis. It is produced from the fermentation of rice by red yeast (Monascus Purpureus) [138, 154]. The available preparations have been reported to have up to 14 active compounds that lower LDL-cholesterol, termed monacolins. Concern has been raised regarding the consistency of the preparations from batch to batch and brand to brand. Recent work has suggested considerable variability among commercially available preparations in monacolin levels, making it difficult to use the preparations adequately for LDL-cholesterol lowering [154].

Vitamin Supplements

In the mid-1990s there was considerable interest in the potential benefit of supplemental doses of vitamins, particularly antioxidant vitamins, and CVD risk reduction [155]. These data came primarily from observational studies. For the most part, a series of randomized controlled intervention trials that followed have failed to demonstrate a benefit of supplemental vitamin E, beta-carotene, vitamin C, or folate on CVD risk reduction [156, 157].

Recently, interest has been focused on the potential effect of supplemental vitamin D in CVD risk reduction. In contrast to the prior vitamins, the relationship between vitamin D and CVD risk is focused on nutrient insufficiency rather than supplemental amounts [156, 158]. Until the results of randomized controlled trials with vitamin D become available, it is premature to make any recommendations.

Physical Activity

Often sidelined when lifestyle issues related to CVD prevention are addressed is the importance of regular physical activity. Physical activity has beneficial effects on body weight, dyslipidemia, hypertension, and diabetes [159, 160, 161]. Importantly, substantial reductions in CVD risk have been observed regardless of whether the physical activity is vigorous or less strenuous, such as walking [160]. A minimum of 30 minutes of physical activity per day is recommended for all adults, and 60 minutes for children [162].

Tobacco Use

Cigarette smoke, both primary and secondary exposure, independently increases CVD risk [163]. Mechanisms of action include increased blood pressure and blood clotting, decreased exercise tolerance and HDL-cholesterol concentrations, and altered lipid metabolism through increased lipolysis, insulin resistance, and tissue lipotoxicity. Prospective investigations have demonstrated a substantial decrease in CVD mortality in former smokers compared with continuing smokers [164]. Progressively lower CVD mortality occurs relatively soon after smoking cessation. Increased intervals since the last cigarette smoked are associated with progressively lower mortality rates [165]. Tobacco use is associated with increased occurrence of angina one year after a myocardial infarction [166].

Case Study 1

A 62-year old woman presents with a 25 lb weight gain since menopause. She has a challenging job as a mid-level administrator in a company that has downsized over the past two years. Her father was treated for type 2 diabetes and had a CVD event at age 54 years; her mother has no history of diabetes or CVD. On exam, her BMI is 29, total cholesterol is 238 mg/dL, LDL-cholesterol is 181 mg/dL, HDL-cholesterol is 27 mg/dL, BP is 140/89 mmHg (untreated), and she smokes cigarettes. Her preference is to avoid cholesterol-lowering medications. She indicates that she avoids "fatty foods," eats out for most of her meals, intends to increase her physical activity but runs out of time at the end of the day, and wants to quit smoking but is too stressed to try.

Multiple-Choice Questions

1 What would you ask the patient regarding the avoidance of "fatty foods"?
   A What does she consider a "fatty food"?
   B What does she use as replacement(s) for "fatty foods"?
   C Where does she purchase most of her food?
   D All of the above.

2 What recommendation would you give the patient regarding her body weight?
   A Think about what factors may have caused your weight gain.
   B Don't worry about the weight gain, take a multivitamin daily.
   C Put more emphasis on cutting down on "fatty foods."
   D A and C.

3 Which aspects of the patient's lifestyle would you recommend she change?
   A Diet.
   B Physical activity.
   C Smoking cessation.
   D All of the above.

Answers provided after the References

Guidelines and Web Links

http://www.cnpp.usda.gov/dgas2010-policydocument.htm
http://www.heart.org/HEARTORG/GettingHealthy/Diet-and-Lifestyle
  -Recommendations_UCM_305855_Article.jsp

http://www.nhlbi.nih.gov/about/ncep/
Dietary Guidelines for Americans, 2010.
National Cholesterol Education Program
The American Heart Association's Diet and Lifestyle Recommendations

References

1 Appel LJ, Moore T, Obarzanek E et al. A clinical trial of the effects of dietary patterns on blood pressure: DASH Collaborative Research Group. *N Engl J Med* 1997; 336(16): 111724.

2 Appel LJ, Sacks FM, Carey VJ et al. Effects of protein, monounsaturated fat, and carbohydrate intake on blood pressure and serum lipids: Results of the OmniHeart randomized trial. *JAMA* 2005; 294: 2455–64.

3 Lichtenstein AH, Appel LJ, Brands M et al. Diet and lifestyle recommendations revision 2006: A scientific statement from the American Heart Association Nutrition Committee. *Circulation* 2006; 114(1): 82–96.

4 Dietary Guidelines for Americans. http://www.cnpp.usda.gov/DGAs2010-DGACReport.htm. 2010. Accessed November 17, 2013.

5 Bantle JP, Wylie-Rosett J, Albright AL et al. Nutrition recommendations and interventions for diabetes: A position statement of the American Diabetes Association. *Diabetes Care* 2008; 31(Suppl 1): S61–S78.

6 American Diabetes Association. Executive summary: Standards of medical care in diabetes – 2012. *Diabetes Care* 2012; 35: s1.

7 Roberts SB, Pi-Sunyer FX, Dreher M et al. Physiology of fat replacement and fat reduction: Effects of dietary fat and fat substitutes on energy regulation. *Nutrition Reviews* 1998; 56(5 Pt 2): S29–S41; discussion S41–S49.

8 Du H, van der A DL, Boshuizen HC et al. Dietary fiber and subsequent changes in body weight and waist circumference in European men and women. *Am J Clin Nutr* 2010; 95: 329–36.

9 Papathanasopoulos A, Camilleri M. Dietary fiber supplements: Effects in obesity and metabolic syndrome and relationship to gastrointestinal functions. *Gastroenterol* 2010; 138: 65–72.

10 Forouhi NG, Sharp SJ, Du H et al. Dietary fat intake and subsequent weight change in adults: Results from the European Prospective Investigation into Cancer and Nutrition cohorts. *Am J Clin Nutr* 2009; 90: 1632–41.

11 Hellerstein MK. Carbohydrate-induced hypertriglyceridemia: Modifying factors and implications for cardiovascular risk. *Curr Opin Lipidol* 2002; 13(1): 33–40.

12 Parks EJ. Changes in fat synthesis influenced by dietary macronutrient concent. *Proc Nutr Soc* 2002; 61: 281–6.

13 Fried SK, Rao SP. Sugars, hypertriglyceridemia, and cardiovascular disease. *Am J Clin Nutr* 2003; 78(4): 873S–880S.

14 Hudgins LC, Seidman CE, Diakun J, Hirsch J. Human fatty acid synthesis is reduced after the substitution of dietary starch for sugar. *Am J Clin Nutr* 1998; 67(4): 631–9.

15 Raben A, Holst JJ, Madsen J, Astrup A. Diurnal metabolic profiles after 14 d of an ad libitum high-starch, high-sucrose, or high-fat diet in normal-weight never-obese and postobese women. *Am J Clin Nutr* 2001; 73(2): 177–89.

16 Mittendorfer B, Sidossis LS. Mechanism for the increase in plasma triacylglycerol concentrations after consumption of short-term, high-carbohydrate diets. *Am J Clin Nutr* 2001; 73(5): 892–9.

17 Chong M, Fielding BA, Frayn KN. Metabolic interaction of dietary sugars and plasma lipids with a focus on mechanisms and de novo lipogenesis. *Proc Nutr Soc* 2007; 66: 52–9.

18 Lin J, Fang DZ, Du J et al. Elevated levels of triglyceride and triglyceride-rich lipoprotein triglyceride induced by a high-carbohydrate diet is associated with polymorphisms of APOA5-1131T>C and APOC3-482C>T in Chinese healthy young adults. *Ann Nutr Metab* 2011; 58: 150–57.

19 Parks EJ, Krauss RM, Christiansen MP, Neese RA, Hellerstein MK. Effects of a low-fat, high-carbohydrate diet on VLDL-triglyceride assembly, production, and clearance. *J Clin Inv* 1999; 104(8): 1087–96.

20 Mancini M, Mattock M, Rabaya E et al. Studies of the mechanisms of carbohydrate-induced lipaemia in normal man. *Atherosclerosis* 1973; 17(3): 445–54.

21 Grundy SM, Nix D, Whelan MF, Franklin L. Comparison of three cholesterol-lowering diets in normolipidemic men. *JAMA* 1986; 256(17): 2351–5.

22 Garg A, Grundy SM, Koffler M. Effect of high carbohydrate intake on hyperglycemia, islet function, and plasma lipoproteins in NIDDM. *Diabetes Care* 1992; 15(11): 1572–80.

23 Lichtenstein AH, Ausman LM, Carrasco W, Jenner JL, Ordovas JM, Schaefer EJ. Short-term consumption of a low-fat diet beneficially affects plasma lipid concentrations only when accompanied by weight loss: Hypercholesterolemia, low-fat diet, and plasma lipids. *Arterioscler Thromb* 1994; 14(11): 1751–60.

24 Kasim-Karakas SE, Almario RU, Mueller WM, Peerson J. Changes in plasma lipoproteins during low-fat, high-carbohydrate diets: Effects of energy intake. *Am J Clin Nutr* 2000; 71(6): 1439–47.

25 Mensink RP, Zock PL, Kester AD, Katan MB. Effects of dietary fatty acids and carbohydrates on the ratio of serum total to HDL cholesterol and on serum lipids and apolipoproteins: A meta-analysis of 60 controlled trials. *Am J Clin Nutr.* 2003; 77(5): 1146–55.

26 Ginsberg HN, Kris-Etherton P, Dennis B et al. Effects of reducing dietary saturated fatty acids on plasma lipids and lipoproteins in healthy subjects: The DELTA Study, protocol 1. *Arterioscler Thromb Vasc Biol* 1998; 18(3): 441–9.

27 Lichtenstein AH. Thematic review series: Patient-oriented research. Dietary fat, carbohydrate, and protein: Effects on plasma lipoprotein patterns. *J Lipid Res* 2006; 47(8): 1661–7.

28 Hooper L, Summerbell CD, Higgins JP et al. Reduced or modified dietary fat for preventing cardiovascular disease. *Cochrane Database Syst Rev* 2011; CD002137.

29 Krauss RM, Blanche PJ, Rawlings RS et al. Separate effects of reduced carbohydrate intake and weight loss on atherogenic dyslipidemia. *Am J Clin Nutr* 2006; 83(5): 1025–31; quiz 1205.

30 Hegsted DM, McGandy RB, Myers ML, Stare FJ. Quantitative effects of dietary fat on serum cholesterol in man. *Am J Clin Nutr* 1965; 17(5): 281–95.

31 Keys A, Anderson JT, Grande F. Serum cholesterol response to change in the diet. *Metab Clin Exp* 1965; 14(7), 747–58.

32 Jakobsen MU, O'Reilly EJ, Heitmann BL et al. Major types of dietary fat and risk of coronary heart disease: A pooled analysis of 11 cohort studies. *Am J Clin Nutr* 2009; 89(5): 1425–32.

33 Siri-Tarino PW, Sun Q, Hu FB, Krauss RM. Saturated fat, carbohydrate, and cardiovascular disease. *Am J Clin Nutr* 2010; 91: 502–9.

34 Mozaffarian D, Micha R, Wallace S. Effects on coronary heart disease of increasing polyunsaturated fat in place of saturated fat: A systematic review and meta-analysis of randomized controlled trials. *PLoS Med* 2010; 7: e1000252.

35 Hu FB, Willett WC. Optimal diets for prevention of coronary heart disease. *JAMA* 2002; 288(20): 2569–78.

36 Shepherd J, Packard CJ, Grundy SM, Yeshurun D, Gotto AM, Jr,, Taunton OD. Effects of saturated and polyunsaturated fat diets on the chemical composition and metabolism of low density lipoproteins in man. *J Lipid Res* 1980; 21(1): 91–9.

37 Matthan NR, Welty FK, Barret HR et al. Dietary hydrogenated fat increases high-density lipoprotein apoA-I catabolism and decreases low-density lipoprotein apoB-100 catabolism in hypercholesterolemic women. *Arterioscler Thromb Vasc Biol* 2004; 24(6): 1092–7.

38 Velez-Carrasco W, Lichtenstein AH, Li Z et al. Apolipoprotein A-I and A-II kinetic parameters as assessed by endogenous labeling with [(2)H(3)]leucine in middle-aged and elderly men and women. *Arterioscler Thromb Vasc Biol* 2000; 20(3): 801–6.

39 Marsh JB, Welty FK, Schaefer EJ. Stable isotope turnover of apolipoproteins of high-density lipoproteins in humans. *Curr Opin Lipidol* 2000; 11(3): 261–6.

40 Kromann N, Green A. Epidemiological studies in the Upernavik district, Greenland: Incidence of some chronic diseases 1950–1974. *Acta Med Scand* 1980; 208(5): 401–6.

41 Dyerberg J, Bang HO. A hypothesis on the development of acute myocardial infarction in Greenlanders. *Scand J Clin Lab Inv Suppl.* 1982; 161: 7–13.

42 Mozaffarian D, Rimm EB. Fish intake, contaminants, and human health: Evaluating the risks and the benefits. *JAMA* 2006; 296(15): 1885–99.

43 Wang C, Harris WS, Chung M et al. n-3 Fatty acids from fish or fish-oil supplements, but not alpha-linolenic acid, benefit cardiovascular disease outcomes in primary- and secondary-prevention studies: A systematic review. *Am J Clin Nutr* 2006; 84(1): 5–17.

44 De Caterina R, Zampolli A. Omega-3 fatty acids, atherogenesis, and endothelial activation. *J Cardiovasc Med* 2007; 8(Suppl 1): S11–S14.

45 Harris WS, Miller M, Tighe AP, Davidson MH, Schaefer EJ. Omega-3 fatty acids and coronary heart disease risk: Clinical and mechanistic perspectives. *Atherosclerosis* 2008; 197(1): 12–24.

46 Nodari S, Triggiani M, Campia U et al. n-3 polyunsaturated fatty acids in the prevention of atrial fibrillation recurrences after electrical cardioversion: A prospective, randomized study. *Circulation* 2011; 124: 1100–6.

47 Musa-Veloso K, Binns MA, Kocenas A et al. Impact of low v. moderate intakes of long-chain n-3 fatty acids on risk of coronary heart disease. *Brit J Nutr* 2011; 106: 1129–41.

48 Kris-Etherton PM, Harris WS, Appel LJ; for the Nutrition Committee. Fish consumption, fish oil, omega-3 fatty acids, and cardiovascular disease. *Circulation* 2002; 106(21): 2747–57.

49 Burdge GC, Calder PC. Conversion of alpha-linolenic acid to longer-chain polyunsaturated fatty acids in human adults. *Reprod Nutr Dev* 2005; 45(5): 581–97.

50 Brenna JT, Salem N, Jr,, Sinclair AJ, Cunnane SC; for the International Society for the Study of Fatty Acids and Lipids, ISSFAL. Alpha-Linolenic acid supplementation and conversion to n-3 long-chain polyunsaturated fatty acids in humans. *Lipids* 2009; 80: 85–91.

51 Deckelbaum RJ, Torrejon C. The omega-3 fatty acid nutritional landscape: Health benefits and sources. *J Nutr* 2012; 142: 587S–591S.

52 Chapman MJ, Ginsberg HN, Amarenco P et al. Triglyceride-rich lipoproteins and high-density lipoprotein Cholesterol in patients at high risk of cardiovascular disease: Evidence and guidance for management. *Eur Heart J* 2011; 23: 1345–61.

53 Bernstein AM, Ding EL, Willett WC, Rimm EB. A meta-analysis shows that docosahexaenoic acid from algal oil reduces serum triglycerides and increases

HDL-cholesterol and LDL-cholesterol in persons without coronary heart disease. *J Nutr* 2012; 142: 99–104.

54 Mensink RP, Katan MB. Effect of dietary trans fatty acids on high-density and low-density lipoprotein cholesterol levels in healthy subjects. *N Engl J Med* 1990; 323(7): 439–45.

55 Lichtenstein AH, Ausman LA, Nelson S, Schaefer EJ. Comparison of different forms of hydrogenated fats on serum lipid levels in moderately hypercholesterolemic female and male subjects. *N Engl J Med* 1999; 340: 1933–40.

56 Ascherio A, Katan MB, Zock PL, Stampfer MJ, Willett WC. Trans fatty acids and coronary heart disease. *N Engl J Med* 1999; 340(25): 1994–8.

57 Mozaffarian D, Katan MB, Ascherio A, Stampfer MJ, Willett WC. Trans fatty acids and cardiovascular disease. *N Engl J Med* 2006; 354(15): 1601–13.

58 Cascio G, Schiera G, Di Liegro I. Dietary fatty acids in metabolic syndrome, diabetes and cardiovascular diseases. *Curr Diabetes* 2012; 8: 2–17.

59 Food and Drug Administration. Food labeling: Trans fatty acids in nutrition labeling, nutrient content claims, and health claims. Final rule. *Federal Register* 2003; 133: 41433–506.

60 Rahkovsky I, Martinez S, Kuchler F. New food choices free of trans fats better align U.S. diets with health recommendations. *Economic Information Bulletin.* 2012; 95.

61 Angell SY, Silver LD, Goldstein GP et al. Cholesterol control beyond the clinic: New York CIty's trans fat restriction. *Ann Inter Med* 2009; 151: 129–34.

62 Vesper HW, Kulper HC, Mirel LB, Johnson CL, Pirkle JL. Levels of plasma trans-fatty acids in non-hispanic white adults in the United States in 2000 and 2009. *JAMA* 2012; 307: 562.

63 Temme EH, Millenaar IL, Van Donkersgoed G et al. Impact of fatty acid food reformulations on intake of Dutch young adults. *Acta Cardiol* 2011; 66: 721–8.

64 Pot GK, Prynne CJ, Stephen AM. National Diet and Nutrition Survey: Fat and fatty acid intake from the first year of the rolling programme and comparison with previous surveys. *Brit J Nutr* 2012; 107: 405–15.

65 Finking G, Hanke H. Nikolaj Nikolajewitsch Anitschkow (1885–1964) established the cholesterol-fed rabbit as a model for atherosclerosis research. *Atherosclerosis* 1997; 135(1): 1–7.

66 Clarke R, Frost C, Collins R, Appleby P, Peto R. Dietary lipids and blood cholesterol: Quantitative meta-analysis of metabolic ward studies. *Brit Med J* 1997; 314(7074): 112–17.

67 Stamler J, Shekelle R. Dietary cholesterol and human coronary heart disease: The epidemiologic evidence. *Arch Path Lab Med* 1988; 112(10): 1032–40.

68 Institute of Medicine. *Dietary Reference Intakes. Energy, Carbohydrate, Fiber, Fat, Fatty Acids, Cholesterol, Protein and Amino Acids*. Washington, DC: National Academy of Sciences. 2005.

69 Brownawell AM, Falk MC. Cholesterol: Where science and public health policy intersect. *Nutr Rev* 2010; 68: 355–84.

70 Expert Panel on Detection Evaluation and Treatment of High Blood Cholesterol in Adults (Adult Treatment Panel III). Executive summary of the third report of the National Cholesterol Education Program (NCEP). *JAMA* 2001; 285: 2486–97.

71 Katan MB, Beynen AC. Characteristics of human hypo- and hyperresponders to dietary cholesterol. *Am J Epidemiol* 1987; 125(3): 387–99.

72 Sahyoun NR, Jacques PF, Zhang XL, Juan W, McKeown NM. Whole-grain intake is inversely associated with the metabolic syndrome and mortality in older adults. *Am J Clin Nutr* 2006; 83: 124–31.

73 de Munter JSL, Hu FB, Spiegelman D, Franz M, van Dam RM. Whole grain, bran, and germ intake and risk of type 2 diabetes: A prospective cohort study and systematic review. *PLoS Med*. 2007; 4(8): e261.

74 Mellen PB, Walsh TF, Herrington DM. Whole grain intake and cardiovascular disease: A meta-analysis. *Nutr Metab Cardiovasc Dis* 2008; 18(4): 283–90.

75 Eshak ES, Iso H, Date C et al. Dietary fiber intake is associated with reduced risk of mortality from cardiovascular disease among Japanese men and women. *J Nutr* 2010; 140: 1445–53.

76 Sun Q, Spiegelman D, van Dam RM et al. White rice, brown rice, and risk of type 2 diabetes in US men and women. *Arch Inter Med* 2010; 170: 961–9.

77 He M, van Dam RM, Rimm E, Hu FB, Qi L. Whole-grain, cereal fiber, bran, and germ intake and the risks of all-cause and cardiovascular disease-specific mortality among women with type 2 diabetes mellitus. *Circulation* 2010; 121: 2162–8.

78 Mellen PB, Liese AD, Tooze JA, Vitolins MZ, Wagenknect LE, Herrington DM. Whole-grain intake and carotid artery atherosclerosis in a multiethnic cohort: The Insulin Resistance Atherosclerosis Study. *Am J Clin Nutr* 2007; 85(6): 1495–502.

79 Lutsey PL, Jacobs DR, Kori S et al. Whole grain intake and its cross-sectional association with obesity, insulin resistance, inflammation, diabetes and subclinical CVD: The MESA Study. *Brit J Nutr* 2007; 98: 397–405.

80 Jacobs DR, Jr., Andersen LF, Blomhoff R. Whole-grain consumption is associated with a reduced risk of noncardiovascular, noncancer death attributed to inflammatory diseases in the Iowa Women's Health Study. *Am J Clin Nutr* 2007; 85: 1606–14.

81 Masters RC, Liese AD, Haffner SM, Wagenknecht LE, Hanley AJ. Whole and refined grain intakes are related to inflammatory protein concentrations in human plasma. *J Nutr* 2010; 140: 587–94.

82 Gaskins AJ, Mumford SJ, Rovner AJ et al. Whole grains are associated with serum concentrations of high sensitivity C-reactive protein among premenopausal women. *J Nutr* 2010; 140: 1669–76.

83 Katcher HI, Legro RS, Kunselman AR et al. The effects of a whole grain-enriched hypocaloric diet on cardiovascular disease risk factors in men and women with metabolic syndrome. *Am J Clin Nutr* 2008; 87: 79–90.

84 Estruch R, Martinez-González D, Corelia D et al. Effects of dietary fibre intake on risk factors for cardiovascular disease in subjects at high risk. *J Epidemiol Comm Health* 2009; 63: 582–8.

85 Marckmann P, Raben A, Astrup A. Ad libitum intake of low-fat diets rich in either starchy foods or sucrose: Effects on blood lipids, factor VII coagulant activity, and fibrinogen. *Metab Clin Exp* 2000; 49(6): 731–5.

86 Chong MFF, Fielding BA, Frayn KN. Metabolic interaction of dietary sugars and plasma lipids with a focus on mechanisms and de novo lipogenesis. *Proc Nutr Soc* 2007; 66(1): 52–9.

87 Ross AB, Bruce SJ, Blondel-Lubrano A et al. A whole-grain cereal-rich diet increases plasma betaine, and tends to decrease total and LDL-cholesterol compared with a refined-grain diet in healthy subjects. *Brit J Nutr* 2011; 105: 1492–502.

88 Brownlee IA, Moore C, Chatfield M, et al. Markers of cardiovascular risk are not changed by increased whole-grain intake: The WHOLEheart study, a randomised, controlled dietary intervention. *Brit J Nutr* 2010; 104(1): 125–34.

89 Esposito K, Kastorini C-M, Panagiotakos DB, Giugliano D. Prevention of type 2 diabetes by dietary patterns: A systematic review of prospective studies and meta-analysis. *Metab Syndr Relat Disord* 2010; 8(6): 471–6.

90 Nettleton JA, McKeown NM, Kanoni S et al. Interactions of dietary whole-grain intake with fasting glucose- and insulin-related genetic loci in individuals of

European descent: A meta-analysis of 14 cohort studies. *Diabetes Care* 2010; 33(12): 2684–91.

91 Bleich SN, Wang YC. Consumption of sugar-sweetened beverages among adults with type 2 diabetes. *Diabetes Care* 2011; 34(3): 551–5.

92 Wolever TMS, Campbell JE, Geleva D, Anderson GH. High-fiber cereal reduces postprandial insulin responses in hyperinsulinemic but not normoinsulinemic subjects. *Diabetes Care* 2004; 27: 1281–5.

93 Andersson A, Tengblad S, Karlstrom B et al. Whole-grain foods do not affect insulin sensitivity or markers of lipid peroxidation and inflammation in healthy, moderately overweight subjects. *J Nutr* 2007; 137: 1401–7.

94 Johnson RK, Appel LJ, Brands M et al. Dietary sugars intake and cardiovascular health: A scientific statement from the American Heart Association. *Circulation* 2009; 120(11): 1011–20.

95 Chandalia M, Garg A, Lutjohann D, von Bergmann K, Grundy SM, Brinkley LJ. Beneficial effects of high dietary fiber intake in patients with type 2 diabetes mellitus. *N Eng J Med* 2000; 342: 1392–8.

96 Pereira MA, Jacobs DR, Jr., Pins JJ et al. Effect of whole grains on insulin sensitivity in overweight hyperinsulinemic adults. *Am J Clin Nutr* 2002; 75: 848–55.

97 Juntunen KS, Laaksonen DE, Poutanen KS, Niskanen LK, Mykkanen HM. High-fiber rye bread and insulin secretion and sensitivity in healthy postmenopausal women. *Am J Clin Nutr* 2003; 77(2): 385–91.

98 Flight I, Clifton P. Cereal grains and legumes in the prevention of coronary heart disease and stroke: A review of the literature. *Eur J Clin Nutr* 2006; 60: 1145–59.

99 Brown L, Rosner B, Willett WW, Sacks FM. Cholesterol-lowering effects of dietary fiber: A meta-analysis. *Am J Clin Nutr* 1999; 69(1): 30–42.

100 Anderson JW, Randles KM, Kendall CW, Jenkins DJ. Carbohydrate and fiber recommendations for individuals with diabetes: A quantitative assessment and meta-analysis of the evidence. *J Am Coll Nutr* 2004; 23: 5–17.

101 Queenan KM, Stewart ML, Smith KN, Thomas W, Fulcher RG, Slavin JL. Concentrated oat beta-glucan, a fermentable fiber, lowers serum cholesterol in hypercholesterolemic adults in a randomized controlled trial. *Nutr J* 2007; 6: 6.

102 Lattimer JM, Haub MD. Effects of dietary fiber and its components on metabolic health. *Nutrients* 2010; 2: 1266–89.

103 Kristensen M, Toubro S, Jensen MG et al. Whole grain compared with refined wheat decreases the percentage of body fat following a 12-week, energy-restricted dietary intervention in postmenopausal women. *J Nutr* 2012; 142: 710–16.

104 Lipsky H, Gloger M, Frishman WH. Dietary fiber for reducing blood cholesterol. *J Clin Pharmacol* 1990; 30(8): 699–70.

105 Erkkila AT, Herrington DM, Mozaffarian D, Lichtenstein AH. Cereal fiber and whole-grain intake are associated with reduced progression of coronary-artery atherosclerosis in postmenopausal women with coronary artery disease. *Am Heart J* 2005; 150(1): 94–101.

106 Steffen LM, Jacobs DR, Jr., Stevens J, Shahar E, Carithers T, Folsom AR. Associations of whole-grain, refined-grain, and fruit and vegetable consumption with risks of all-cause mortality and incident coronary artery disease and ischemic stroke: The Atherosclerosis Risk in Communities (ARIC) Study. *Am J Clin Nutr* 2003; 78(3): 383–90.

107 Liu S, Manson JE, Stampfer MJ et al. Whole grain consumption and risk of ischemic stroke in women: A prospective study. *JAMA* 2000; 284(12): 1534–40.

108 Malik V, Popkin BM, Bray GA, Després J-P, Hu FB. Sugar-sweetened beverages, obesity, type 2 diabetes mellitus, and cardiovascular disease risk. *Circulation* 2010; 121: 1356–64.

109 Malik, V.S., Popkin BM, Bray GA, Després J-P, Willett WC, Hu FB. Sugar-sweetened beverages and risk of metabolic syndrome and type 2 diabetes: A meta-analysis. *Diabetes Care* 2010; 33: 2477–83.

110 Levy DT, Friend KB, Wang YC. A review of the literature on policies directed at the youth consumption of sugar sweetened beverages. *Adv Nutr* 2011; 2: 182S–200S.

111 Bray GA, Nielsen SJ, Popkin BM. Consumption of high-fructose corn syrup in beverages may play a role in the epidemic of obesity. *Am J Clin Nutr* 2004; 79(4): 537–43.

112 Stanhope KL, Griffen SC, Bair BR, Swarbrick MM, Keim NL, Havel PJ. Twenty-four-hour endocrine and metabolic profiles following consumption of high-fructose corn syrup-, sucrose-, fructose-, and glucose-sweetened beverages with meals. *Am J Clin Nutr* 2008; 87(5): 1194–203.

113 Sunehag AL, Toffolo G, Campioni M, Bier DM, Haymond MW. Short-term high dietary fructose intake had no effects on insulin sensitivity and secretion or glucose and lipid metabolism in healthy, obese adolescents. *J Pediatr Endocrinol Metab* 2008; 21: 225–35.

114 Sievenpiper JL, de Souza RJ, Mirrahimi A et al. Effect of fructose on body weight in controlled feeding trials: A systematic review and meta-analysis. *Ann Intern Med* 2012; 156: 291–304.

115 Wolf A, Bray GA, Popkin BM. A short history of beverages and how our body treats them. *Obes Rev* 2008; 9(2): 151–64.

116 Pan A, Hu FB. Effects of carbohydrates on satiety: differences between liquid and solid food. *Curr Opin Clin Nutr Metab Care* 2011; 14: 385–90.

117 The Expert Panel. Report of the National Cholesterol Education Program Expert Panel on Detection, Evaluation, and Treatment of High Blood Cholesterol in Adults. *Arch Intern Med* 1988; 148(1): 36–9.

118 The Expert Panel. Summary of the second report of the National Cholesterol Education Program (NCEP) Expert Panel on Detection, Evaluation, and Treatment of High Blood Cholesterol in Adults (Adult Treatment Panel II). *JAMA* 1993; 269(23): 3015–23.

119 Krauss RM, Deckelbaum RJ, Ernst N et al. Dietary guidelines for healthy American adults: A statement for health professionals from the Nutrition Committee, American Heart Association. *Circulation* 1996; 94(7): 1795–800.

120 Krauss RM, Eckel RH, Howard B et al. AHA Dietary Guidelines: Revision 2000: A statement for healthcare professionals from the Nutrition Committee of the American Heart Association. *Circulation* 2000; 102(18): 2284–99.

121 Carroll KK, Kurowska EM. Soy consumption and cholesterol reduction: Review of animal and human studies. *J Nutr* 1995; 125(3 Suppl): 594S–597S.

122 Vega-Lopez S, Lichtenstein AH. Dietary protein type and cardiovascular disease risk factors. *Prev Cardiol* 2005; 8(1): 31–40.

123 Anderson JW, Johnstone BM, Cook-Newell ME. Meta-analysis of the effects of soy protein intake on serum lipids. *N Engl J Med* 1995; 333(5): 276–82.

124 Clifton PM. Protein and coronary heart disease: The role of different protein sources. *Curr Atheroscler Rep* 2011; 13: 493–8.

125 Kreijkamp-Kaspers S, Kok L, Grobbee DE et al. Effect of soy protein containing isoflavones on cognitive function, bone mineral density, and plasma lipids in postmenopausal women: A randomized controlled trial. *JAMA* 2004; 292: 65–74.

126 Sacks FM, Lichtenstein A, Van Horn L, Harris W, Kris-Etherton P, Winston P; for the AHA Nutrition Committee. Soy protein, isoflavones, and cardiovascular health:

A summary of a statement for professionals from the American Heart Association Nutrition Committee. *Arterioscler Thromb Vasc Biol* 2006; 26(8): 168–992.

127 Dewell A, Hollenbeck PL, Hollenbeck CB. Clinical review: A critical evaluation of the role of soy protein and isoflavone supplementation in the control of plasma cholesterol concentrations. *J Clin Endocrinol Metab* 2006; 91(3): 772–80.

128 Balk E, Chung M, Chew P et al. Effects of Soy on Health Outcomes. Evidence Report/Technology Assessment No. 126. (Prepared by Tufts-New England Medical Center Evidence-based Practice Center under Contract No. 290-02-0022.) AHRQ Publication No. 05-E024-2. Rockville, MD: Agency for Healthcare Research and Quality. 2005.

129 Anderson JW, Bush HM. Soy protein effects on serum lipoproteins: A quality assessment and meta-analysis of randomized, controlled studies. *J Am Coll Nutr* 2011; 30: 79–91.

130 Plat J, Mensink RP. Effects of plant stanol esters on LDL receptor protein expression and on LDL receptor and HMG-CoA reductase mRNA expression in mononuclear blood cells of healthy men and women. *FASEB* 2002; 16(2): 258–60.

131 Katan MB, Grundy SM, Jones P, Law M, Miettinen T, Paoletti R; Stresa Workshop Participants. Efficacy and safety of plant stanols and sterols in the management of blood cholesterol levels. *Mayo Clin Proc* 2003; 78(8): 965–78.

132 Ostlund RE, Jr., Phytosterols and cholesterol metabolism. *Curr Opin Lipidol* 2004; 15(1): 37–41.

133 de Jong A, Plat J, Mensink RP. Metabolic effects of plant sterols and stanols. *J Nutr Biochem* 2003; 14(7): 362–9.

134 Musa-Veloso K, Poon TH, Elliot JA, Chung C. A comparison of the LDL-cholesterol lowering efficacy of plant stanols and plant sterols over a continuous dose range: Results of a meta-analysis of randomized, placebo-controlled trials. *Prostaglandins Leukot Essent Fatty Acids* 2011; 85: 9–28.

135 Rocha M, Banuls C, Bellod L, Jover A, Victor VM, Hernandez-Mijares A. A review on the role of phytosterols: New insights into cardiovascular risk. *Curr Pharm Des* 2011; 17: 4061–75.

136 AbuMweis SS, Jones PJ. Cholesterol-lowering effect of plant sterols. *Curr Atheroscler Rep* 2008; 10: 467–72.

137 Scholle JM, Baker WL, Talati R, Coleman CI. The effect of adding plant sterols or stanols to statin therapy in hypercholesterolemic patients: Systematic review and meta-analysis. *J Am Coll Nutr* 2009; 28: 517–24.

138 Nijjar PS, Burke FM, Bloesch A, Rader DJ. Role of dietary supplements in lowering low-density lipoprotein cholesterol: A review. *J Clin Lipidol* 2010; 4: 248–58.

139 Talati R, Sobieraj DM, Makanji SS, Phung OJ, Coleman CI. The comparative efficacy of plant sterols and stanols on serum lipids: A systematic review and meta-analysis. *J Am Dietetic Assoc* 2010; 110(5): 719–26.

140 Patch CS, Tapsell LC, Williams PG, Gordon M. Plant sterols as dietary adjuvants in the reduction of cardiovascular risk: Theory and evidence. *Vasc Health Risk Manag* 2006; 2(2): 157–62.

141 Gylling H, Miettinen TA. The effect of plant stanol- and sterol-enriched foods on lipid metabolism, serum lipids and coronary heart disease. *Ann Clin Biochem* 2005; 42(Pt 4): 254–63.

142 Wilund KR, Yu L, Xu F et al. No association between plasma levels of plant sterols and atherosclerosis in mice and men. *Arterioscler Thromb Vasc Biol* 2004; 24(12): 2326–32.

143 Weingartner O, Lütjohann D, Ji S et al. Vascular effects of diet supplementation with plant sterols. *J Am Coll Cardiol* 2008; 51(16): 1553–61.

144 Reiner Z, Tedeschi-Reiner E. Rice policosanol does not have any effects on blood coagulation factors in hypercholesterolemic patients. *Collegium Antropologicum* 2007; 31(4): 1061–4.

145 Lin Y, Rudrum M, van der Wielen RP et al. Wheat germ policosanol failed to lower plasma cholesterol in subjects with normal to mildly elevated cholesterol concentrations. *Metab Clin Exp* 2004; 53(10): 1309–14.

146 Varady KA, Wang Y, Jones PJ. Role of policosanols in the prevention and treatment of cardiovascular disease. *Nutr Rev* 2003; 61(11): 376–83.

147 Gouni-Berthold I, Berthold HK. Policosanol: Clinical pharmacology and therapeutic significance of a new lipid-lowering agent. *Am Heart J* 2002; 143(2): 356–65.

148 Chen JT, Wesley R, Shamburek RD, Pucino F, Csako G. Meta-analysis of natural therapies for hyperlipidemia: Plant sterols and stanols versus policosanol. *Pharmacotherapy* 2005; 25(2): 171–83.

149 Cubeddu LX, Hoffmann IS, Jimenez E et al. Comparative lipid-lowering effects of policosanol and atorvastatin: A randomized, parallel, double-blind, placebo-controlled trial. *Am Heart J* 2006; 152(5): 982.e1-5.

150 Kassis AN, Marinangeli CP, Jain D, Ebine N, Jones PJ. Lack of effect of sugar cane policosanol on plasma cholesterol in Golden Syrian hamsters. *Atherosclerosis* 2007; 194(1): 153–8.

151 Dulin MF, Hatcher LF, Sasser HC, Barringer TA. Policosanol is ineffective in the treatment of hypercholesterolemia: A randomized controlled trial. *Am J Clin Nutr* 2006; 84(6): 1543–8.

152 Greyling A, De Witt C, Oosthuizen W, Jerling JC. Effects of a policosanol supplement on serum lipid concentrations in hypercholesterolaemic and heterozygous familial hypercholesterolaemic subjects. *Brit J Nutr* 2006; 95(5): 968–75.

153 Berthold HK, Unverdorben S, Degenhardt R, Bulitta M, Gouni-Berthold I. Effect of policosanol on lipid levels among patients with hypercholesterolemia or combined hyperlipidemia: A randomized controlled trial. *JAMA* 2006; 295(19): 2262–9.

154 Gordon RY, Cooperman T, Obermeyer W, Becker DJ. Marked variability of monacolin levels in commercial red yeast rice products: Buyer beware! *Arch Intern Med* 2010; 170: 1722–7.

155 Kris-Etherton P, Lichtenstein AH, Howard BV et al. Antioxidant vitamin supplements and cardiovascular disease. *Circulation* 2004; 110: 637–41.

156 Lichtenstein AH. Nutrient supplements and cardiovascular disease: A heartbreaking story. *J Lipid Res* 2009; 50: S429–S433.

157 Tinkel J, Hassanain H, Khouri SJ. Cardiovascular antioxidant therapy: A review of supplements, pharmacotherapies, and mechanisms. *Cardiol Rev* 2012; 20: 77–83.

158 Elamin MB, Abu Elnour NO, Elamin KB et al. Vitamin D and cardiovascular outcomes: A systematic review and meta-analysis. *J Clin Endocrinol Metab* 2011; 96: 1931–42.

159 Albright C, Thompson DL. The effectiveness of walking in preventing cardiovascular disease in women: A review of the current literature. *J Women's Health* 2006; 15(3): 271–80.

160 Hamer M, Chida Y. Walking and primary prevention: A meta-analysis of prospective cohort studies. *Brit J Sports Med* 2008; 42(4): 238–43.

161 Kelley GA, Kelley KS. Impact of progressive resistance training on lipids and lipoproteins in adults: A meta-analysis of randomized controlled trials. *Prev Med* 2009; 48: 9–19.

162 Physical Activity Guidelines for Americans, http://www.health.gov/paguidelines /. 2008. Accessed November 17, 2013.

163 Barnoya J, Glantz SA. Cardiovascular effects of second-hand smoke help explain the benefits of smoke-free legislation on heart disease burden. *J Cardiovasc Nurs* 2006; 21(6): 457–62.

164 Gastaldelli A, Folli F, Maffei S. Impact of tobacco smoking on lipid metabolism, body weight and cardiometabolic risk. *Curr Pharm Des* 2010; 16: 2526–30.

165 Ockene IS, Miller NH. Cigarette smoking, cardiovascular disease, and stroke: A statement for healthcare professionals from the American Heart Association. American Heart Association Task Force on Risk Reduction. *Circulation* 1997; 96(9): 3243–7.

166 Maddox TM, Reid KJ, Rumsfeld JS, Spertus JA. One-year health status outcomes of unstable angina versus myocardial infarction: A prospective, observational cohort study of ACS survivors. *BMC Cardiovasc Disord* 2007; 7: 28.

Answers to Multiple-Choice Questions for Case Study 1

1 D

2 A

3 D

CHAPTER 10

Management of Acute Coronary Syndrome

Christopher M. Huff and A. Michael Lincoff
Cleveland Clinic, Cleveland, OH, USA

Key Points

- Diabetes is a major risk factor for coronary atherosclerosis.
- Acute coronary syndrome is a leading cause of morbidity and mortality in patients with diabetes.
- Acute coronary syndrome is a spectrum of unstable atherosclerotic coronary disease that includes UA, NSTEMI, and STEMI.
- The focus of treatment for STEMI is emergent myocardial reperfusion, which is preferably done mechanically with percutaneous coronary intervention (PCI).
- Patients with STEMI who present to a non-PCI-capable facility should be transferred for emergent PCI.
- If anticipated transfer for PCI is >120 minutes and there are no contraindications, STEMI patients should receive thrombolysis.
- Because UA and NSTEMI are the result of only partial vessel occlusion, emergent reperfusion is usually not indicated.
- Patients with UA and NSTEMI should not receive thrombolysis, but rather be managed conservatively or referred for coronary angiography based on a variety of factors, including patient risk and preference, PCI capability at the presenting facility, and initial response to medical therapy.
- Unless contraindicated, dual antiplatelet therapy (DAPT) and a parenteral antithrombin agent should be given to all patients with ACS.

Introduction and Epidemiology of Acute Coronary Syndrome

Cardiovascular disease is the most common cause of mortality. Each year it accounts for 30% of deaths worldwide and 38.5% in the United States and Western Europe [1]. Although the incidence of cardiovascular disease is decreasing in high-income countries due to education and advancement in

---

Managing Cardiovascular Complications in Diabetes, First Edition.
Edited by D. John Betteridge and Stephen Nicholls.
© 2014 John Wiley & Sons, Ltd. Published 2014 by John Wiley & Sons, Ltd.

medical therapy, it is rapidly rising in middle- and low-income countries as they become increasingly industrialized and urbanized [1]. Acute coronary syndrome (ACS) is a spectrum of unstable cardiovascular disease that includes unstable angina (UA), non-ST-elevation myocardial infarction (NSTEMI), and ST-elevation myocardial infarction (STEMI), and is often the initial clinical presentation for coronary artery disease (CAD). The major risk factors for ACS include tobacco abuse, family history of CAD, advanced age, hypertension, hyperlipidemia, and diabetes mellitus.

   This chapter focuses on the management of ACS in patients with diabetes. Diabetics are more likely than nondiabetics to experience ACS, and diabetes is an independent predictor for mortality in ACS. Diabetics are also more likely to develop complications of ACS and its management such as heart failure and bleeding. With a few exceptions, the management of ACS is similar in patients with and without diabetes. In patients with diabetes, management does not differ between patients who are insulin dependent and patients who do not require insulin. Although intensive treatment of hyperglycemia, dyslipidemia, and hypertension can reduce cardiovascular and microvascular events in diabetics by as much as 50%, diabetes remains a major risk factor for ACS [2].

Pathophysiology

The initiating event in ACS is rupture or erosion of an atherosclerotic plaque within the coronary endothelium. This exposes the lumen of the coronary artery to subendothelial matrix, leading to the activation of platelets and eventual thrombus formation. ACS is a dynamic process, during which there is cyclical transition among partial vessel occlusion, complete occlusion, and reperfusion. In UA, plaque rupture results in severe obstruction of coronary blood flow and subsequent ischemic symptoms, at times associated with electrocardiographic ST depressions or T-wave inversions without elevation of cardiac biomarkers. NSTEMI is defined by obstruction that leads to infarction without electrocardiographic ST elevation. Plaque rupture that results in complete and prolonged coronary artery occlusion usually leads to ST elevation and subsequent myocardial infarction.

Clinical Presentation

Classically, patients with ACS present with substernal chest pain characterized as "vice-like" or "pressure." The pain often radiates to the left shoulder or jaw, but can radiate to the right arm, back, neck, and/or epigastrium. Associated symptoms include nausea, vomiting, diaphoresis, palpitations, dyspnea, dizziness, and/or confusion. The chest discomfort associated with STEMI is usually more severe than the discomfort experienced with UA/NSTEMI. Also, chest pain in the setting of STEMI is less likely to be relieved by nitroglycerine. Atypical symptoms or silent ischemia (with associated symptoms such as cardiac dysrhythmias or heart failure) are more common in diabetics, women, and the elderly. Appropriate therapy for ACS is dependent on early recognition of symptoms by the patient, as delayed medical evaluation can result in cardiogenic shock and sudden cardiac death. While physical examination is unlikely to aid in the diagnosis of ACS, it is important in risk stratification, excluding alternate diagnoses, and determining whether mechanical complications of myocardial infarction (MI) are present.

Differential Diagnosis

Other diagnoses that cause chest pain can be mistaken for ACS. Gastrointestinal disorders such as gastroesophageal reflux disease (GERD), esophageal spasm, and esophageal hyperalgesia can mimic ischemic chest pain. GERD and CAD can coexist, and it is not uncommon for patients with ACS to mistake their symptoms as reflux. Given this, it is prudent to exclude ACS before proceeding with further evaluation for gastrointestinal disease.

Acute pericarditis causes pleuritic chest pain that is worse when supine and relieved by sitting up and leaning forward. It is usually associated with diffuse ST-segment elevation and concomitant PR-segment depression. If there is myocardial involvement (myocarditis), the cardiac biomarkers may be elevated and transthoracic echocardiogram (TTE) may reveal a regional wall motion abnormality. It can be distinguished from acute MI by the lack of reciprocal ST depression. Also, the ST elevations in acute pericarditis are usually concave, as opposed to the convex ST elevations seen in acute MI.

Aortic dissection typically causes sharp, tearing chest pain with radiation to the back. It is often most severe at onset, as opposed to ischemic chest pain, the severity of which increases over time. Aortic dissection is usually distinguished from ACS based on symptoms, though physical examination can assist in the diagnosis. Examination in patients with aortic dissection may reveal a difference between right and left upper extremity blood flow, detected by comparing the pulse and blood pressure. The diastolic murmur of aortic insufficiency may also be present. If the aorta is enlarged, the chest radiograph will show a widened mediastinum. A TTE may reveal the dissection flap, but the diagnosis is usually made by transesophageal echocardiogram (TEE), computerized tomography (CT), or magnetic resonance imaging (MRI).

Acute onset of pleuritic chest pain and shortness of breath in the absence of pathology on chest radiography suggests pulmonary embolism (PE). The ECG most often shows sinus tachycardia, but may demonstrate right ventricular strain. Although cardiac biomarkers can be slightly elevated with acute PE, TTE can be performed to rule out a left ventricular wall motion abnormality and identify right ventricular dysfunction.

Diagnosis

The diagnosis of ACS should be suspected in any patient with chest pain and risk factors for CAD. The most important initial investigation is a 12-lead electrocardiogram (ECG). This will help distinguish STEMI from UA or NSTEMI. If the ECG reveals ST-segment elevation in a pattern that would suggest MI, the focus of care should shift to emergent myocardial reperfusion. By definition, there should be 1-mm ST-segment elevation in two or more contiguous leads. In acute MI, the ST-segment elevations are usually convex. It is important to be aware of other diagnoses that may cause ST-segment elevation without concomitant ischemia. These diagnoses are listed in Table 10.1.

There are a few situations in which the patient presents with an acute MI but the ECG does not reveal classic ST-segment elevation. The first is posterior MI due to circumflex coronary artery occlusion, which because of its location causes anterior ST-segment depression and tall R waves. It is also possible for a posterior MI to be electrically silent, and thus patients with an occluded left circumflex artery can have a normal ECG [4]. Another situation in which classic ST-segment elevation may be absent is left bundle branch block (LBBB). LBBB "not known to be chronic" in the appropriate clinical setting is considered a STEMI equivalent for two reasons. First, in the setting of proximal left anterior descending (LAD) coronary artery occlusion, new LBBB can occur because of lack of blood flow to the left

Table 10.1 Nonischemic causes of electrocardiographic ST-segment elevation. (Source: Adapted from Wang et al. 2003 [3].)

Early repolarization
Left ventricular hypertrophy
Left bundle branch block
Male pattern
Hyperkalemia
Acute pericarditis
Brugada syndrome
Pulmonary embolism
Postcardioversion

bundle through the first septal perforator. Next, an existing LBBB due to conduction disease can impair the diagnosis of subsequent MI. If the diagnosis of MI is in question, a TTE can assist the clinician by identifying a regional wall motion abnormality. Once the diagnosis of STEMI is made, eligible patients should receive emergent reperfusion without waiting for results of cardiac biomarker testing. Post-reperfusion cardiac biomarkers can aid in determining the size of myocardial infarction.

By definition, the ECG in UA and NSTEMI does not show ST-segment elevation. Rather, the ECG may be normal or show ST-segment depression and/or T-wave inversion. UA and NSTEMI cannot be differentiated based on ECG changes, but instead by cardiac biomarker analysis. In UA cardiac biomarkers are within normal limits, whereas with NSTEMI these markers are elevated. After the onset of MI, it can take up to four hours for these biomarkers to be released into the blood stream. Thus, a patient who presents with MI two hours after the onset of chest pain may have initially normal cardiac biomarkers. In patients with UA and NSTEMI, it is therefore important to check at least two sets of biomarkers (preferably three) drawn a minimum of four hours apart. The most commonly used cardiac biomarkers and their timing of release are shown in Figure 10.1. Troponin T and I are highly sensitive and available at most healthcare facilities. A troponin T measured 72 hours after acute MI may predict infarct size [5, 6, 12]. Because of its high sensitivity, troponin elevation can occur in the setting of other conditions such as PE and congestive heart failure (CHF). Creatinine kinase (CK) and creatinine kinase myocardial band (CK-MB) are also elevated in myocardial infarction. Like troponin, CK is helpful in determining the size of myocardial infarction. CK is also important for

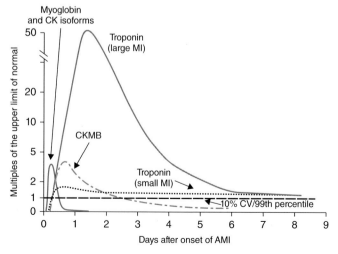

Figure 10.1 Timing of cardiac biomarker release after myocardial infarction. (Source: Anderson et al. 2007 [5]. Reproduced with permission of Elsevier.)

determining reinfarction as it normalizes 24 hours after MI, unlike CK-MB and troponin, which may remain elevated for several days.

Risk Stratification

Estimating risk of death is useful in patients with ACS, as it can aid in treatment decisions and in the counseling of patients and their families. Risk models have been developed to assist the clinician in risk prediction. The Global Registry of Acute Coronary Events (GRACE) score predicts in-hospital mortality in all patients with ACS [9]. Calculation involves multiple variables, including age, heart rate, Killip class (Table 10.2), systolic blood pressure, creatinine level, presence or absence of cardiac arrest on admission, presence or absence of cardiac biomarkers, and ST-segment changes. A score of 250 or greater predicts a >50% chance of in-hospital death.

In STEMI, the most important risk factor for 30-day mortality is age, followed by systolic blood pressure, Killip classification, heart rate, and location of MI (Table 10.3). The thrombolysis in myocardial infarction (TIMI) risk model (Table 10.4) for patients with STEMI incorporates these and other variables obtained from the history, physical exam, and ECG. A TIMI risk score of 9 or greater predicts a 30-day mortality of 35%. By comparison, 30-day mortality is <2% in STEMI patients with a score of 0 to 1.

There is also a TIMI risk score for patients with UA and NSTEMI (Table 10.5). The score consists of seven variables extracted from the patient's history, ECG, and cardiac biomarker analysis. A score of 6 or

Table 10.2 Killip class and estimated 30-day mortality. (Source: Adapted from Lee et al. 1995 [7]. Reproduced with permission of Wolters Kluwer Health).

Killip class	Characteristics	Mortality rate (%)
I	No signs of heart failure	5.1
II	Rales, JVD, S3 gallop	13.6
III	Pulmonary edema	32.2
IV	Cardiogenic shock	57.8

JVD, jugular venous distention.

Table 10.3 Location of myocardial infarction and mortality. (Source: Adapted from Topol 1998 [6]. Reproduced with permission of Lippincott Williams & Wilkins.)

Location	30-day mortality rate (%)	1-year mortality rate (%)
Proximal LAD	19.6	25.6
Mid LAD	9.2	12.4
Distal LAD	6.8	10.2
Proximal RCA or LCx	6.4	8.4
Distal RCA or LCx	4.5	6.7

LAD, Left anterior descending; LCx, Left circumflex; RCA, Right coronary artery.

Table 10.4 TIMI risk model for prediction of 30-day mortality in patients with ST-segment elevation myocardial infarction. (Source: Adapted from Morrow 2000 [9]. Reproduced with permission of Wolters Kluwer Health.)

History	Points
65–74 years old	2
≥75 years old	3
Angina or DM/HTN	1
Physical Exam	
HR >100 bpm	2
SBP <100 mmHg	3
Killip class II–IV	2
Weight <67 kg	1
Presentation	
Time to treatment >4 hrs	1
Anterior ST elevation or LBBB	1
TIMI risk score = (0–14) points	

DM, diabetes mellitus; HR, heart rate; HTN, hypertension; SBP, systolic blood pressure.

Table 10.5 TIMI risk model for predicting 14-day outcomes in patients with UA/NSTEMI. (Source: Data from Antman 2000 [10].)

Characteristics	Points
≥1 mm ST deviation on ECG	1
≥2 episodes of angina in the preceding 24 hours	1
≥3 risk factors for CAD	1
Elevated cardiac biomarkers	1
≥50% stenosis on prior left heart catheterization	1
≥65 years of age	1
Use of aspirin in the past 7 days	1
TIMI risk score = (0–7) points	

greater predicts a 41% incidence of all-cause mortality, MI, or severe recurrent ischemia requiring revascularization. The ischemic complication event rate with a score of 0 to 1 is 4.7%. Not only can this risk model be used to predict outcomes in patients with UA/NSTEMI, but it can also serve as a clinical decision-making tool for determining which patients should receive early coronary angiography. In the TACTICS-TIMI 18 (Treat Angina with Aggrastat and Determine Cost of Therapy with an Invasive or Conservative Strategy-Thrombolysis in Acute Myocardial Infarction) trial, a TIMI risk score of 3 or greater favored an early (within 48 hours) invasive strategy, whereas patients with a score of 2 or less had better outcomes with conservative therapy [13].

Table 10.6 Absolute and relative contraindications to thrombolysis in patients with ST elevation myocardial infarction. (Source: Adapted from Van de Werf et al. 2008 [15]. Reproduced with permission of Oxford University Press.)

Absolute contraindications
Known intracranial neoplasm
Any prior intracranial hemorrhage
Suspected aortic dissection
Active bleeding (Excluding menses)
Known cerebral vascular lesion
Ischemic stroke within the past 3 months
Severe closed head or facial trauma within the past 3 months
Relative contraindications
Blood pressure on presentation >180/110
History of chronic, severe, poorly controlled hypertension
History of ischemic stroke greater than 3 months before presentation, dementia, or other intracranial pathology not listed as an absolute contraindication
Traumatic or prolonged CPR
Internal bleeding within the past 2–4 weeks
Pregnancy
Use of anticoagulation
Active peptic ulcer disease
Vascular punctures at noncompressible sites

Management

With the exception of reperfusion timing, patients across the spectrum of ACS are managed similarly. The major difference is that STEMI patients need emergent reperfusion, whereas patients with UA and NSTEMI can be risk stratified to early coronary angiography or conservative management. The following discussion will include medical management and reperfusion strategies in patients with ACS. The management of patients with and without diabetes is similar, with a few exceptions that will be discussed below.

Initial Medical Therapy
Anti-ischemic Therapy
The three classes of drugs used to reduce myocardial ischemia in patients presenting with ACS are beta-blockers, nitrates, and calcium channel blockers. Beta-blockers reduce myocardial oxygen demand by reducing blood pressure, heart rate, and contractility [11]. Although the benefit of long-term beta-blocker therapy in ACS patients has been well established by clinical trials, there are no randomized data in the era of percutaneous coronary intervention (PCI) to suggest that early administration of beta-blocker therapy reduces mortality [14, 15].The COMMIT/CCS-2 (Clopidogrel and Metoprolol in Myocardial Infarction Trial/Second

Chinese Cardiac Study) trial randomized 45,852 patients with acute MI to intravenous metoprolol followed by oral administration until discharge, or, if prolonged hospitalization, a maximum of four weeks [14]. While there was a reduction in reinfarction and ventricular fibrillation (VF), there was no improvement in mortality, mainly due to an increase in cardiogenic shock [14]. Based on these results, current European Society of Cardiology (ESC) and American Heart Association (AHA) guidelines caution against early administration of beta-blocker therapy in STEMI patients at risk for developing cardiogenic shock [15, 16]. In patients with UA and NSTEMI, in-hospital administration of these agents may prevent progression of ACS and reduce mortality [11]. For instance, the CRUSADE (Can Rapid Risk Stratification of Unstable Angina Patients Suppress Adverse Outcomes with Early Implementation of the ACC/AHA Guidelines) registry demonstrated that patients with UA and NSTEMI who received beta-blockade had a 34% reduction in in-hospital mortality (3.9% vs. 6.9%, $p < 0.001$) [17]. Because of confounding that exists in nonrandomized analyses, these data should be interpreted carefully. Similar to STEMI patients, guidelines caution against aggressive early administration of these agents in UA/NSTEMI patients at risk for developing cardiogenic shock.

Nitrates reduce myocardial oxygen demand through venodilatation, which reduces myocardial preload and thus ventricular wall stress [11, 18]. Nitroglycerine also causes vasodilatation of normal and atherosclerotic coronary arteries, thus improving myocardial blood flow [11, 18]. Although no randomized, placebo-controlled trials have been performed to assess the efficacy of nitroglycerine in improving symptoms or reducing cardiac events, these agents are commonly administered on the basis of observational data. Nitrates are particularly useful in the setting of persistent chest pain, hypertension, or congestive heart failure (CHF). Nitroglycerine can be administered orally, topically, or intravenously. Intravenous nitroglycerine is preferred in patients with persistent ischemic symptoms, because it is easily titratable. The dose is 10 to 20 mcg/min with 5–10 mcg/min increases every 5–10 minutes. Nitrates should be used with caution in STEMI patients suspected of having right ventricular infarction, as these patients are preload dependent. Patients taking phosphodiesterase-5 inhibitors (sildenafil, vardenafil, tadalefil) should not receive nitroglycerine, as this combination of therapy may result in profound hypotension [11, 18].

Calcium channel blockers improve myocardial ischemia by reducing vascular smooth muscle contractility, which results in coronary artery vasodilatation. These agents are not first line for the treatment of ischemia, but are rather given to patients with persistent symptoms despite therapy with beta-blockers and nitrates [11, 18]. As they are contraindicated in the setting of CHF or impaired left ventricular function, calcium channel blockers are rarely used in patients with STEMI. In patients with UA and NSTEMI, diltiazem and verapamil are the preferred agents, as their efficacy in reducing myocardial ischemia is similar compared to beta-blockers [19, 20]. Because of reflex sympathetic activation, nifedipine and other dihydropiridine calcium channel blockers should be avoided in patients with ACS unless combined with a beta-blocker [11, 18, 21].

Antiplatelet Therapy

According to both ESC and AHA guidelines, all patients with ACS should receive dual antiplatelet therapy (DAPT) [11, 16, 17, 18, 22, 23]. One of the antiplatelet agents should be aspirin at an oral dose of 150–325 mg. Nonenteric coated aspirin is preferred for more rapid absorption [11]. Current options for the second antiplatelet agent include an oral platelet $P2Y_{12}$ receptor antagonist or an intravenous platelet glycoprotein IIb/IIIa receptor inhibitor (GPI). There are three $P2Y_{12}$ receptor antagonists currently available for use in ACS. Clopidogrel and prasugrel are thienopyridines that irreversibly bind the platelet $P2Y_{12}$ receptor, and ticagrelor is a triazolopyrimidine that reversibly inhibits the same platelet receptor [11, 16, 17, 18, 22].

Clopidogrel is a pro-drug that is poorly metabolized to its active metabolite. Because of this, it is the least potent of the $P2Y_{12}$ receptor antagonists. The benefit of clopidogrel in ACS has been extensively studied in randomized trials. In the large, randomized CURE (Clopidogrel in Unstable Angina to Prevent Recurrent Events) trial, patients who received clopidogrel had a significant reduction in the primary composite endpoint of cardiovascular death, MI, and stroke (9.3% vs. 11.4%, $p < 0.001$). The benefit persists in patients who receive PCI. A subset analysis, PCI-CURE, compared outcomes in the 2,658 patients who received PCI and found a significant reduction in cardiovascular death, MI, and urgent target vessel revascularization in the patients treated with clopidogrel (4.5% vs. 6.4%, $p = 0.03$) [24]. Clopidogrel is given as a loading dose of 300–600 mg, and continued at a dose of 75 mg daily. The 600 mg loading dose has improved onset of action and platelet inhibition, and in patients undergoing PCI is associated with improved ischemic outcomes compared to 300 mg [11, 16, 17, 18, 22, 23]. The CURRENT-OASIS 7 (Committee members of the Clopidogrel and Aspirin Optimal Dose Usage to Reduce Recurrent Events – Seventh Organization to Assess Strategies in Ischemic Syndromes) trial compared a 300 mg clopidogrel loading dose to a 600 mg loading dose in patients with ACS. Although the higher loading dose did not reduce the primary composite endpoint of cardiovascular death, MI, or stroke in the overall study population, it did significantly reduce the primary endpoint in patients who received PCI (3.9% vs. 4.5%, $p = 0.04$) [25]. Clopidogrel should be discontinued five days prior to major surgery [11].

Prasugrel is a pro-drug with more complete and rapid metabolism to active drug, and thus is superior to clopidogrel in onset of action and strength of platelet inhibition. It is given as a loading dose of 60 mg and maintained at a dose of 10 mg daily. Prasugrel was compared to clopidogrel in the TRITON-TIMI 38 (Trial to Assess Improvement in Therapeutic Outcomes by Optimizing Platelet Inhibition with Prasugrel–Thrombolysis In Myocardial Infarction) trial, which randomized ACS patients to either 300 mg of clopidogrel or 60 mg of prasugrel for up to 15 months [26]. The primary outcome of cardiovascular death, MI, or stroke was reduced in patients who received prasugrel (9.9% vs. 12.1%, $p < 0.001$), which was driven mainly by a reduction in MI (7.3% vs. 9.5%, $p < 0.001$) [26]. Patients who received prasugrel had an increase in major bleeding, particularly patients greater than 75 years of age or with body weight less than 60 kg. In addition, post hoc analysis showed worse outcomes in patients with a history of transient ischemic attack (TIA) or stroke, and thus prasugrel should be avoided in these patients [26]. A subgroup analysis showed a substantially greater treatment effect of prasugrel compared to clopidogrel in diabetics compared to nondiabetics (primary outcome in diabetics: 12.2% vs. 17%, HR 0.70, $p < 0.001$; in nondiabetics: 9.2% vs. 10.6%, HR 0.80, $p = 0.02$). These results should be interpreted carefully, as they are subject to the same potential for spurious findings as with any subgroup analysis. Prasugrel should be discontinued seven days before major surgery [11].

Ticagrelor is the newest of the platelet $P2Y_{12}$ inhibitors. It is given as a loading dose of 180 mg and continued at a dose of 90 mg twice daily. Because it is administered in active form, the onset of action is rapid (30 minutes) and the platelet inhibition is consistent [11]. Ticagrelor is the only $P2Y_{12}$ inhibitor that has been shown in a randomized trial to provide mortality benefit in ACS [27]. The PLATO (Platelet Inhibition and Patient Outcomes) trial compared ticagrelor to clopidogrel for 12 months in 18,624 patients presenting with all forms of ACS [27]. The primary composite endpoint of death from vascular causes, MI, and stroke was significantly reduced in patients who received ticagrelor (9.8% vs. 11.7%, $p < 0.001$). The individual endpoints of death from vascular causes (4.0% vs. 5.1%, $p = 0.001$) and death from any cause (4.5% vs. 5.9%, $p < 0.001$) were decreased with ticagrelor compared to clopidogrel. There was no difference in overall major bleeding, although nonsurgical major bleeding was more common in patients who received ticagrelor (4.5% vs. 3.8%, $p = 0.03$) [27]. A quarter of patients in each treatment arm were diabetic, though outcomes were not specifically reported for this group. Post hoc analysis of the PLATO trial, specifically the US patient cohort, demonstrated worse outcomes in patients who were maintained on high-dose aspirin in conjunction with ticagrelor. Based on this, a maintenance aspirin dose higher than 100 mg is not recommended [23]. Ticagrelor should be discontinued five days prior to major surgery [11].

Current AHA guidelines for the management of STEMI and UA/NSTEMI do not yet recommend one agent over another except in certain situations. As mentioned previously, prasugrel should be avoided in patients with a history of TIA or stroke due to the increased risk of intracranial hemorrhage (ICH). After thrombolysis, clopidogrel is the preferred agent based on results from the CLARITY-TIMI 28 (Clopidogrel as Adjunctive Reperfusion Therapy-Thrombolysis in Acute Myocardial Infarction) trial. The addition of clopidogrel to thrombolytic therapy in CLARITY resulted in a 36% reduction in the composite endpoint of an occluded infarct-related artery, death, or recurrent MI prior to angiography [28]. The recommended dose of clopidogrel with thrombolysis is 300 mg [23]. There are no data showing efficacy or safety of prasugrel or ticagrelor with fibrinolytic therapy. The ESC also recommends clopidogrel in patients treated with thrombolysis. Otherwise, ESC guidelines recommend ticagrelor as the preferred agent for moderate-to high-risk ACS patients, if the coronary anatomy is unknown. Prasugrel is the preferred agent in $P2Y_{12}$ inhibitor naïve patients (especially diabetics) after the coronary anatomy has been defined to rule out the need for coronary artery bypass grafting (CABG) [11].

The three GPIs currently approved for use in ACS include abciximab, a monoclonal antibody fragment, and the small molecules eptifibatide and tirofiban [11, 16, 17, 18, 21, 22]. Although there are extensive data demonstrating the benefit of GPI therapy in ACS, most of these studies were performed in an era before dual oral antiplatelet therapy. A few trials have evaluated the effectiveness of GPI therapy in addition to contemporary antiplatelet and antithrombin therapy in STEMI patients. The BRAVE-3 (Bavarian Reperfusion Alternatives Evaluation-3) and ON-TIME 2 (Ongoing Tirofiban in Myocardial Infarction Evaluation) trials evaluated the efficacy of adding GPI therapy to heparin and 600 mg of clopidogrel in patients presenting with STEMI. Neither of these trials showed an improvement in ischemic outcomes when compared to placebo. The HORIZONS-AMI (Harmonizing Outcomes With Revascularization and Stents in Acute Myocardial Infarction) study evaluated the benefit of GPI therapy compared with more contemporary anticoagulation with bivalirudin. Patients with STEMI presenting for PCI were randomized to UFH plus a GPI (abciximab or double-bolus eptifibatide) or bivalirudin alone with provisional GPI therapy. All patients received aspirin and a thienopyridine. Bivalirudin treatment was associated with noninferior protection against ischemic events, but substantially reduced bleeding compared with UFH plus GPI. Although rates of acute stent thrombosis were higher with bivalirudin, there were no net differences in thrombosis rates by 30 days; mortality was significantly reduced by bivalirudin by one year [29]. Based on the above, STEMI patients treated with a $P2Y_{12}$ antagonist who receive anticoagulation with either heparin or bivaliruidn derive minimal benefit from the addition of GPI therapy.

The benefit of GPI therapy has also been established in patients with UA and NSTEMI; however, as with the STEMI data, efficacy was determined before contemporary therapy with platelet $P2Y_{12}$ antagonists and bivalirudin [30]. In the current era UA/NSTEMI patients most likely to benefit from GPI therapy are high-risk patients undergoing PCI with UFH. This was demonstrated in the ISAR-REACT 2 (Intracoronary Stenting and Antithrombotic Regimen: Rapid Early Action for Coronary Treatment) trial, which examined the efficacy of adding abciximab to 600 mg of clopidogrel and heparin during PCI. High-risk patients who received abciximab had a significant reduction in the primary composite endpoint of death, MI, and urgent target vessel revascularization (13.1% vs. 18.3%, $p = 0.02$) [31]. The benefit of GPI therapy in UA/NSTEMI appears isolated to PCI, as the EARLY ACS (Early Glycoprotein IIb/IIIa Inhibition in Patients With Non–ST-Segment Elevation Acute Coronary Syndrome) trial showed no further benefit of routine early administration prior to PCI [32]. The ACUITY (Acute Catheterization and Urgent Intervention Triage strategy) study investigated whether GPI therapy would provide added benefit to UA/NSTEMI patients treated with clopidogrel and the novel anticoagulant bivalirudin. Patients with UA/NSTEMI were randomly assigned to UFH plus a GPI, bivalirudin plus a GPI, or bivalirudin alone. Bivalirudin alone was noninferior to UFH plus a GPI in reducing ischemic endpoints and was associated with a significant decrease in major bleeding [33].

Based on the above data, current guidelines for the management of patients with UA/NSTEMI state that treatment with GPI therapy during PCI is reasonable in high-risk patients (elevated troponin or diabetes) who have received a platelet $P2Y_{12}$ antagonist and UFH [11, 23, 30]. In patients treated with bivalirudin, it is reasonable to omit GPI therapy [30]. Because of the risk of bleeding, routine early administration of a GPI prior to coronary angiography or in patients being managed conservatively is not recommended [11, 23, 30].

Antithrombin Therapy

All patients with ACS should receive antithrombin therapy. Current options include UFH, bivalirudin, low molecular weight heparin (LMWH), and fondaparinux. The anticoagulant that has been studied the most in clinical trials is UFH. UFH is given intravenously as a 60 U/kg bolus (maximum 4000 U) and continued at 12 U/kg/hr (maximum 1000 U/hr) with a goal partial thromboplastin time (PTT) of 50 to 70 seconds [18]. In patients who are referred for PCI, the goal intraprocedural activated clotting time (ACT) is based on whether GPI therapy is planned. If GPI therapy is planned, the goal ACT is 200 to 250 seconds. If concurrent GPI therapy is not planned, the goal ACT is 250 to 300 seconds [23]. After PCI, UFH should be discontinued to avoid bleeding complications. For ACS patients who are managed conservatively (without coronary angiography), UFH should be continued for 48 hours [30]. UFH is the preferred agent prior to CABG [18].

Bivalirudin is a direct thrombin inhibitor used for anticoagulation in patients undergoing PCI. It has been evaluated in all forms of ACS. When compared with the combination of heparin and GPI therapy, bivalirudin reduces bleeding without compromising protection against ischemic events. The use of bivalirudin in STEMI patients was investigated in the HORIZONS-AMI trial. As discussed previously, this study compared treatment with bivalirudin versus the combination of UFH and a GPI in patients undergoing PCI for STEMI. Treatment with bivalirudin was associated with a decrease in cardiac death and a reduction in major bleeding [29]. The ACUITY and ISAR-REACT 4 (Intracoronary Stenting and Antithrombotic Regimen: Rapid Early Action for Coronary Treatment) trials compared bivalirudin to heparin plus GPI therapy in patients with Non-ST-Segment Elevation ACS (NSTE-ACS) [33, 34]. In both studies, bivalirudin was non-inferior to heparin plus GPI in reducing ischemic events and significantly reduced major bleeding. Based on the above data, bivalirudin is preferred over UFH and a GPI in patients undergoing PCI who are at high risk for bleeding. Bivalirudin has not been studied in conservative management of ACS and therefore other agents are preferred in this situation. For PCI, the dose of bivalirudin is a 0.75 mg/kg bolus followed by an infusion at 1.75 mg/kg/hr [22, 23].

LMWHs are obtained through chemical and enzymatic depolymerization of UFH [18]. The three most investigated forms of LMWH are dalteparin, nadroparin, and enoxaparin. Enoxaparin has been studied in STEMI, particularly in the setting of thrombolysis. The ASSENT-3 (Assessment of the Safety and Efficacy of a New Thrombolytic-3) trial compared enoxaparin to UFH in STEMI patients receiving thrombolysis with weight-based tenecteplase. The combination of enoxaparin and tenecteplase was superior to UFH and tenecteplase in reducing the primary composite endpoint of death, reinfarction, or refractory ischemia [35]. The ExTRACT-TIMI 25 (Enoxaparin and Thrombolysis Reperfusion for Acute Myocardial Infarction Treatment – Thrombolysis in Myocardial Infarction) trial also investigated the efficacy of enoxaparin in the setting of thrombolysis. STEMI patients undergoing thrombolysis were randomized to UFH for 48 hours or enoxaparin throughout the index hospitalization. Compared to UFH, patients who received enoxaparin had a significant reduction in the primary endpoint of death and nonfatal MI through 30 days (12.0% vs. 9.9%, $p < 0.001$). The reduced primary endpoint with enoxaparin was entirely due to a decrease in reinfarction, as there was no difference in mortality between the two groups [34]. This reduction in reinfarction came at the risk of increased major bleeding.

Several studies have compared LMWH to UFH in patients with UA/NSTEMI. Trials involving the use of dalteparin and nadroparin demonstrate similarity to UFH in reducing rates of death and nonfatal MI [18]. There is, however, data to suggest that enoxaparin may be superior to UFH in patients with UA/NSTEMI. In the ESSENCE (Efficacy and Safety of Subcutaneous Enoxaparin in Non-Q-Wave Coronary Events) trial, patients who received enoxaparin had a lower incidence of death, MI, or recurrent angina at 30 days when compared to UFH (19.8% vs. 23.3%, $p = 0.016$) [37]. Similarly, in the TIMI 11B trial, patients with UA/NSTEMI who received enoxaparin had a significant reduction in the primary composite endpoint of death, MI, and urgent revascularization at 43 days compared to patients treated with UFH (17.3% vs. 19.7%, $p = 0.048$) [38]. Both ESSENCE and TIMI 11B were performed at a time when an invasive strategy was not routine. A more contemporary study, the SYNERGY (Superior Yield of the New Strategy of Enoxaparin, Revascularization and Glycoprotein IIb/IIIa Inhibitors) trial, compared enoxaparin to UFH in high-risk UA/NSTEMI patients undergoing PCI. In this study the primary endpoint of death or MI did not differ between enoxaparin and UFH, but there was an increase in TIMI major bleeding in the patients treated with enoxaparin (9.1% vs. 7.6%, $p = 0.008$) [39].

Based on the above data, enoxaparin should be considered a first-line anticoagulant in STEMI patients undergoing thrombolysis and for patients with UA/NSTEMI who are managed conservatively. It may be used in the setting of PCI, but is not superior to UFH. The dose of enoxaparin is 1 mg/kg subcutaneously every 12 hours. If it is used as the primary anticoagulant for patients undergoing PCI, additional dosing in the cardiac catheterization lab is based on the time at which the last dose was given. If the last dose was given within 8 hours, no additional therapy is necessary. If 8–12 hours have elapsed since the last dose, an intravenous dose of 0.3 mg/kg should be administered. If 12 hours have passed since the last dose, the patient should receive 1 mg/kg subcutaneously [23]. LMWH is not recommended in patients greater than 75 years of age or with significant renal dysfunction [23].

Fondaparinux is a synthetic heparin pentasaccharide that selectively inhibits clotting factor Xa. Its efficacy in STEMI was investigated in the OASIS-6 (Organization for the Assessment of Strategies for Ischemic Syndromes-6) trial. This study examined the efficacy of fondaparinux in STEMI patients treated with either thrombolysis or PCI. In the patients who received thrombolysis, fondaparinux compared to placebo resulted in a significant reduction in death or reinfarction at 30 days without an increase in bleeding. In the patients who received PCI, fondaparinux resulted in worse outcomes compared to UFH, in part related to an increase in guiding catheter thrombosis, coronary dissection, no reflow, and abrupt vessel closure [40]. The use of fondaparinux in the management of UA/NSTEMI was evaluated in the OASIS-5 study. This trial randomized patients with UA and NSTEMI to treatment with fondaparinux or enoxaparin. There was no difference in the primary endpoint of death, MI, or refractory ischemia at 9 days; however, treatment with fondaparinux significantly reduced major bleeding (2.2% vs 4.1%, $p < 0.001$). There was also a decrease in the number of deaths at 30 days ($p = 0.02$) and 180 days ($p = 0.05$) in the patients who received fondaparinux. Of the patients who underwent PCI, guiding catheter thrombosis was increased with fondaparinux [41].

Based on the above, fondaparinux is not the preferred anticoagulant in patients undergoing primary PCI for STEMI because of the increased risk of guiding catheter thrombosis [15, 23]. However, it is reasonable to administer fondaparinux in patients undergoing thrombolysis [15]. In patients with UA/NSTEMI who are being managed conservatively, fondaparinux should be considered as a first-line agent due to its favorable efficacy–safety profile [11]. Patients with UA/NSTEMI receiving PCI may be treated with fondaparinux, but an additional anticoagulant with anti-IIa activity such as heparin or bivalirudin should be administered. The dose of fondaparinux is 2.5 mg per day given subcutaneously.

Coronary Reperfusion

As discussed previously, the initial acute management of ACS hinges on whether or not the patient needs immediate coronary reperfusion (STEMI or equivalent). The decision for early coronary angiography versus conservative management in patients with UA/NSTEMI is based on a variety of factors, including patient risk and preference, PCI capability at the presenting facility, and initial response to medical therapy. Once a decision has been made regarding the need for reperfusion, this can be accomplished with thrombolysis, percutaneous coronary intervention, or coronary artery bypass grafting. The preferred approach depends on time to presentation, anticipated time to PCI, extent of coronary artery disease, hemodynamic status, left ventricular function, and comorbid disease. The different options for coronary reperfusion are discussed below.

Thrombolysis

Extensive research has documented the benefit of thrombolytic therapy in STEMI, which includes improved survival and left ventricular function. This clinical benefit has not been observed in patients with UA/NSTEMI; accordingly, thrombolysis should not be used in this setting. The benefit of

Table 10.7 High-risk features in patients with
UA/NSTEMI. (Source: Adapted from Hamm 2011
[11]. With permission of Oxford University Press
(UK) © European Society of Cardiology.
www.escardio.org/guidelines.)

Elevated troponin
Dynamic ST- or T-wave changes on the ECG
Diabetes mellitus
Renal insufficiency (eGFR <60 mL/min/1.73 m^2)
LVEF <40%
Early postinfarction angina
Recent PCI
Prior CABG
Intermediate to high GRACE risk score

---

eGFR, estimated glomerular filtration rate.

thrombolysis in STEMI declines with time, with the maximum treatment effect within one hour of symptom onset and little to no benefit after 12 hours of symptoms. If a decision is made for thrombolysis and there are no contraindications (Table 10.6), it should be performed within 30 minutes of first medical contact (FMC). Available thrombolytic agents include streptokinase, alteplase, reteplase, and tenecteplase.

Streptokinase (SK) is a first-generation thrombolytic that acts against clot-bound fibrin and circulating fibrinogen. Because it is not fibrin specific, concomitant heparin administration is not required. In general, the rate of intracranial hemorrhage (ICH) is lower with SK compared to fibrin-specific thrombolytics, making it a preferred agent in patients with risk factors or intracranial bleeding, such as elderly patients with cerebrovascular disease. Allergic reactions are common with streptokinase, and thus re-exposure to this agent should be avoided.

Alteplase (tPA) is a fibrin-specific thrombolytic agent that was compared to SK in the GUSTO 1 (Global Use of Strategies to Open Occluded Coronary Arteries) trial. This study compared tPA to SK in patients with STEMI. Compared to SK, patients who received an accelerated regimen of tPA had a 15% reduction in 30-day mortality and increased TIMI 3 flow on coronary angiogram (54% vs 31%, $p < 0.001$) [42]. The currently accepted accelerated regimen of tPA is administered as an intravenous bolus dose of 15 mg followed by 0.75 mg/kg (up to 50 mg) infused over 30 minutes and then 0.5 mg/kg infused over 60 minutes.

Reteplase (rPA) is a thirt-generation thrombolytic that is less fibrin specific than alteplase. It was compared to tPA in the GUSTO III trial, which showed no mortality benefit with rPA over tPA [43]. It is administered in two 10 mg boluses given 30 minutes apart. Its ease of administration may make it a preferable agent to tPA.

Tenecteplase (TNK) is another third-generation thrombolytic that is more fibrin specific than rPA. It was compared to tPA in the ASSENT-2 trial. In this study there was no mortality difference between tPA and TNK, although TNK was associated with a significant reduction in noncerebral bleeding (26.4% vs. 29.0%, $p = 0.0003$) [44]. TNK is administered as a single weight-adjusted bolus of 30–50 mg. Its primary advantage is bolus administration.

Percutaneous Coronary Intervention

Percutaneous coronary intervention (PCI) is the preferred method of coronary reperfusion in patients presenting with STEMI. Once the infarct-related artery has been identified, mechanical reperfusion is accomplished through the use of various catheters, wires, balloons, and stents. In the current era, the two approaches to PCI in the setting of STEMI are primary PCI and a pharmacoinvasive strategy. Facilitated PCI, an approach that involves routine thrombolysis of all STEMI patients before PCI, is no longer recommended given the lack of efficacy in randomized trials [45]. Rescue PCI, which refers to PCI in patients who have failed thrombolysis, has been replaced by the pharmacoinvasive strategy [22, 23]. As discussed previously, patients with UA/NSTEMI do not require emergent PCI.

In primary PCI, patients with STEMI are referred for emergent PCI without having received thrombolysis. This is the preferred approach for reperfusion if it can be performed within 120 minutes of FMC [23]. There are considerable data showing the benefit of primary PCI over thrombolysis. A 23-trial meta-analysis of STEMI patients who were randomized to primary PCI or thrombolysis showed a significant reduction in mortality and nonfatal MI with primary PCI. Primary PCI was also associated with a significant reduction in stroke due to a decrease in ICH [46]. Primary PCI is superior to thrombolysis even if it requires transferring the patient to a PCI-capable facility. In the DANAMI-2 (Danish Multicenter Randomized Study on Thrombolytic Therapy Versus Acute Coronary Angioplasty in Acute Myocardial Infarction-2) trial, patients who were randomized to transfer for PCI had a significant reduction in 30-day mortality compared to patients who received thrombolysis (8.5% vs. 14.3%, $p = 0.002$) [47]. The benefit of transfer extends to high-risk STEMI patients. The Air-PAMI (Air-Primary Angioplasty in Myocardial Infarction) trial compared transfer for primary PCI to onsite thrombolysis in high-risk STEMI patients. Patients who were transferred for PCI had a significant reduction in hospital stay (6.1 days vs. 7.5 days, $p = 0.015$) and ischemia (12.7% vs. 31.8%, $p = 0.007$) [48].

In a pharmacoinvasive strategy, patients who present to a non-PCI-capable facility with an expected transfer time of >120 minutes receive thrombolysis and are then immediately transferred for PCI. This management strategy was evaluated in the CARESS-in-AMI (Combined Abciximab REteplase Stent Study in Acute Myocardial Infarction) and TRANSFER-AMI (Trial of Routine Angioplasty and Stenting after Fibrinolysis to Enhance Reperfusion in Acute Myocardial Infarction) trials. In CARESS-in-AMI, patients who received high-dose thrombolytics and abciximab were randomized to immediate transfer for PCI or standard treatment with the possibility of rescue PCI. Patients who were immediately transferred for PCI had a significant reduction in the primary endpoint of death, reinfarction, or refractory ischemia at 30 days (4.4% vs. 10.7%, $p = 0.004$) [49]. Similarly, the TRANSFER-AMI study randomized high-risk STEMI patients who received thrombolysis at a non-PCI-capable facility to either immediate transfer for PCI or standard therapy (including rescue PCI). The primary composite endpoint of death, reinfarction, recurrent ischemia, new or worsening heart failure, and cardiogenic shock was significantly less in the patients who were transferred for PCI (11% vs. 17.2%, $p = 0.004$) [50].

Based on factors discussed previously, patients with UA/NSTEMI can be managed either conservatively with medical therapy or invasively with coronary angiography. Most trials comparing conservative management to an early invasive strategy demonstrate improved outcomes with early coronary angiography. An exception to this is the ICTUS (Invasive versus Conservative Treatment in Unstable Coronary Syndromes) trial, which compared early angiography to initial medical therapy in patients with NSTE-ACS. In this study, there was no benefit of early angiography compared to initial medical management, even in troponin-positive patients [51]. If an invasive strategy is chosen, there does not appear to be an advantage to very early angiography (<24 hrs) except possibly in very high-risk patients. The large, multicenter TIMACS (Timing of Intervention in Acute Coronary Syndromes) trial compared angiography within 24 hours to delayed angiography (≥36 hrs) in patients with UA/NSTEMI. Overall, the primary endpoint of death, new MI, or stroke did not significantly differ between the two groups. However, when patients were analyzed in groups according to risk, high-risk patients had a significant reduction in the primary endpoint by receiving angiography within 24 hrs (13.9% vs. 21%, $p = 0.006$) [52].

Based on the above data, if a patient with STEMI can receive PCI within 120 minutes of FMC, this is the preferred approach. If the anticipated time to PCI is >120 minutes and there are no contraindications, thrombolysis should be performed [23]. After thrombolysis, patients should be transferred to a PCI-capable facility for coronary angiography and subsequent PCI if needed. In high-risk (Table 10.7) patients with UA/NSTEMI, coronary angiography within 24 hours of presentation is reasonable, although a conservative approach is acceptable in patients who stabilize on initial medical therapy.

Coronary Artery Bypass Grafting

The logistical difficulties of mobilizing operating personnel within 90-120 minutes to achieve emergent reperfusion has limited the utility of CABG in STEMI, but it should be strongly considered for STEMI patients with failed PCI, severe left main artery stenosis, and complications of MI such as lateral wall or papillary muscle rupture. Compared to patients with STEMI, patients with UA/NSTEMI are more likely to have multivessel CAD. Fortunately, because these patients require urgent rather than emergent reperfusion, they can be referred for CABG in a timely manner if coronary anatomy is suitable without the concern for decreased myocardial salvage. CABG is a particularly important revascularization strategy in patients with diabetes. A meta-analysis from 10 randomized trials shows that diabetics with multivessel CAD have a significant reduction in long-term (5.9 years) mortality with CABG as compared to PCI (23% vs. 29%, $p = 0.05$) [55].

Late Hospital and Post-Discharge Management
Diabetes Management

There are conflicting data regarding the strategy for glycemic control in the setting of ACS. In the DIGAMI (Diabetes, Insulin Glucose Infusion in Acute Myocardial Infarction) trial, tight glycemic control in STEMI patients using intravenous insulin therapy was associated with a 30% reduction in one-year mortality [56]. Unfortunately, the DIGAMI 2 trial did not confirm these findings, and more recent data suggest increased hypoglycemic events in patients allocated to tight glucose control [15]. The current recommendation is that patients with ACS be treated according to American Diabetes Association (ADA) guidelines with a target blood glucose level of <180 mg/dL [11, 30]. After discharge, the goal HbA1c is <6.5–7% [15, 30].

Antiplatelet Therapy

It is recommended that patients with ACS receive DAPT for one year regardless of whether or not they received PCI [15, 22, 23, 30]. Aspirin should be continued indefinitely at a dose of 81–162 mg. The second antiplatelet agent should be one of the three $P2Y_{12}$ inhibitors at the maintenance doses mentioned above. If ticagrelor is the second antiplatelet agent, the aspirin dose should be no higher than 100 mg [23]. Patients who are allergic to aspirin should be treated indefinitely with 75 mg of clopidogrel [15, 22, 30]. One year of DAPT therapy is not always reasonable due to financial difficulties, bleeding complications, or concomitant warfarin therapy. If these issues exist, and the patient either did not receive coronary artery stenting or received a bare metal stent (BMS), the $P2Y_{12}$ inhibitor can be discontinued after one month. Patients who received a drug-eluting stent (DES) should be treated with 12 months of DAPT to prevent stent thrombosis [23].

Beta-Blockade

The use of beta-blocker therapy in the acute setting was discussed previously. Indefinite beta-blocker therapy is indicated in all patients recovering from ACS, unless there is a contraindication. The beneficial effects of beta-blocker therapy include a reduction in ischemia, arrhythmias, and reduced dilation of the left ventricle. If the patient has moderate to severe left ventricular dysfunction, the beta-blocker should be started at a low dose and titrated up slowly to prevent the development of cardiogenic shock.

Inhibition of the Renin-Angiotensin-Aldosterone System

Angiotensin-converting enzyme inhibitor (ACEI) therapy is indicated for all patients with ACS who have clinical heart failure or a left ventricular ejection fraction (LVEF) $\leq 40\%$. ACEI should also be given to ACS patients with a preserved LVEF who have diabetes, hypertension, or chronic kidney disease [15, 22, 30]. In addition, ESC and AHA guidelines state that it is reasonable to start an ACEI in any patient who presents with ACS. For patients who are intolerant to ACEI therapy, an angiotensin receptor blocker (ARB) can be used. Candesartan and valsartan are the preferred ARBs, because they have demonstrated efficacy in ACS patients.

AMI patients with a LVEF of <40% and either clinical heart failure or diabetes receive added benefit from the addition of aldosterone blockade to an ACEI or ARB. Compared to placebo, the addition of eplerenone decreases mortality and hospitalization for heart failure [57]. Current guidelines recommend the addition of an aldosterone antagonist to any patient with diabetes who presents with ACS and a LVEF <40%, assuming the patient is already receiving therapeutic doses of an ACEI [11, 15, 18]. Eplerenone is not recommended for patients with significant renal dysfunction (GFR ≤ 30) or a serum potassium >5.

Lipid Management

Unless contraindicated, all ACS patients should be treated with an HMG-CoA reductase inhibitor (statin). Furthermore, large-scale clinical trials demonstrate improved ischemic outcomes with intensive compared to standard statin therapy. For example, in the PROVE IT-TIMI 22 (Pravastatin or Atorvastatin Evaluation and Infection Therapy–Thrombolysis in Myocardial Infarction) study, treatment with high-dose lipitor offered a 16% greater reduction in the primary composite endpoint of death, MI, UA, revascularization, and stroke compared to treatment with moderate dose pravastatin [58]. For patients with ACS, the target LDL cholesterol (LDL-C) is <100 mg/dL and preferably <70 mg/dL.

Blood Pressure Control
To help prevent future cardiovascular events, it is important that patients with a history of ACS remain normotensive. This should be accomplished with the combination of an ACEI, beta-blocker, and, if the LVEF is reduced, an aldosterone antagonist. Additional agents may be necessary to reach this goal.

Stress Testing
In ACS patients who do not receive a left heart catheterization, stress testing to assess for myocardial ischemia should be performed prior to or early after discharge. While exercise treadmill testing is preferred, patients with a history of ACS often have baseline ECG abnormalities that prevent the interpretation of ischemia based on ECG alone. In these patients echocardiography or nuclear imaging can aid in the diagnosis of ischemia.

Assessment of Left Ventricular Function
Appropriate prognosis and therapy in ACS patients depend on adequate assessment of the LVEF. This can be accomplished with a TTE. If concurrent disease or patient body habitus prevents adequate assessment of the LVEF by surface echocardiogram, nuclear imaging can be performed.

Prevention of Sudden Cardiac Death
The development of left ventricular scar after myocardial infarction increases the risk for ventricular arrhythmia and sudden cardiac death (SCD). The risk of SCD is inversely proportional to the ejection fraction. Multiple studies have shown a reduction in mortality by the insertion of an implantable cardioverter defibrillator (ICD) in patients who are at high risk for SCD. Current guidelines recommend ICD insertion in patients with an EF ≤35% and NYHA class II–III heart failure or an EF ≤30% and NYHA class I–II heart failure. Because these studies did not show mortality benefit if the ICD was inserted immediately after MI, insertion should be delayed for at least 40 days after infarction and 90 days in patients who received CABG [59]. In the interim, the patient should be managed medically with a beta-blocker, ACEI, and aldosterone antagonist. These therapies may improve the LVEF and eliminate the need for ICD insertion. Assuming that there is no residual ischemia, patients who have hemodynamically significant sustained VT or VF at least 48 hours after MI should receive an ICD without delay [58].

Smoking Cessation

Smoking cessation may be the most effective secondary prevention measure, with the potential to reduce mortality by 33% over 10 years [15]. Before hospital discharge, patients with ACS should receive counseling regarding the hazards of smoking and the benefits of cessation. Counseling should then continue in the outpatient setting. Nicotine supplementation and/or antidepressant therapy can be prescribed to assist patients in their effort to quit smoking.

Weight Control

Weight loss should be encouraged to achieve a goal body mass index (BMI) between 18.5 and 24.9 kg/m^2. The goal waist circumference is <40 inches in men and <35 inches in women. Weight loss should be achieved through a balance of increased physical activity and decreased caloric intake for an initial reduction in body weight of 10%.

Physical Activity

Assuming that there is no residual ischemia, patients can begin exercise training 1–2 weeks after hospital discharge. Patients who are at high risk (multiple comorbidities, reduced LVEF, etc.) may benefit from supervised exercise training in a cardiac rehabilitation program. Under supervision, the target heart rate is 70–85% of the maximum predicted. The target heart rate for unsupervised exercise training is 60–75% of the maximum predicted. Patients should be encouraged to exercise for 30 to 60 minutes at least five days per week.

Conclusion

Patients with diabetes are at high risk for developing coronary artery disease and subsequent ACS. The management of ACS begins with determining the appropriate timing for coronary artery reperfusion. Patients with STEMI or an equivalent should receive emergent reperfusion, preferably with PCI. Patients with UA/NSTEMI can be risk stratified to determine the appropriate timing for coronary angiography. In these patients angiography is used to decide if medical therapy, PCI, or CABG is the preferred treatment strategy. All patients with ACS should be treated with antiplatelet and antithrombin therapy, as well as adjuvant therapy with a statin, ACEI, and beta-blocker. Prior to discharge the focus of care should shift to aggressive risk factor modification, and outpatient follow-up is necessary to ensure that secondary prevention goals are met. Overall, the management of patients with and without diabetes is similar, though the preferred choice of antiplatelet, antithrombin, and reperfusion therapy may differ.

Case Study 1

A 67-year-old female with a history of noninsulin-dependant diabetes mellitus and hypertension presents to your office with episodes of tightness in the center of her chest that began three days prior. She has noted similar discomfort in the past while climbing stairs or steep hills. Three days ago she began feeling chest discomfort while walking around her house. Today the chest discomfort occurred while driving to your office. Physical exam reveals a blood pressure of 160/90 mmHg and a heart rate of 90 bpm. There is no jugular venous distention. She has a soft systolic ejection murmur at the right upper sternal border and her lungs are clear. There is no peripheral edema. An ECG performed in the office reveals normal sinus rhythm with T-wave inversions in the lateral precordial leads. The patient is given four baby aspirin, which she is asked to chew. EMS is called and the patient is transported to the emergency room, where her cardiac biomarkers are within normal limits. She is given the diagnosis of unstable angina and treated with 180 mg of ticagrelor, 80 mg of atorvastatin, intravenous heparin, and a nitroglycerine infusion. She is admitted to the coronary care unit for further observation. Overnight, she continues to have mild, intermittent chest pain, though there is no elevation in her cardiac biomarkers. The next day she is referred for coronary angiography, which reveals thrombus in the proximal left circumflex artery and a resultant 80% stenosis. Otherwise there is moderate, diffuse coronary artery disease, involving the left anterior descending artery and right coronary artery. The patient receives a drug-eluting stent to the proximal left circumflex artery without complication. She is discharged home the following day.

Case Study 2

A 45-year-old male with type 1 diabetes mellitus and hyperlipidemia is shoveling snow from his driveway when he develops crushing, substernal chest pain with radiation to his left jaw. Over 20 minutes, the pain increases in severity and is accompanied by nausea, diaphoresis, and shortness of breath. The patient asks his wife to call a rescue squad, which arrives ten minutes later. When they arrive, the patient is in acute distress, tachypneic, and confused. Vital signs reveal a blood pressure of 85/40 mmHg and a heart rate of 110 bpm. He is given oxygen, 325 mg of aspirin, and transferred to the emergency room. A 12-lead ECG is obtained within five minutes of arrival to the hospital, and reveals 2 mm of ST elevation in leads V1-V5, I, and aVL. The patient is given 60 mg of prasugrel, 4,000 units of intravenous heparin, and taken emergently to the cardiac catheterization lab. Coronary angiography reveals an occluded proximal left anterior descending artery and otherwise normal coronary vessels. He is started on bivalirudin and percutaneous intervention is performed. He receives aspiration thrombectomy, which extracts red thrombus and exposes a severe stenosis. A drug-eluting stent is placed, with subsequent improvement in the patient's hemodynamics. He is admitted to the cardiac intensive care unit for further evaluation and management.

Multiple-Choice Questions

1 Which of the following locations for a myocardial infarction is least likely to cause ST elevation?

   A Anterior

    B Posterior

    C Inferior

    D Lateral

2 What is the strongest predictor of mortality during an ST-elevation myocardial infarction?Prior myocardial infarction

    A Age

    B Insulin-dependent diabetes mellitus

    C Systolic blood pressure >90 mmHg

    D Killip Class

3 Which of the following antiplatelet agents should not be given to patients with a history of stroke?

    A Clopidogrel

    B Ticagrelor

    C Prasugrel

    D Abciximab

Answers provided after the References

Guidelines

Hamm CW, Bassand J, Agewall S et al. ESC Guidelines for the management of acute coronary syndromes in patients presenting without persistent ST-segment elevation: The Task Force for the management of acute coronary syndromes (ACS) in patients presenting without persistent ST-segment elevation of the European Society of Cardiology (ESC). *Eur Heart J* 2011; 32: 2999–3054.

Kushner FG, Hand M, King SB et al. 2009 focused updates: ACC/AHA guidelines for the management of patients with ST-elevation myocardial infarction (updating the 2004 guideline and 2007 focused update) and ACC/AHA/SCAI guidelines on percutaneous coronary intervention (updating the 2005 guideline and 2007 focused update). *J Am Coll Cardiol* 2009; 54: 2205–41.

Levine GN, Bates ER, Blankenship JC et al. 2011 ACCF/AHA/SCAI guideline for percutaneous coronary intervention. A report of the American College of Cardiology Foundation/American Heart Association Task Force on Practice Guidelines and the society for cardiovascular angiography and interventions. *J Am Coll Cardiol* 2011; 58: e44–e122.

Van de Werf F, Bax J, Betrio A et al. Management of acute myocardial infarction in patients presenting with persistent ST-segment elevation. The Task Force on the management of ST-segment elevation acute myocardial infarction of the European Society of Cardiology. *Eur Heart J* 2008; 29: 2909–45.

Wright RS, Anderson JL, Adams CD et al. 2011 ACCF/AHA focused update of the guidelines for the management of patients with unstable angina/non-ST-elevation myocardial infarction (updating the 2007 guideline): A report of the American College of Cardiology Foundation/American Heart Association Task Force on Practice Guidelines developed in collaboration with the American College of Emergency Physicians, Society for Cardiovascular Angiography and Interventions, and Society of Thoracic Surgeons. *J Am Coll Cardiol* 2011; 57: 1920–59.

References

1 Ridker PM, Libby P. Risk factors for atherothrombotic disease. In: Libby P (ed.), *Braunwald's Heart Disease: A Textbook of Cardiovascular Medicine*, 8th edn. Philadelphia: Saunders Elsevier, 2008: 1003–26.

2 Gaede P, Vedel P, Larsen N et al. Multifactorial intervention and cardiovascular disease in patients with type 2 diabetes. *N Engl J Med* 2003; 348: 383–93.

3 Wang K, Asinger RW, Marriott HJ. ST-segment elevation in conditions other than acute myocardial infarction. *N Engl J Med* 2003; 349: 2128–35.

4 Krishnaswamy A, Lincoff AM, Menon V. Magnitude and consequences of missing the acute infarct-related circumflex artery. *Am Heart J* 2009; 158: 706–12.

5 Anderson JL, Adams CD, Antman EM et al. ACC/AHA 2007 Guidelines for the Management of Patients with Unstable Angina/Non-ST-Elevation Myocardial Infarction: A Report of the American College of Cardiology/American Heart Association Task Force on Practice Guidelines (Writing Committee to Revise the 2002 Guidelines for the Management of Patients with Unstable Angina/Non-ST- Elevation Myocardial Infarction). *J Am Coll Cardiol* 2007; 50: e1–157.

6 Topol EJ, Van de Werf FJ. Acute myocardial infarction: Early diagnosis and management. In: Topol EJ, ed. *Textbook of Cardiovascular Medicine*. New York: Lippincott-Raven, 1998.

7 Granger CB, Goldberg RJ, Dabbous O, Pieper KS, Eagle KA, Cannon CP, Van De Werf F, Avezum A, Goodman SG, Flather MD, Fox KA. Predictors of hospital mortality in the Global Registry of Acute Coronary Events. *Arch Intern Med* 2003;163:2345–2353.

8 Lee KL, Woodlief LH, Topol EJ, et al. Predictors of 30-day mortality in the era of reperfusion for acute myocardial infarction. Results from an international trial of 41,021 patients. GUSTO-I Investigators. *Circulation* 1995;91:1659–1668.

9 Morrow DA, Antman EM, Charlesworth A et al. TIMI risk score for ST-elevation myocardial infarction: A convenient, bedside, clinical score for risk assessment at presentation: An intravenous nPA for treatment of infarcting myocardium early II trial substudy. *Circulation* 2000; 102: 2031–7.

10 Antman EM, Cohen M, Bernink P et al. The TIMI risk score for unstable angina/non-ST elevation MI: A method for prognostic and therapeutic decision making. *JAMA* 2000; 284: 835–42.

11 Hamm CW, Bassand J, Agewall S et al. ESC guidelines for the management of acute coronary syndromes in patients presenting without persistent ST-segment elevation: The Task Force for the management of acute coronary syndromes (ACS) in patients presenting without persistent ST-segment elevation of the European Society of Cardiology (ESC). *Eur Heart J* 2011; 32: 2999–3054.

12 Licka M, Zimmermann R, Zehelein J et al. Troponin T concentrations 72 hours after myocardial infarction as a serological estimate of infarct size. *Heart* 2002; 87: 520–4.

13 Cannon CP, Weintraub WS, Demopoulos LA et al. Comparison of early invasive and conservative strategies in patients with unstable coronary syndromes treated with the glycoprotein IIb/IIIa inhibitor tirofiban. *N Engl J Med* 2001; 344: 1879–87.

14 Chen ZM, Pan HC, Chen YP et al. Early intravenous than oral metoprolol in 45,852 patients with acute myocardial infarction: Randomised placebo-controlled trial. *Lancet* 2005; 366: 1622–32.

15 Van de Werf F, Bax J, Betrio A et al. Management of acute myocardial infarction in patients presenting with persistent ST-segment elevation. The Task Force on the management of ST-segment elevation acute myocardial infarction of the European Society of Cardiology. *Eur Heart J* 2008; 29: 2909–45.

16 Antman EM, Hand M, Armstrong PW et al. 2007 Focused Update of the ACC/AHA 2004 Guidelines for the Management of Patients with ST-Elevation Myocardial Infarction. *J Am Coll Cardiol* 2008; 51: 210–47.

17 Miller CD, Roe MT, Mulgund J et al. Impact of acute beta-blocker therapy for patients with non-ST-segment elevation myocardial infarction. *Am J Med* 2007; 120: 685–92.

18 Anderson JL, Adams CD, Antman EM et al. ACC/AHA 2007 Guidelines for the Management of Patients with Unstable Angina/Non-ST-Elevation Myocardial Infarction: A Report of the American College of Cardiology/American Heart Association Task Force on Practice Guidelines (Writing Committee to Revise the 2002 Guidelines for the Management of Patients with Unstable Angina/Non-ST-Elevation Myocardial Infarction). *J Am Coll Cardiol* 2007; 50: e1e157.

19 Theroux P, Taeymans Y, Morissette D et al. A randomized study comparing propranolol and diltiazem in the treatment of unstable angina. *J Am Coll Cardiol* 1985; 5: 717–22.

20 Parodi O, Simonetti I, Michelassi C et al. Comparison of verapamil and propranolol therapy for angina pectoris at rest: A randomized, multiple-crossover, controlled trial in the coronary care unit. *Am J Cardiol* 1986; 57: 899–906.

21 Antman EM, Anbe DT, Armstrong PW et al. ACC/AHA guidelines for the management of patients with ST-elevation myocardial infarction – executive summary. A report of the American College of Cardiology/American Heart Association Task Force on Practice Guidelines (Writing Committee to revise the 1999 guidelines for the management of patients with acute myocardial infarction). *J Am Coll Cardiol* 2004; 44: 671–719.

22 Kushner FG, Hand M, King SB et al. 2009 focused updates: ACC/AHA guidelines for the management of patients with ST-elevation myocardial infarction (updating the 2004 guideline and 2007 focused update) and ACC/AHA/SCAI guidelines on percutaneous coronary intervention (updating the 2005 guideline and 2007 focused update). *J Am Coll Cardiol* 2009; 54: 2205–41.

23 Levine GN, Bates ER, Blankenship JC et al. 2011 ACCF/AHA/SCAI guideline for percutaneous coronary intervention. A report of the American College of Cardiology Foundation/American Heart Association Task Force on Practice Guidelines and the society for cardiovascular angiography and interventions. *J Am Coll Cardiol* 2011; 58: e44–e122.

24 Mehta SR, Yusuf S, Peters RJ et al. Effects of pretreatment with clopidogrel and aspirin followed by long-term therapy in patients undergoing percutaneous coronary intervention: The PCI-CURE study. *Lancet* 2001; 358: 527–33.

25 Mehta SR, Tanguay JF, Eikelboom JW et al. Double-dose versus standard-dose clopidogrel and high dose versus low-dose aspirin in individuals undergoing percutaneous coronary intervention for acute coronary syndromes (CURRENT-OASIS 7): A randomised factorial trial. *Lancet* 2010; 376: 1233–43.

26 Wiviott SD, Braunwald E, McCabe CH et al. Prasugrel versus clopidogrel in patients with acute coronary syndromes: From the TRITON-TIMI 38 investigators. *N Engl J Med* 2007; 357(20): 2001–15.

27 Wallentin L, Becker RC, Budaj A et al. for the PLATO Investigators. Ticagrelor versus clopidogrel in patients with acute coronary syndromes. *N Engl J Med* 2009; 361: 1045–57.

28 Sabatine MS, Cannon CP, Gibson CM et al. Addition of clopidogrel to aspirin and fibrinolytic therapy for myocardial infarction with ST-segment elevation. *N Engl J Med* 2005; 352: 1179–89.

29 Stone GW, Witzenbichler B, Guagliumi G et al. Bivalirudin during primary PCI in acute myocardial infarction. *N Engl J Med* 2008; 358: 2218–30.

30 Wright RS, Anderson JL, Adams CD et al. 2011 ACCF/AHA Focused Update of the Guidelines for the Management of Patients with Unstable Angina/Non-ST-Elevation Myocardial Infarction (Updating the 2007 Guideline): A Report of the American College of Cardiology Foundation/American Heart Association Task Force on Practice Guidelines developed in Collaboration with the American College of Emergency Physicians, Society for Cardiovascular Angiography and Interventions, and Society of Thoracic Surgeons. *J Am Coll Cardiol* 2011; 57: 1920–59.

31 Kastrati A, Mehilli J, Neumann FJ et al. Abciximab in patients with acute coronary syndromes undergoing percutaneous coronary intervention after clopidogrel pretreatment: The ISAR-REACT 2 randomized trial. *JAMA* 2006; 295: 1531–8.

32 Giugliano RP, White JA, Bode C et al. Early versus delayed, provisional eptifibatide in acute coronary syndromes. *N Engl J Med* 2009; 360: 2176–90.

33 Stone GW, Bertrand ME, Moses JW et al. Routine upstream initiation vs deferred selective use of glycoprotein IIb/IIIa inhibitors in acute coronary syndromes: The ACUITY Timing trial. *JAMA* 2007; 297: 591–602.

34 Kastrati A, Neumann F, Schulz S et al. Abciximab and Heparin versus Bivalirudin for non–ST-elevation myocardial infarction. *N Engl J Med* 2011; 365: 1980–89.

35 ASSENT-3 investigators. Efficacy and safety of tenecteplase in combination with enoxaparin, abciximab, or unfractionated heparin: The ASSENT-3 randomised trial in acute myocardial infarction. *Lancet* 2001; 358: 605–13.

36 Antman EM, Morrow DA, McCabe CH et al. Enoxaparin versus unfractionated heparin with fibrinolysis for ST-elevation myocardial infarction. *N Engl J Med* 2006; 354: 1477–88.

37 Cohen M, Demers C, Gurfinkel EP et al. A comparison of low-molecular-weight heparin with unfractionated heparin for unstable coronary artery disease. Efficacy and Safety of Subcutaneous Enoxaparin in Non-Q-Wave Coronary Events Study Group. *N Engl J Med* 1997; 337: 447–52.

38 Antman EM, McCabe CH, Gurfinkel EP et al. Enoxaparin prevents death and cardiac ischemic events in unstable angina/non-Q-wave myocardial infarction: Results of the Thrombolysis In Myocardial Infarction (TIMI) 11B trial. *Circulation* 1999; 100: 1593–601.

39 Ferguson JJ, Califf RM, Antman EM et al. Enoxaparin vs unfractionated heparin in high-risk patients with non-ST-segment elevation acute coronary syndromes managed with an intended early invasive strategy: Primary results of the SYNERGY randomized trial. *JAMA* 2004; 292: 45–54.

40 Yusuf S, Mehta SR, Chrolavicius S et al. Effects of fondaparinux on mortality and reinfarction in patients with acute STE-segment elevation myocardial infarction: The OASIS-6 randomized trial. *JAMA* 2006; 295: 1519–30.

41 Yusuf S, Mehta SR, Chrolavicius S et al. Comparison of fondaparinux and enoxaparin in acute coronary syndromes. *N Engl J Med* 2006; 354: 1464–76.

42 The GUSTO investigators. An international randomized trial comparing four thrombolytic strategies for acute myocardial infarction. *N Engl J Med* 1993; 329: 673–82.

43 The Global Use of Strategies to Open Occluded Coronary Arteries (GUSTO III) Investigators. A comparison of reteplase with alteplase for acute myocardial infarction. *N Engl J Med* 1997; 337: 1118–23.

44 Van De Werf F, Adgey J, Ardissino D et al. Single-bolus tenecteplase compared with front-loaded alteplase in acute myocardial infarction: The ASSENT-2 double-blind randomised trial. *Lancet* 1999; 354: 716–22.

45 Primary versus tenecteplase-facilitated percutaneous coronary intervention in patients with ST-segment elevation acute myocardial infarction (ASSENT-4 PCI): Randomised trial. *Lancet* 2006; 367: 569–78.

46 Keeley EC, Boura JA, Grines CL. Primary angioplasty versus intravenous thrombolytic therapy for acute myocardial infarction: A quantitative review of 23 randomised trials. *Lancet* 2003; 361: 13–20.

47 Andersen HR, Nielsen TT, Rasmussen K et al. A comparison of coronary angioplasty with fibrinolytic therapy in acute myocardial infarction. *N Engl J Med* 2003; 349: 733–742.

48 Grines CL, Westerhausen DR, Jr,, Grines LL et al. A randomized trial of transfer for primary angioplasty versus on-site thrombolysis in patients with high-risk myocardial infarction: The Air Primary Angioplasty in Myocardial Infarction study. *J Am Coll Cardiol* 2002; 39: 1713–19.

49 Di Mario C, Dudek D, Piscione F et al. Immediate angioplasty versus standard therapy with rescue angioplasty after thrombolysis in the Combined Abciximab REteplase Stent Study in Acute Myocardial Infarction (CARESS-in-AMI): An open, prospective, randomised, multicentre trial. *Lancet* 2008; 371: 559–68.

50 Cantor WJ, Fitchett D, Borgundvaag B et al. Routine early angioplasty after fibrinolysis for acute myocardial infarction. *N Engl J Med* 2009; 360: 2705–18.

51 de Winter RJ, Windhausen F, Cornel JH et al. Early invasive versus selectively invasive management of acute coronary syndromes. *N Engl J Med* 2005; 353: 1095–104.

52 Mehta SR, Granger CB, Boden WE et al. Early versus delayed invasive intervention in acute coronary syndromes. *N Engl J Med* 2009; 360: 2165–75.

53 Serruys PW, Morice MC, Kappetein AP et al. Percutaneous coronary intervention versus coronary-artery bypass grafting for severe coronary artery disease. *N Engl J Med* 2009; 360: 961–72.

54 Weintraub WS, Grau-Sepulveda MV, Weiss JM et al. Comparative effectiveness of revascularization strategies. *N Engl J Med* 2012; 366: 1467–76.

55 Hlatky MA, Boothroyd DB, Bravata DM et al. Coronary artery bypass surgery compared with percutaneous coronary interventions for multivessel disease: A collaborative analysis of individual patient data from ten randomised trials. *Lancet* 2009; 373: 1190–97.

56 Malmberg K. Prospective randomised study of intensive insulin treatment on long term survival after acute myocardial infarction in patients with diabetes mellitus. DIGAMI (Diabetes Mellitus, Insulin Glucose Infusion in Acute Myocardial Infarction) Study Group. *Brit Med J* 1997; 314: 1512–15.

57 Pitt B, Remme W, Zannad F et al. Eplerenone, a selective aldosterone blocker, in patients with left ventricular dysfunction after myocardial infarction. *N Engl J Med* 2003; 348: 1309–21.

58 Cannon CP, Braunwald E, McCabe CH et al. intensive versus moderate lipid lowering with statins after acute coronary syndromes. *N Engl J Med* 2004; 350: 1495–504.

59 Epstein AE, DiMarco JP, Ellenbogen KA et al. ACC/AHA/HRS 2008 guidelines for device-based therapy of cardiac rhythm abnormalities: Executive summary. *Circulation* 2008; 117: 2820–40.

Answers to Multiple-Choice Questions

1 B

2 A

3 C

CHAPTER 11

Management of Peripheral Arterial Disease

Rüdiger Egbert Schernthaner[1], Gerit Holger Schernthaner[1] and Guntram Schernthaner[2]

[1] *Medical University of Vienna, Vienna, Austria*
[2] *Rudolfstiftung Hospital Vienna, Vienna, Austria*

Key Points

- Immediate revascularization in highly qualified high-throughput centers for patients with stage III or IV (ischemia, ulcer, gangrene) of peripheral arterial disease.

- Careful planning of interventions in patients with stage II (if only one vessel runoff is identified in preinterventional screening with CT- or MR angiography, an interdisplinary board should discuss the treatment options).

- No surgical procedures in the lower extremity in patients with PAD and diabetes prior to morphological (CT- or MR angiography) and hemodynamical (ABI, toe pressures) assessements.

- Primary amputations only in a leg-for-life situation, after consideration with the patient (bad prognosis after major amputation in patients especially above 80 years of age).

- A high cardiovascular morbidity and mortality rate requires intensified screening for coronary heart disease and cerebral ischmia.

- Strict multimodal pharmacotherapy.

Introduction

The aim of this chapter is to focus on the complex diagnostic and therapeutic stragegies that are necessary to inhibit cardiovascual events, amputations, and life loss. The following case may enlighten the various problems.

A 61-year-old female patient with type 2 diabetes mellitus presents at the outpatient department with a reduced walking distance of 100 meters due to pain in the right calf, corresponding to peripheral arterial disease (PAD)

Managing Cardiovascular Complications in Diabetes, First Edition.
Edited by D. John Betteridge and Stephen Nicholls.
© 2014 John Wiley & Sons, Ltd. Published 2014 by John Wiley & Sons, Ltd.

in stage IIb. The PAD of the patient was already treated in the past with two stents in the right proximal superficial femoral artery. The patient is obese, has hypertension, and suffers from diabetic polyneuropathy and chronic venous insufficiency grade 1. Smoking history shows 80 pack-years (of cigarettes). In addition to her PAD, the patient has undergone cardiac bypass grafting five years ago, had already had a minor stroke, and is on anticoagulant therapy for atrial fibrillation.

Patients with type 2 diabetes have a substantially higher risk of mortality, primarily from cardiovascular disease, than the general population [1]. PAD, referring to atherosclerotic occlusive disease of the lower limb arteries is a common, debilitating complication that correlates with cardiovascular disease mortality [2].

Diabetes is a significant independent risk factor for PAD (odds ratio of 2–3) [3], together with hypertension, cardiovascular disease, hyperlipidemia, smoking, and obesity [3, 4]. The prevalence of PAD in patients with type 2 diabetes has been estimated at 23.5% in a UK population [5], and is strongly dependent on the duration of diabetes [6, 7]. Compared with men without diabetes, the adjusted relative risk of PAD among men with diabetes increased from 1.39 with diabetes duration of 1–5 years' to 4.53 for diabetes of >25 years' duration [7]. Remarkably, a very high prevalence (71%) of PAD was recently reported in 1,462 elderly patients with diabetes (>70 years) in Spain as evaluated by a pathological ABI (ankle-brachial index) [8].

Diabetes Is an Important Risk Factor for Lower-Extremity Amputation

Amputation of the lower limb is one of the most feared adverse health outcomes among patients with diabetes. The result is frequently devastating in terms of social functioning and mood. Amputations are usually preceded by a foot ulcer and the most important factors predicting a poor outcome of these ulcers are the extent of tissue loss, infection, peripheral arterial disease (PAD), and comorbidity [2, 3, 4]. The reasons for a major amputation are limited; the most frequent reasons are critical limb ischemia with rest pain or progressive infection in a leg that cannot be successfully revascularized [5]. Sometimes an immediate amputation is performed because of life-threatening infection or infection with massive tissue loss. In addition, a minor amputation is frequently performed for a forefoot abscess, osteomyelitis, or gangrene of a toe. If other options are exhausted or undesirable, amputation can therefore be a treatment and not a failure.

A prospective study identifying risk factors for lower-extremity amputation (LEA) of 776 US veterans in Seattle shows that peripheral sensory neuropathy, PAD, foot ulcers (particularly if they appear on the same side as the eventual LEA), former amputation, and treatment with insulin are independent risk factors for LEA in patients with diabetes [6]. A recent meta-analysis [7] including 94,640 participants and 1,227 LEA cases reported in 14 studies demonstrated a substantial increase in the risk of LEA associated with glycemia in individuals with diabetes. The overall risk reduction (RR) for LEA was 1.26 (95% CI 1.16–1.36) for each percentage point increase in HbA1c. The estimated RR was 1.44 (95% CI 1.25–1.65) for type 2 diabetes and 1.18 (95% CI 1.02–1.38) for type 1 diabetes. Remarkably, the risk for LEA was not different in patients with diabetes duration < or >10 years.

The presence of PAD is a very important predictor of amputation in patients presenting with the diabetic foot syndrome (DFS). In a recent study [3] investigating a large cohort of diabetic foot patients ($n = 1,088$) treated at centers of excellence in 10 different European countries, the major amputation rate among patients with PAD during a 12-month follow-up was 8%, compared to only 2% among patients without PAD ($p < 0.001$). In two recent studies [4, 9], severe PAD (ankle pressure <50 mmHg or toe pressure <30 mmHg) was a predictor of increased major amputation risk in diabetic patients with neuroischemic or ischemic foot ulcers.

Poor Prognosis of Patients with Diabetes after Amputation

A Scottish study showed that after LEA diabetic subjects had a 55% greater risk of death than those without diabetes [10]. Median time to death (Figure 11.1) was 27.2 months with diabetes versus 46.7 months without diabetes ($p < 0.01$) and survival rate 10 years after amputation was 22.9% in nondiabetic patients but only 8.4% in diabetic patients ($p = 0.0007$). In a recent 10-year follow-up study [11], a first major amputation occured in 38 of 257 (15.4%) patients with diabetic foot ulcers. All but one of these patients had evidence of PAD at inclusion in the study, and 51.4% had severe PAD (ABI <0.4). Cumulative mortalities at year 1, 3, 5, and 10 were 15.4, 33.1, 45.8, and 70.4%, respectively. Significant predictors for death were age, male sex, chronic renal insufficiency, dialysis, and PAD. Thus, although long-term limb salvage in this current series of diabetic foot patients is favorable, long-term survival remains poor, especially among patients with PAD or renal insufficiency.

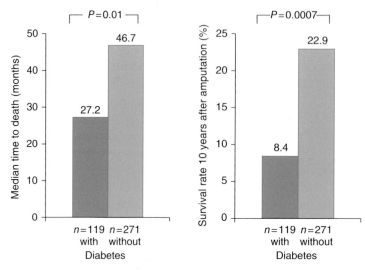

Figure 11.1 Mortality rates of patients with and without diabetes mellitus after amputation. (Source: Data from Schofield 2006 [10].)

Decrease in the Amputation Rates in Patients with Diabetes

For years, the diabetic foot syndrome did not achieve the promise of the 1989 St. Vincence Declaration. In contrast to asthonishing advances in the treatment of diabetic nephropathy, retinopathy, and coronary events, for years the amputation rates remained high.

In very recent years (after 2000) several studies in Scotland [12] and the USA [13, 14] showed a dramatic decrease in amputation rates in patients with diabetes mellitus. The incidence of major amputations in Tayside, Scotland [12] decreased from 5.1 [95% CI 3.8–6.4] to 2.9 (95% CI 1.9–3.8) per 1,000 patients with diabetes ($p < 0.05$) over a seven-year period (2000–06). From 1996 to 2008, the age-adjusted nontraumatic LEA rates among US residents aged ≥ 40 years [14] decreased in diabetic patients by 67% ($p < 0.001$; Figure 11.2). Despite a much greater decrease in LEA rates, the age-adjusted LEA rate in the diabetic population was still about eight times the rate of the nondiabetic population in 2008 (3.9 vs. 0.5 per 1,000 persons). A five-year follow-up of veterans' health administration healthcare system users with diabetes and without prior amputations in 2000 ($n = 405,580$) and in 2004 ($n = 739,377$) showed that the age- and sex-standardized LEA rates decreased by 34% during the five-year period from 2000 to 2005 [14]. Of major amputations, below-knee rates decreased by 19% and above-knee decreased by 49% (Figure 11.3).

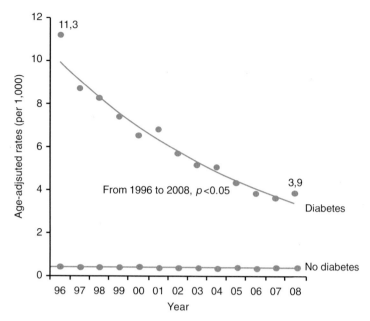

Figure 11.2 Nontraumatic amputations of lower extremities, age-adjusted per 1,000 patients after 40 years of age from 1996–2008 in the USA. (Source: Data from Li 2012 [14].)

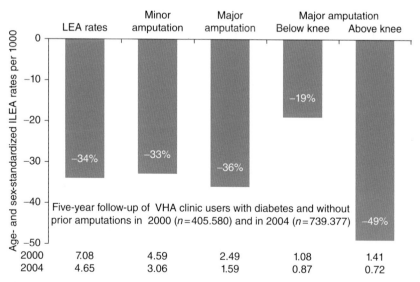

Figure 11.3 Decrease of various amputations from 2000 to 2004 among Veterans' Health Administration health care system users. (Source: Tseng et al. 2011 [13].)

Patients with Type 2 Diabetes and Peripheral Arterial Disease in the PROactive Study

The PROactive study [15] is a double blind interventional study evaluating the effect of pioglitazone versus placebo as add-on therapy to many other cardiovascular preventive drugs. In total 5,238 patients with type 2 diabetes and a history of macrovascular disease were included and followed up for 34.5 months. At baseline, 1,274 patients had PAD and 3,964 had no previous PAD [16]. The PROactive study is a major follow-up study of patients with type 2 diabetes and PAD. Patients with PAD at baseline were older and had a longer median duration of diabetes (10 years versus 8 years in patients with no PAD at baseline). Due to the selection criteria, only 26% and 10% of patients with PAD had a previous myocardial infarction (MI) or stroke, whereas 53% and 22% of patients without PAD had a previous MI or stroke, respectively. Nevertheless, patients with diabetes and PAD at baseline (Figure 11.4) had significantly higher rates of primary and secondary composite cardiovascular disease endpoints, together with higher all-cause mortality and stroke (HR = 1.5–2.0; $p < 0.0001$) compared to those with no PAD. The cardiovascular disease event risk in patients with baseline PAD alone (i.e., with no other macrovascular disease) was similar to that in patients with MI alone. The amputation rate during the 2.8 years' follow-up was 2.7% in the diabetic patients with PAD at baseline versus only 0.4% in those without PAD at baseline (HR = 6.69; $p < 0.0001$).

In the PROactive study [16], pioglitazone did not alter the macrovascular event rate in patients with PAD at baseline; it is unclear why additional PAD modified the treatment effect. Leg revascularization occurred more

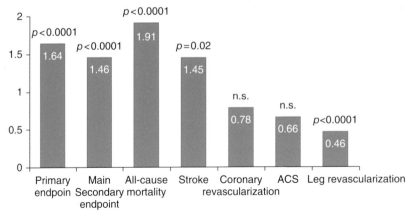

Figure 11.4 Despite strict pharmacotherapy, patients with PAD had higher rates of endpoints compared to those without. (Source: Dormandy et al. 2005 [15]. Reproduced with permission of Elsevier.)

commonly in the pioglitazone group than in the placebo group. The difference in leg revascularization occurred only in patients with PAD at baseline; there was no difference in leg revascularization between the pioglitazone and placebo group in patients who did not have PAD at entry. Moreover, the difference in leg revascularization occurred entirely in the first year.

Remarkably, a very recent secondary analysis [17] of the Bypass Angioplasty Revascularization Investigation 2 Diabetes (BARI 2D) trial showed very promising results, indicating that the risk of new PAD is significantly decreased when insulin-sensitizing drugs (thiazolidinediones or metformin or both) are used instead of insulin-providing drugs (insulin or sulfonylurea or meglitinide). A total of 1,479 BARI 2D participants with normal ABI (0.91–1.30) were eligible for analysis. The following PAD-related outcomes were evaluated: new low ABI ≤0.9, lower-extremity revascularization, lower-extremity amputation, and a composite of the three outcomes. During an average of 4.6 years of follow-up, 303 participants experienced one or more of the outcomes listed above. Incidence of the composite outcome was significantly lower (Figure 11.5) among participants assigned to insulin-sensitizing (IS) therapy than those assigned to insulin-providing (IP) therapy (16.9% vs. 24.1%; p = 0.001). The difference was significant in time-to-event analysis (hazard ratio 0.66 [95% CI 0.51–0.83], p = 0.001) and remained significant after adjustment for in-trial HbA1c (HR 0.76 [95% CI 0.59–0.96], p = 0.02).

As discussed earlier, diabetic patients presenting with PAD have the highest risk for cardiovascular mortality/morbidity. A very new analysis of the association between rosiglitazone use and cardiovascular events among 2,368 patients with diabetes mellitus and coronary artery disease (CAD) in BARI 2D [18] showed totally unexpected results, which started a critical

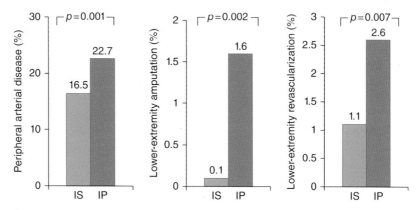

Figure 11.5 These findings clearly indicate the superiority of insulin-sensitizing (IS) versus an insulin-providing (IP) medical therapy for patients with diabetes mellitus and peripheral arterial disease. (Source: Data from Althouse 2013 [17].)

reevaluation of this drug by both the US Food and Drug Administration (FDA) and the European Medicines Agency (EMA). Total mortality, composite death, myocardial infarction, and stroke, the individual incidence of death, myocardial infarction, stroke, congestive heart failure, and fractures, were compared during 4.5 years of follow-up among patients treated with rosiglitazone versus patients not receiving a thiazolidinedione (TZD) by use of Cox proportional hazards and Kaplan–Meier analyses that included propensity matching. After multivariable adjustment among patients treated with rosiglitazone, mortality was similar (HR 0.83; 95% CI 0.58–1.18), whereas a lower incidence of composite death, myocardial infarction, and stroke (HR 0.72; 95% CI 0.55–0.93) and stroke (HR 0.36; 95% CI 0.16–0.86) and a higher incidence of fractures (HR 1.62; 95% CI 1.05–2.51) was observed. The incidence of myocardial infarction (HR 0.77; 95% CI 0.54–1.10) and congestive heart failure (HR 1.22; 95% CI 0.84–1.82) did not differ significantly. Among propensity-matched patients, rates of major ischemic cardiovascular events and congestive heart failure were not significantly different. The authors concluded that among patients with T2DM and CAD in the BARI 2D trial, neither on-treatment nor propensity-matched analysis supported an association of rosiglitazone treatment with an increase in major ischemic cardiovascular events.

Decrease in Mortality in Patients with Peripheral Arterial Disease

Blinc et al. [19] analyzed the survival of 811 patients with PAD (defined by an ABI <0.9) in comparison with 778 control subjects in a two-year follow-up study. Mean age was 65 (SD 9) years at inclusion, with a male/female ratio of 3/2. Diabetes was present in 34% of the PAD patients, but in only 18% of the controls. All patients were treated according to the European guidelines on cardiovascular disease prevention and evaluated yearly for occurrence of death, nonfatal acute coronary syndrome, stroke, or critical limb ischemia (major events) and revascularization procedures (minor events). At baseline, classical risk factors were significantly more prevalent in the PAD group and protective cardiovascular medication was prescribed to patients with PAD more frequently than to control subjects. The overall two-year mortality was only 3.2% in the PAD group and 1.8% in the control group ($p = 0.059$), which is substantially lower than described in a review including older studies of patients with PAD [20]. The groups differed in two-year major event-free survival: 93.5% in PAD vs. 97.1% in controls ($p < 0.017$), as well as in event-free survival: 79.9% in PAD vs. 96.4% in controls ($p < 0.001$). Thus, patients with PAD had a borderline higher risk of all-cause death and a significantly higher risk of major and minor nonfatal cardiovascular events compared to control subjects. However, treatment according to the European guidelines on cardiovascular disease prevention resulted in encouragingly low absolute mortality and morbidity. Unfortunately, the authors did not report data for the diabetic subgroup.

Diagnosis of Peripheral Arterial Disease in Patients with Diabetes

The clinical stage of symptomatic PAD can be classified using the Fontaine staging system [21]. Fontaine stage I represents those who have PAD but are asymptomatic; stages IIa and IIb include patients with mild and moderate-to-severe intermittent claudication, respectively; those with ischemic rest pain are classified in Fontaine stage III; and patients with distal ulceration and gangrene represent Fontaine stage IV.

Diagnosing PAD in patients with diabetes is of clinical importance for two reasons. The first is to identify a patient who has a high risk of subsequent MI or stroke regardless of whether symptoms of PAD are present. Indeed, patients with diabetes and PAD have a fivefold increased risk compared to the presence of either disease alone [22, 23, 24, 25]. An observational study less then ten years ago demonstrated that patients with diabetes and PAD stage IV (=ulcer) have a 100% mortality within six years [26].

The second reason is to elicit and treat symptoms of PAD, which may be associated with functional disability and limb loss. PAD is responsible for the majority of amputations in patients with diabetic foot syndrome in the Western world [6, 27, 28]; in other hemispheres infections, neuropathy, and diabetes per se are still the leading cause. Overall, if PAD is present in patients with diabetic foot syndrome, the likelihood of amputation is four times elevated [23].

PAD is often more subtle in its presentation in patients with diabetes than in those without diabetes. In contrast to the focal and proximal atherosclerotic lesions of PAD found typically in other high-risk patients, in diabetic patients the lesions are more likely to be more diffuse and distal [29, 30, 31]. Importantly, PAD in individuals with diabetes is usually accompanied by peripheral neuropathy with impaired sensory feedback. Thus, a classic history of claudication symptoms may be less common. In addition, diabetic autonomous neuropathy is present as well, so that arterious-venous shunts are opened and severe ischemic legs present warm with rose skin, although their low perfusion (toe pressure < 30 mmHg) should render them pale and cold. Furthermore, Moenkeberg's mediasclerosis – incompressibility of the distal lower arteries – is frequently present in subjects with PAD and diabetes (up to 35%), resulting in false high ankle pressures and thus in a false high ABI. Johnansson et al. demonstrated that severe PAD is nearly doubled if ankle pressures are not measured alone but accompanied by toe pressure measurements [32].

Adler et al. [33] demonstrated the dilemma of a difficult diagnosis when they investigated 2,398 patients of the UKPDS for prevalent PAD. Of the classical trias for PAD, an ABI <0.8, missing distal pulses and claudication, all three were present in only 10 of the 61 patients with later PAD; in other words, in only 16%. Thus a careful inspection of the legs in patients with diabetes is mandatory and screening procedures should include toe pressure measurements.

Ankle-Brachial Index

The ankle-brachial index (ABI), a primary noninvasive screening test for PAD, is an objective measure and a risk-assessment tool with a level of sensitivity that suggests that the method may have greater utility than questionnaires and other noninvasive tools for evaluating PAD [34]. The American College of Cardiology/American Heart Association (ACC/AHA) guidelines recommend that resting ABI should be used to establish PAD diagnosis in patients with suspected PAD (subjects with exertional leg symptoms), with nonhealing wounds, and in those aged ≥70 years or ≥50 years with a history of smoking or diabetes [35, 36].

The ABI is essentially a ratio of Doppler-recorded systolic blood pressure (BP) in the lower and upper extremities and can be easily calculated. Systolic BP is measured using a Doppler stethoscope and BP cuffs on each arm and each ankle [37]. The ACC/AHA guidelines recommend selecting the higher of the two arm pressures (brachial) and the higher of the two ankle pressures (anterior tibial/dorsalis pedis or posterior tibial) to calculate the ABI [35, 36]. Thus, the right ABI = higher right ankle pressure/higher arm pressure; the left ABI = higher left ankle pressure/higher arm pressure. The index leg is generally defined as the leg with the lower ABI.

It is important to note that, because this technique for ABI calculation uses the higher pressure in the lower extremity instead of the lower pressure, it may potentially miss distal disease, thus underestimating the severity and prevalence of PAD. Therefore, several working groups have argued for using the lower of the two ankle pressures. Obviously, such a strategy improves sensitivity but lowers specifity. Nevertheless, in addition to its utility as a screening tool for PAD, where a normal ABI falls in the range of 0.91–1.30, a low ABI at rest (<0.90) indicates a high risk of PAD and provides significant evaluative and prognostic information on cardiovascular risk [38].

As it is a simple, rapid, inexpensive, and reliable method of screening asymptomatic patients for PAD, the ABI test is ideal for implementation in the primary care physician's office. An ABI <0.9 is accepted as an indication of the presence of PAD, while values <0.5 and <0.3 indicate severe disease and critical ischemia respectively [31].

Values >1.4 may be associated with arterial incompressibility due to Mönckeberg's sclerosis, which can be seen in diabetic patients as well as in patients with chronic renal insufficiency.

With any suspicion of incompressibility at the ankle level, the toe brachial index (the ratio of the systolic pressure of the toe to that of the arm) should be used.

Visualization of Peripheral Arterial Disease

As mentioned before, PAD is a clinical diagnosis, based on the patient's history and ankle-brachial index measurement. However, visualization of the peripheral arteries is necessary for the therapeutic management of PAD. As recommended by the TASC II group [38], this visualization should not be limited to the localization of the target lesion itself; instead, the complete peripheral arterial tree, including the in- and out-flow, should be depicted. This is necessary to detect additional yet unknown lesions on one hand, and to identify distal runoff arteries suitable for bypass surgery on the other hand.

For several decades, digital subtraction angiography (DSA) served as the standard diagnostic modality for the visualization of patients with PAD, although it has certain disadvantages: it is an invasive and expensive examination with exposure of both the investigator and the patient to ionizing radiation [39]; moreover, DSA can visualize only the vessel lumen – the composition of vessel plaques and the surrounding structures cannot be evaluated [40].

Duplex Ultra Sonography

The first modality for noninvasive mapping of peripheral arteries was duplex ultrasound, first described in 1985 [41]. Duplex ultrasonography is a safe (no radiation or contrast agent) and cost-effective method to accurately determine the severity and location of stenosis and differentiating stenosis from occlusion [42]. B-mode or grayscale imaging displays a two-dimensional image of the artery wall and lumen, permitting a rough evaluation of the lesion and atheroma characteristics. Color-flow Doppler and pulsed-wave Doppler allow an estimation of stenosis severity on the basis of Doppler-derived velocity criteria [42, 43]. Duplex ultrasonography is an accurate method for determining the degree of stenosis or length of occlusion of the arteries supplying the lower extremity [42, 43, 44].

Although ultrasound is inexpensive and widely available, it is of limited value, being strongly dependent on investigator expertise. In addition, with the improvement in read-out MR and CT angiography, as well as fewer complications due to technical developments (less radiation, better contrast agents), duplex sonography is now considered a better pre-interventional screening technique. Before complex interventional procedures (and this is normally the case in a patient with diabetes and PAD or even a full-blown diabetic foot syndrome), CT or MR angiographies are now mandatory in order to safely plan a crural intervention in the catheterization laboratory or a femoral-pedal bypass graft. Furthermore, the sensitivity of stenosis detection was shown to decrease in the presence of additional stenosis in adjacent vessel segments [45, 46], but multiple stenoses are the normal finding in patients with diabetes and PAD [23].

Magnetic Resonance Angiography

The next noninvasive modality for the depiction of peripheral arteries is magnetic resonance (MR) angiography, which vastly improved with the development of rapid [47, 48], gadolinium-enhanced acquisition sequences, as well as multistation and hybrid protocols [49, 50] and surpassed duplex ultrasound sonography with regard to stenosis detection sensitivity [51].

Despite the rare occurrence of nephrogenic systemic fibrosis (NSF) in patients with renal failure after exposition to MR contrast media containing gadolinium chelates [52], contrast-enhanced MR angiography can still be performed in such patients using certain macro-cyclic gadolinium chelates, as recommended by the ESUR [53]. In addition, thanks to a recently developed MR sequence, nonenhanced MR angiography was shown to be as accurate as enhanced MR angiography [54]. However, this study consisted only of 25 patients; larger patient cohort studies need to be performed to confirm these results.

Finally, the use of MR angiography is limited by other contraindications such as certain cardiovascular devices (e.g. pacemakers) [55] present in a high percentage of diabetic patients due to cardiovascular comorbidities.

The quality of MR angiography has improved so that it has replaced diagnostic angiography in determining what type of intervention is feasible. The accuracy of MR angiography in identifying small runoff vessels meets or exceeds that of traditional catheter-based angiography [56]. With current technology, contrast-enhanced three-dimensional MR angiography has a sensitivity of approximately 90% and a specificity of approximately 97% in the detection of hemodynamically significant stenoses in any of the lower-extremity arteries as compared to digital subtraction angiography [57].

Computed Tomographic Angiography

The latest noninvasive modality for evaluation of patients with PAD is computed tomography (CT) angiography, which became useful with the clinical availability of multidetector CT scanners [58] and yielded highly accurate stenosis detection comparable to DSA [59].

Compared to MR angiography, CT angiography provides higher image resolution and faster image acquisition [60], both being very important for the artefact-free depiction of the lower-leg arteries of diabetic patients with severe PAD and restless legs syndrome, the latter being highly associated with diabetes mellitus type 2 [61]. Consequently, insufficient depiction of peripheral arteries is more common in MR angiography (Figure 11.6), particularly in the lower leg [62] and in the presence of endovascular stents [63], although it seems that the depiction of the in-stent lumen in MR angiography might improve with the use of blood-pooling contrast agents [64]. On the other hand, vessel wall calcifications that are highly associated with diabetes mellitus [65] decrease the diagnostic sensitivity of CT angiography (Figure 11.7). However, the information on the presence of calcification is highly important for surgical procedures such as bypass grafting, in particular in the area of the landing zone of the distal anastomosis and the clamping of the original vessel. One promising solution to this problem might be dual-energy CT scanning, which is currently under evaluation [66].

In addition, CT angiography has been shown to be more cost-effective than MR angiography [67] and DSA [68], although postprocessing for the generation of 3D reformations is mandatory [69], such as bone segmentation for maximum-intensity projections (MIP) and vessel tracking for multipath curved planar reformations (mpCPR) [70]. The main disadvantage of CT angiography is the use of ionizing radiation and potentially nephrotoxic contrast agents, the latter being particularly important in diabetic patients with nephropathy. At the moment, there are several efforts to reduce the required dose of radiation and contrast agents while maintaining diagnostic image quality by using automatic dose modulation and iterative reconstruction algorithms [71]. For the time being, CT angiography may be considered the gold standard for planning of peripheral crural interventions or bypass grafts [72].

Treatment Strategies in Diabetic Patients with Peripheral Arterial Disease

The aims in the management of the diabetic patient with PAD is to improve symptoms and to prevent cardiovascular morbidity and mortality.

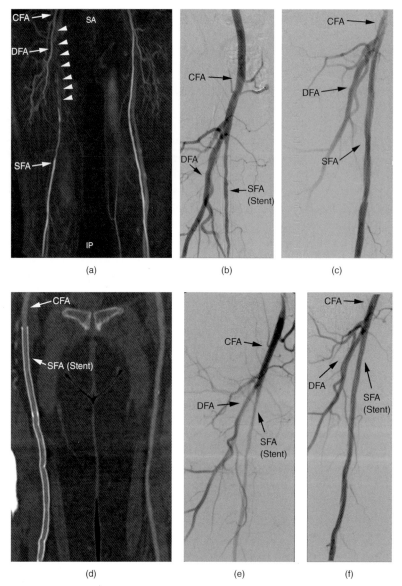

Figure 11.6 Although the patient described at the beginning of this chapter had already been treated with two stents in the symptomatic extremity, an MR angiography was performed, where the in-stent lumen (white arrowheads) was not assessable and seemed occluded (a). At DSA a few days later, the in-stent lumen presented with high-grade stenosis, but patent (b). The in-stent stenosis was treated with percutaneous transluminal angioplasty (PTA) (c). Due to the chronic progressive nature of PAD, the patient returned one year later, again with a reduced walking distance of 150 meters due to pain in the right calf. This time, CT angiography was performed. The curved planar reformations accurately depicted the in-stent-stenosis (d), which was confirmed at DSA (e) prior to PTA (f) a few days later. CFA, common femoral artery; DFA, deep femoral artery; SFA, superficial femoral artery.

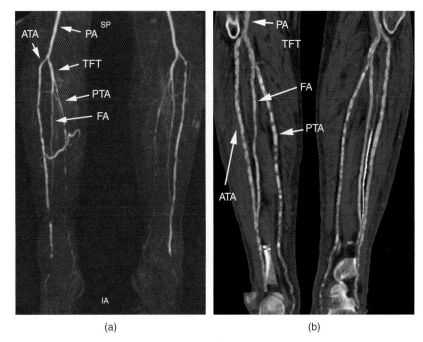

(a)   (b)

Figure 11.7 A 66-year-old male diabetic patient with chronic renal failure and hypertension presents at the outpatient department with PAD stage IV. The fourth toe on the right side was amputated in the past, and now the patient presents with ulceration at the amputation margin. MR angiography (a) clearly depicts the vessels on the lower leg, whereas the reformations of the CT angiography performed one month later (b) are of limited usability due to severe vessel wall calcifications. ATA, anterior tibial artery; FA, fibular artery; PA, popliteal artery; PTA, posterior tibial artery; TFT, tibiofibular trunk.

Treatment of PAD consists of three stages: lifestyle and risk factor modifications, drug therapy, and vascular interventions.

Lifestyle Modifications

Lifestyle modifications are the first step to improve metabolic and lipid abnormalities. Smoking cessation is very important, since cigarette smoking is the single most important risk factor for the development of atherosclerosis. Physical exercise improves exercise tolerance and most of the studies have shown at least a doubling in walking distance [73]. It is noteworthy that these changes were found without significant improvement in blood flow, but exercise increases cardiovascular fitness, oxidative enzyme activities, nitric oxide production, and insulin sensitivity, enhances utilization of fatty acids in calf muscles, and improves walking biomechanics as well as blood rheology. Exercise training leads to modest reductions in blood pressure, cholesterol, and glucose levels.

Rationale for Aggressive Treatment of cardiovascular Risk Factors in Peripheral Arterial Disease: Many Patients have Atherosclerosis in Other Vascular Beds

The majority of patients with early PAD are either asymptomatic or have atypical leg symptoms, with "classical" claudication in only 10–35%, therefore detection is elusive unless actively sought. Given shared risk factors, it is axiomatic that there exists a high coprevalence of atherosclerosis in other vascular beds, including the coronary arteries in PAD patients [74]. The prevalence of CAD in PAD patients ranged from 14% to 90%, which clearly reflects differences in sensitivity of the detection technique for CAD. CAD was present in 19% to 47% of PAD patients in studies using clinical history plus ECG; in 62% to 63% using stress tests (modified stress ECG or dipyridamole-stress thallium); and in 90% of subjects when coronary angiography was used [74]. Similarly, the prevalence of cerebrovascular disease (CVD) in PAD is a direct function of the sensitivity of CVD assessment. Thus, comorbid carotid stenosis >30% was reported in 51% to 72% of subjects with PAD and stenosis >70% in 25% of patients with PAD [74].

In the more advanced stage of PAD, patients may experience a multitude of problems, such as claudication, ischemic rest pain, ischemic ulcerations, repeated hospitalizations, revascularizations, and limb loss. This may lead to a poor quality of life and a high rate of depression. From the standpoint of the limb, the prognosis of patients with PAD is favorable in that the claudication remains stable in 70–80% of patients over a 10-year period. However, the rate of myocardial infarction, stroke, and cardiovascular death in patients with both symptomatic and asymptomatic PAD is markedly increased.

Recommendations for Secondary Prevention and CV Risk Reduction in PAD

As outlined earlier, patients with PAD are at a high risk of cardiovascular events and therefore benefit from aggressive secondary prevention. Current guidelines for secondary prevention and risk-reduction therapy in patients with type 2 diabetes and PAD (Table 11.1) recommend antihypertensive therapy to achieve a systolic blood pressure <140 mmHg, lipid-lowering therapy with statins to achieve a goal low-density lipoprotein (LDL) <100 mg/dl (or <70 mg/dl in high-risk patients), lowering of HbA1c to <7.0%, and antiplatelet therapy. Despite these guidelines, many cross-sectional studies, registries, and surveys have consistently shown that utilization of proven cardioprotective medication for secondary prevention in patients with PAD significantly lags behind CAD. The reasons for this gap in treatment aggressiveness for atherosclerosis in the periphery remain unclear.

Table 11.1 Secondary prevention to reduce cardiovascular events in PAD.

Lipid-lowering	Treatment with statin for all PAD patients to target LDL therapy cholesterol <100 mg/dl
	Target LDL cholesterol <70 mg/dl for high-risk patients
Hypertension treatment	Treat to target blood pressure <140/90 mmHg
	Consider ACE inhibitor in hypertensive patients
	Use of beta-blockers is not contraindicated in PAD
Diabetes control	Target HbA1c <7.0% (or 7.5% in elderly patients with comorbidity)
Smoking cessation	Provide comprehensive smoking intervention program
	Consider pharmacotherapy to support smoking cessation
Antiplatelet therapy	Treat with aspirin 75–325 mg or clopidogrel 75 mg
	Treat with aspirin plus thienopyridine in patients with acute coronary syndrome or coronary or peripheral stent

Underutilization of Cardioprotective Drugs in Patients with Peripheral Arterial Disease

Many studies have documented that secondary prevention is underused in patients with PAD [75, 76, 77, 78, 79, 80]. In a Danish population-based follow-up study between 1997 and 2003, only 26% of patients with lower-limb PAD ($n = 3,424$) used antiplatelet drugs, 10% statins, 22% ACE inhibitors/AT-II receptor antagonists, and 13% beta-blockers compared with 55%, 46%, 42%, and 78% respectively among patients with MI ($n = 1,927$) within 180 days after hospital discharge [75]. The authors concluded that efforts to further increase secondary prevention among patients with PAD are urgently needed.

In the REACH Registry [76], risk factor (RF) management was analyzed in >68,000 outpatients with established atherothrombotic disease. RF control was less frequent in patients with PAD ($n = 8,322$), compared to those presenting with either CAD or CVD (but no PAD, $n = 47,492$). Patients with isolated PAD received a statin in 50% and antiplatelet medication in 76% versus 70% and 84% of patients in the other high-risk disease groups. The use of ACE inhibitors was even lower, prescribed in only 33% of PAD patients versus 45–50% in other groups.

The use of cardioprotective medications was recently analyzed [77] in a very large longitudinal Danish population-based study (2000–07) by comparing three groups of patients: PAD alone ($n = 34,160$), PAD with history of CAD ($n = 9,570$), and patients with incident CAD alone ($n = 154,183$). Use of medications improved temporally among both groups: for PAD alone, any antiplatelet use increased from 29% to 59% from 2000 to 2007 ($p < 0.0001$), while statin use increased sixfold (9% to 56%, $p < 0.0001$). However, use of these therapies at 18 months after incident diagnosis for both PAD groups remained modest and lower compared to

CAD alone. Relative to CAD alone, patients with PAD alone were less likely to use any antiplatelet therapy (adjusted odds ratio [OR] 0.50; 95% CI 0.49–0.52), statins (adjusted OR 0.50; 95% CI 0.48–0.52) or ACE inhibitors (adjusted OR 0.51; 95% CI 0.49–0.53) at 18 months. The authors concluded that despite improvement in use of cardioprotective medications over time, patients with PAD alone remain less likely than those with CAD alone to use these agents.

A recent analysis of the National Health and Nutrition Examination Survey (NHANES) 1999–2004 indicated that millions of US adults with PAD, defined as an ABI <0.90, are not receiving secondary prevention therapies, despite treatment with multiple therapies being associated with reduced all-cause mortality [78]. Of 7,458 eligible participants >40 years, weighted PAD prevalence was 5.9%, corresponding to about 7.1 million US adults with PAD. Statin use was reported in only 30.5%, ACE/ARB use in 24.9%, and aspirin use in 35.8%, corresponding to 5.0 million adults with PAD not taking statins, 5.4 million not taking ACE/ARB, and 4.5 million not receiving aspirin. Remarkably, among PAD subjects without known CAD, the use of multiple preventive therapies was associated with 65% lower all-cause mortality (HR 0.35; $p = 0.02$). In a recent large retrospective cohort study [81] of 83,953 patients with type I and type 2 diabetes mellitus, 217 (0.3%) patients experienced a major lower-extremity amputation (LEA) and 11,716 (14.0%) patients experienced an LEA or death (treatment failure) after a mean follow-up of 4.6 years. Compared to patients who did not use cholesterol-lowering agents, statin users were 35% to 43% less likely (Figure 11.8) to experience LEA (HR 0.65; 95% CI 0.42–0.99) and treatment failure (HR 0.57; 95% CI 0.54–0.60). Users of other cholesterol-lowering medications were not significantly different in LEA risk (HR 0.95; 95% CI 0.35–2.60), but had a 41% lower risk of treatment failure (HR 0.59; 95% CI 0.51–0.68). This is the first study to report a significant association between statin use and diminished amputation risk among patients with diabetes.

PROactive [16] was the first "diabetes" study that gave information about the use of cardiovascular protective drugs focused on patients with type 2 diabetes and presenting with or without PAD. Table 11.2 summarizes the findings of 1,274 patients with PAD versus 3,964 patients without PAD but with CAD (53%) or stroke (23%) at baseline of PROactive. Antiplatelet drugs and aspirin as well as statins were significantly less used in patients with PAD versus those presenting with other vascular diseases but not with PAD (statins 34% vs. 46%, $p < 0.001$; aspirin 63% vs. 76%, $p < 0.001$). The low utilization rate of cardioprotective drugs in type 2 diabetic patients with PAD in PROactive may be partially explained by the fact that almost 60% of the patients recruited for PROactive came from Eastern European countries.

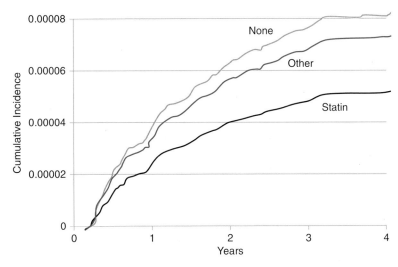

Figure 11.8 Despite the very mild diabetogenic effects of statins, patients with statin therapy for lipid management are at lowest risk for amputation compared to no or other lipid-lowering treatments. (Source: Sohn et al. 2013 [81]. Reproduced with permission of Elsevier.)

Table 11.2 Use of cardioprotective drugs in type 2 diabetic patients with PAD or with no PAD at baseline of PROactive. (Source: Dormandy JA et al. 2009 [16]. Reproduced with permission of Elsevier.)

	PAD at baseline	No PAD at baseline	p value
n	1,274	3,964	
Cardiovascular medication (%)	90	96	<0.0001
Beta-blockers (%)	38	60	<0.0001
ACE inhibitors (%)	63	63	NS
Angiotension II antagonists (%)	7	7	NS
Calcium channel blockers (%)	36	35	NS
Nitrates (%)	26	44	<0.0001
Thiazide diuretics (%)	17	16	NS
Loop diuretics (%)	14	14	NS
Antiplatelet medication (%)	76	86	<0.0001
Aspirin (%)	63	76	<0.0001
Lipid-lowering medication (%)	45	54	<0.0001
Statins (%)	34	46	<0.0001
Fibrates (%)	14	10	<0.0001

A nationwide Spanish study [79] in tertiary diabetes centers demonstrated very similar findings in patients with type 2 diabetes mellitus. Patients with undiagnosed PAD had higher LDL-cholesterol (2.9 ± 0.83 vs. 2.4 ± 0.84 mmol/l; $p < 0.001$) and systolic BP (150 ± 20 vs. 145 ± 21 mmHg; $p < 0.001$) compared to the CAD/CVD group. In addition, they were less likely to take statins (56.9 vs. 71.6%; $p < 0.001$), antihypertensive agents (75.9 vs. 90.1%, $p = 0.001$), and antiplatelet agents (aspirin, 28.7 vs. 57.2%; $p < 0.001$; clopidogrel, 5.6 vs. 20.9%; $p < 0.001$), and more likely to smoke (21.0 vs. 9.2%; $p < 0.001$).

Observational Outcome Data of Cardiovascular Risk Factor Control Show Benefit in Patients with Peripheral Arterial Disease

In the post hoc analysis of the ABCD trial [80], intensive (128/75 mmHg) versus moderate (137/81 mmHg) blood pressure lowering was effective in reducing the risk of cardiovascular events in normotensive diabetic patients with PAD, irrespective of whether a calcium channel blocker or an ACE inhibitor was used. However PAD, defined as an ABI <0.90 at baseline visit, was diagnosed in only 53 of the 480 normotensive patients with type 2 diabetes. In patients with PAD, three cardiovascular events occured (13.6%) with intensive treatment compared with 12 events (38.7%) on moderate treatment ($p = 0.046$). The recently performed post hoc analysis of the INVEST study [82] confirmed the particularly high risk of diabetic patients with PAD, as previously reported in the PROactive study [16]. A J-shaped relationship was observed among 2,599 PAD patients (41% had diabetes) and average treated blood pressure, which was most evident with systolic blood pressure (Figure 11.9). The best outcomes (lowest HR for the primary outcome) were observed with a systolic blood pressure of 135–145 mmHg and a diastolic blood pressure of 60–90 mmHg. Although few data exist,

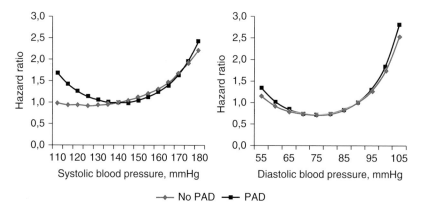

* All-cause death, nonfatal myocardial infarction, or nonfatal stroke

Figure 11.9 Whereas in patients without peripheral arterial disease, the lowest systolic but not diastolic blood pressure seems to be justified, in patients with peripheral arterial disease, too low systolic *and* diastolic blood pressure goals seem to be unjustified. (Source: Bavry et al. 2010 [82]. Reproduced with permission of Wolters Kluwer Health.)

recent guidelines advocate treating hypertension among patients with PAD to a target blood pressure of 130/80 mmHg [83]. These results may challenge the earlier recommendation; however, only a randomized trial can adequately answer this question.

In an Irish prospective study [84], HbA1c was measured in 165 consecutive patients (26% with and 74% without diabetes) undergoing emergency and elective vascular surgical procedures over a six-month period. In patients without diabetes, those with suboptimal HbA1c levels (6–7%) had a significantly higher incidence of overall 30-day morbidity compared to patients with HbA1c levels <6% (56.5 vs 15.7%; $p < 0.001$). Similarly, for patients with diabetes, those with suboptimal HbA1c levels (HbA1c >7%) had a significantly higher incidence of 30-day morbidity compared to those with HbA1c levels <7% (59.1% vs 19%; $p = 0.018$).

Very recently, a large 10-year Japanese follow-up study [85] demonstrated a strong impact of diabetes and glycaemic control on PAD in 1,513 patients with end-stage renal disease (ESRD), who had just begun hemodialysis therapy. As expected, the 10-year event-free rate for development of PAD and lower-limb amputation was significantly higher in the diabetes group than in the nondiabetes group (60% vs 83%, HR 2.99; $p <$ 0.0001 and 94% vs 99%, HR 5.59; $p = 0.0005$ for PAD and lower-limb amputation, respectively). In patients with diabetes, quartile analysis of HbA1c levels showed that the highest-quartile group ($\geq$6.8%) had significant development of PAD and lower-limb amputation compared with lower-quartile groups (PAD: HR 1.63; $p = 0.0038$; lower-limb amputation: HR 2.99; $p = 0.023$). Thus, diabetes was a strong predictor of PAD after initiation of hemodialysis therapy in patients with ESRD. In addition, higher HbA1c levels were associated with increased risk of developing PAD and requiring limb amputation in the Japanese diabetic ESRD population.

In the PREVENT III [86] cohort, 1,404 patients with CLI who underwent lower-extremity bypass grafting were followed up in a prospective trial over a period of one year. In this cohort 636 patients (45%) were taking statins, 835 (59%) were taking beta-blockers, and 1,121 (80%) were taking antiplatelet drugs. Statin use was associated with a significant survival advantage at one year of 86% vs. 81% (HR 0.71; $p = 0.03$), whereas use of beta-blockers and antiplatelet drugs had no appreciable impact on survival. None of the drug classes was associated with graft patency measures at one year. Significant predictors of one-year mortality were statin use (HR 0.67; $p = 0.001$), age >75 (HR 2.1; $p = 0.001$), CAD (HR 1.5; $p = 0.001$), and chronic kidney disease stage 4 (HR 2.0; $p = 0.001$).

These findings are consistent with other observational studies that have examined the effects of statins in PAD populations. In the largest study by Feringa et al. [87], in which 1,374 patients with PAD were monitored for a mean duration of 6.4 years, a strong independent association was observed between statin use and all-cause mortality (HR 1.41 for nonusers; $p < 0.0001$).

A subgroup analysis of the Heart Protection Study (HPS) focusing specifically on 6,748 patients with documented PAD [88] did not include mortality data. However, the authors demonstrated a significant relative reduction of 22% in the rate of a first major vascular event in the simvastatin treatment arm ($p = 0.0001$) compared with placebo.

A Cochrane review about lipid lowering by different drugs for PAD (of the lower limb) published in 2007 [89] included 10,049 participants from 18 trials. The pooled results from all 18 trials indicated that lipid-lowering therapy had no statistically significant effect on overall mortality (OR 0.86; 95% CI 0.49–1.50) or on total cardiovascular events (OR 0.8; 95% CI 0.59–1.09).

However, subgroup analysis with the exclusion of the Probucol Quantitative Regression Swedish Trial (PQRST) [90] showed that lipid-lowering therapy significantly reduced the risk of total CV events (OR 0.74; 95% CI 0.55–0.98) and of total coronary events (OR 0.76; 95% CI 0.67–0.87).

Pooling of the results from trials indicated an improvement in total walking distance and pain-free walking distance, but no significant impact on ankle brachial index. The failure of probucol to affect femoral atherosclerosis despite LDL-cholesterol lowering in PRST may be explained by lowering of HDL2b [91].

How Aggressively Should We Lower Blood Pressure and LDL-Cholesterol Levels in Patients with Type 2 Diabetes and PAD?

Because diabetes increases cardiovascular disease risk by two to three times [92], most hypertension and diabetes practice guidelines have recommended aggressive goals for drug treatment in patients with diabetes and hypertension of 130/80 mmHg [93, 94]. Although observational studies suggest that lower blood pressure is associated with a lower risk for cardiovascular disease, lowering of blood pressure with drugs might not reduce the risk to that of people with lifelong low blood pressure. Very recently, the ACCORD-BP (Action to Control Cardiovascular Risk in Diabetes Blood Pressure) study [95] has clearly shown that only a few patients benefit from lowering systolic blood pressure below 120 mmHg, although those who do reach this goal reduce their risk of stroke, the most devastating and feared complication of hypertension. However, the ADVANCE (Action in Diabetes and Vascular Disease: Preterax and Diamicron Modified-Release Controlled Evaluation) trial [96] suggested goals of around 135/85 mmHg for patients with diabetes. Guidelines will probably go for the more conservative approach, and recommend achieving blood pressures of lower than 140/90 mmHg, preferably around

135/85 mmHg, and for the higher-risk patients close to 130/80 mmHg, but not lower [97]. For those at high risk of stroke, lower blood pressure goals might be recommended. However, aggressive BP lowering to under 120 mmHg was associated with a significant increase of mortality and cardiovascular events in high-risk patients with type 2 diabetes [98, 99].

A recent metaanalysis [100] of 37,736 patients with type 2 diabetes in 13 randomized controlled trials in the period between 1965 and 2010 demonstrated that intensive BP lowering (<130 mmHg) versus standard BP lowering (<140 mmHg) decreased all-cause mortality by 10% (OR 0.90; 95% CI 0.83–0.98) and stroke by 17% (OR 0.83; 95% CI 0.73–0.95) during a follow-up period of about five years. However, intensive BP lowering had no effect on myocardial infarction, heart failure, or ESRD. Remarkably, more intensive BP control (≤130 mmHg) was associated with a 40% increase in serious adverse events(OR 1.40; 95% CI 1.19–1.64; $p < 0.01$).

The Effect of Antiplatelet Drugs Cardiovascular Outcomes in Patients with Peripheral Artery Disease

Antiplatelet drugs that have been shown to reduce the incidence of vascular death, nonfatal myocardial infarction, and nonfatal stroke in patients with PAD are aspirin, ticlopidine, and clopidogrel [101]. Aspirin plus dipyridamole has not been proven to be more efficacious than aspirin alone in the treatment of patients with PAD [101]. The Antithrombotic Trialists' Collaboration Group (ATCG) reported a meta-analysis of 26 randomized studies of 6,263 patients with intermittent claudication due to PAD [101]. At follow-up, the incidence of vascular death, nonfatal myocardial infarction, and nonfatal stroke was 6.4% in patients randomized to antiplatelet drugs vs. 7.9% in the control group. A significant reduction of 23% caused by antiplatelet therapy. The ATCG also reported a meta-analysis of 12 randomized studies of 2,497 patients with PAD undergoing peripheral arterial grafting [101]. At follow-up, the incidence of vascular death, nonfatal myocardial infarction, and nonfatal stroke was 5.4% in patients randomized to antiplatelet drugs vs. 6.5% in the control group, a significant reduction of 22% caused by antiplatelet therapy. Furthermore, the ATCG reported a meta-analysis of four randomized studies of 946 people with PAD undergoing peripheral angioplasty [101]. At follow-up, the incidence of vascular death, nonfatal myocardial infarction, and nonfatal stroke was 2.5% in patients randomized to antiplatelet drugs vs. 3.6% in the control group, a significant reduction of 29% due to by antiplatelet therapy. These data favor the use of aspirin in men and women with PAD [101].

A post hoc analysis of the 3,096 patients with PAD in the Clopidogrel for High Atherothrombotic Risk and Ischemic, Management, and Avoidance (CHARISMA) trial, a primary prevention study, showed that the primary endpoint of cardiovascular death or nonfatal myocardial infarction or non-fatal stroke was insignificantly reduced, by 15% from 8.9% in patients treated with aspirin plus placebo to 7.6% in patients treated with aspirin plus clopidogrel [102]. In the Clopidogrel vs. Aspirin in Patients at Risk for Ischaemic Events (CAPRIE) trial, a secondary prevention study, about 12,000 patients with PAD were randomized to either clopidogrel 75 mg or aspirin 325 mg daily [103]. At 1.9-year follow-up, the annual incidence of vascular death, nonfatal myocardial infarction, and nonfatal stroke was 3.7% in patients randomized to clopidogrel vs. 4.9% in those randomized to aspirin, a 24% significant decrease with the use of clopidogrel [103].

The Scottish POPADAD trial [104], tested whether aspirin and antioxidant therapy, combined or alone, are more effective than placebo in reducing the development of cardiovascular events in patients with diabetes mellitus and asymptomatic PAD. In total, 1,276 adults with type 1 or type 2 diabetes and an ABI <0.99 or less but no symptomatic cardiovascular disease were included. The results obtained in the POPADAD trial do not provide evidence to support the use of aspirin or antioxidants in primary prevention of cardiovascular events and mortality in diabetic patients with asymptomatic PAD.

Similarly, the Aspirin for Asymptomatic Atherosclerosis trial showed in 3,350 patients without clinical cardiovascular disease who had an ABI ≤0.95 based on screening that compared to placebo, aspirin 100 mg daily did not reduce vascular events [105].

Antiplatelet and Anticoagulant Drugs for Prevention of Restenosis/Reocclusion Following Peripheral Endovascular Treatment

Very recently a Cochrane review [106] analyzed whether any antithrombotic drug is more effective in preventing restenosis or reocclusion after peripheral endovascular treatment, compared to another antithrombotic drug, no treatment, placebo, or other vasoactive drugs. In total, 22 trials with 3,529 patients were included. At six months' postintervention, a statistically significant reduction in reocclusion was found for high-dose acetylsalicylic acid (ASA) combined with dipyridamole (DIP; OR 0.40; 95% CI 0.19–0.84), but not for low-dose ASA combined with DIP (OR 0.69; 95% CI 0.44–1.10; $p = 0.12$), nor in major amputations for lipo-ecraprost (OR 0.89; 95% CI 0.44–1.80). At 12 months postintervention, no statistically significant difference in reocclusion/restenosis was detected for any of the following comparisons: high-dose ASA versus low-dose ASA (OR 0.98; $p = 0.91$), ASA/DIP versus vitamin K antagonists (VKA), clopidogrel and aspirin versus low molecular weight heparin (LMWH) plus warfarin (OR 0.31; 95% CI 0.06–1.68; $p = 0.18$), suloctidil versus VKA: reocclusion (OR 0.59; 95% CI 0.20–1.76; $p = 0.34$), restenosis (OR 1.87; 95%

CI 0.66–5.31; $p = 0.24$), and ticlopidine versus VKA (OR 0.71; 95% CI 0.37–1.36; $p = 0.30$). Treatment with cilostazol resulted in statistically significantly fewer reocclusions than ticlopidine (OR 0.32; 95% CI 0.13–0.76; $p = 0.01$). Compared to aspirin alone, LMWH plus aspirin significantly decreased occlusion/restenosis (by up to 85%) in patients with critical limb ischemia (OR 0.15; 95% CI 0.06–0.42; $p = 0.0003$), but not in patients with intermittent claudication (OR 1.73; 95% CI 0.97–3.08; $p = 0.06$), and batroxobin plus aspirin reduced restenosis in diabetic patients (OR 0.28; 95% CI 0.13–0.60).

Revascularization

Vascular imaging with ultrasonography, CT angiography, and MR angiography has replaced catheter-based techniques in the initial diagnostic evaluation of patients in most circumstances. Despite a paradigm shift away from catheter-based angiography as a purely diagnostic technique, its importance in intervention has increased dramatically. The major advantage of digital subtraction angiography is the ability to selectively evaluate individual vessels, obtain physiological information such as pressure gradients, and image the layers of the blood vessel wall with intravascular ultrasonography and as a platform for percutaneous intervention. Exposure to ionizing radiation, use of iodinated contrast agents, and risks related to vascular access and catheterization are limitations of this technique.

Before scheduling patients with diabetes and PAD, the disease stage, prognosis, and the so-called peripheral runoff have to be carefully considered.

For stage I of PAD after Fontaine, no exercise training nor any interventional procedures are indicated [21, 35, 36, 38].

For stage II of PAD, an interventional procedure that provides symptom relief (from claudication), but does not improve overall prognosis, may be considered [21, 35, 36, 38]. In patients with diabetes in stage II of PAD, the peripheral runoff has to be evaluated prior to any interventional or surgical procedure. If three (which would be the normal report) crural vessels – the A. tibialis anterior, the A. interossea, and the A. tibialis posterior – are identified, a PTA (for example) of the proximal A. femoralis superficialis could be done with an acceptable risk. However, if only one-vessel runoff is present, and the thrombotic material gets lost during the intervention in the distal periphery, the A. femoralis superficialis might be open after PTA, but the leg lost because of occlusion of all three crural vessels as a "classic" catheter lab complication.

For stages III (very rare in patients with diabetes) and IV of PAD, immediate revascularization is now the treatment of choice [36, 38].

Recent reports suggest that up to 50% of patients with diabetes with a foot ulcer have signs of PAD (= stage IV of PAD), which has a major impact on ulcer healing and the risk of lower-leg amputation [3, 4]. Early reports on the effectiveness of revascularization in patients with diabetes and PAD were not encouraging and led some researchers to suggest that diabetes was associated with a characteristic occlusive small-vessel disease, consequently leading to a nihilistic attitude toward revascularization.

The International Working Group on the Diabetic Foot therefore established a multidisciplinary working group to evaluate the effectiveness of revascularization of the ulcerated foot in patients with diabetes and PAD. A systematic search was performed to evaluate therapies to revascularize the ulcerated foot in patients with diabetes and PAD from 1980 to June 2010 [107]. The major outcomes following endovascular or open-bypass surgery were broadly similar among the studies. After open surgery, the one-year limb-salvage rates were a median of 85% (interquartile range of 80–90%); after endovascular revascularization, these rates were 78% (70.5–85.5%). At one-year follow-up, >60% of ulcers had healed following revascularization with either open bypass surgery or endovascular revascularization. Studies demonstrated improved rates of limb salvage associated with revascularization compared to medically treated patients in the literature.

Compared to patients with intermittent claudication (IC; stage II of PAD), patients with critical limb ischemia (CLI; stages III and IV after Fontaine) are in a more difficult situation: while amputation is rather infrequently necessary in patients with IC [108], amputation rates of 23% at 12 months were reported in patients with CLI [109]. In patients with CLI, the incidence of diabetes mellitus and chronic renal insufficiency is 70.4% and 27.8%, respectively [109]. Thus, patients with CLI are in the majority among patients with diabetes; other, but rarer causes of CLI are arterial embolism, or rheumatological disorders such as sclerodermia [38].

The prevalence of gangrene is about 20 to 30 times higher in patients with diabetes mellitus [110]. Due to a reduced primary patency rate after endovascular therapy [111], repeated treatment is required in diabetic patients. Since diabetics benefit from early revascularization, close surveillance is mandatory [112]. With aggressive interdisciplinary treatment, diabetic patients achieve limb-salvage and mortality rates not significantly different from those of nondiabetic patients [113], but only in high-throughput and experienced – at best – excellence centers. In particular in stage IV PAD, a high patency rate over a longer period (> one year) per se is still not a realistic goal of treatment, but ulcer healing. A rather short-term – about six months – augmentation of peripheral blood pressures (ankle from 50–80 mmHg and toe 30–50 mmHg) is often sufficient for ulcer healing [114].

Very recently, Pedrajas et al. [115] have summarized several studies showing good results and patency rates after percutaneous transluminal balloon angioplasty (PTA) for diabetic critical limb ischemia (Table 11.3). In 2005, Faglia et al. [116] reported very positive findings of 993 diabetic patients from the Milan center who had a mean follow-up of 26 months

Table 11.3 Summary of recent studies of endovascular therapy for diabetic critical limb ischemia . (Source: Dormandy JA et al. 2005 [15]. Reproduced with permission of Elsevier.)

First author/Year	n	Diabetic (%)	CLI (%)	PTA somplication	Patency	Limb salvage	Mortality
Faglia et al. [114]	993	100	100	3.4% complication rate	88% 5y	1.7% amputation after 5 y	5-year survival 74%
Giles et al. [115]	176	72	100	93% technical success	51% 2 y	84% 2 y	5% mortality 30d
Conrad et al. [116]	144	66	86	95% technical success	62% primary patency 90% assist patency	86.2% 40 mos	54% survival, 46 mos
Haider et al. [118]	198	29	100	92% technical success	Femoropopliteal 75% 2 y Below the Knee (BTK) 60% 2 year	Femoropopliteal 90% 2 y BTK 76% 2 y	82% survival, 2y
Faglia et al. [117]	420	100				5.2% amputation 30d	67% 1 y
Faglia et al. [30]	191	100				5.2% amputation 30d	
Dick et al. [119]	119	100				80% 1 y	

after PTA as first-line therapy. The five-year primary patency was 88%, and a major amputation rate of only 1.7% was observed. Another study from the same center [30] focused on 221 diabetic patients with ischemic foot ulcers. PTA was feasible and effective for foot revascularization, with infrapopliteal intervention included. Clinical recurrence was infrequent and the procedure could be repeated successfully in most cases. In subjects treated successfully with PTA, the above-the-ankle amputation rate was low (<5%).

Giles et al. [117] reported the experience with infrapopliteal angioplasty stratified by TASC (Inter-Society Consensus for the Management of PAD) lesion classification in 176 patients with CLI. They observed a 93% technical success rate, a 30-day mortality of 5%, a two-year primary patency of 51%, and limb salvage of 84%. The freedom from reintervention, amputation, or restenosis was 35%. Within two years, 15% of patients underwent bypass and 18% had repeated PTA.

Conrad et al. [118] have treated 144 CLI patients with PTA and demonstrated a primary patency of 62% and limb salvage of 86% at 40 months.

In another study by Faglia et al. [119], runoff was a key factor in limb salvage in 420 diabetics with CLI who underwent tibial angioplasty. Those who had no open tibial arteries at the end of the study suffered a 62.5% limb-amputation rate, compared with a 1.7% amputation rate in patients with at least one open vessel to the foot.

In a comparison of results for above-the-knee versus below-the-knee (BTK) angioplasty in CLI patients, two-year primary patency and limb salvage were 75% and 90%, respectively, for femoropopliteal angioplasty and 60% and 76% for BTK angioplasty [120].

A prospective study by Dick et al. [121] assessed the efficacy of tailored endovascular-first versus surgical-first revascularization stratified for the presence of diabetes, with 383 patients (45.7% had diabetes) presenting 426 limbs with chronic CLI. Success with primary revascularization was significantly worse in diabetic patients as compared with nondiabetic patients. Repeat endovascular procedures significantly improved clinical success, which became equivalent between diabetic and nondiabetic patients (HR 1.02; 95% CI 0.7–1.4). Cumulative one-year mortality was 30%, with a trend toward increased mortality in patients with diabetes, and limb-salvage rates were similar in treatment cohorts. Choice of initial revascularization modality seemed not to influence clinical success in this study.

Conclusion

Recent advantages demonstrate that rapid acute therapy and intensified medical support for a long period can dramatically lower the burden of diabetic foot syndrome, the horrifying combination of PAD and diabetes.

Blinc et al. [19] have clearly shown that in patients with various stages of PAD (II–IV), a stringent therapy setting lowers the two-year mortality to 3.2%, which is only about double the amount of a control group without PAD (1.8%). However, the rate of patients with stage IV during the study is not stated.

Faglia et al. [122] suggested a systematic interventional and medical approach in patients with stage IV PAD (= ulcer, gangrene) and tested this in a study, which when published in 2009 was provocative for many scientists and clinicians:

- All patients and relatives were educated in the treatment of an ulcerated and nonulcerated diabetic foot.
- All patients underwent a detailed investigation program, which analyzed all factors of the diabetic foot syndrome (neuropathy, osteoarthropathy, infection, and PAD).
- All patients received dual platelet inhibition throughout the study (six years).
- All patients were agressively treated for all other cardiovasdcular risk factors (diabetes, hypertension, hyperlipidemia).
- All patients were primarily treated endovascularly (even TASC C and D), and surgical procedures were the second choice.

Faglia's multimodal aggressive approach resulted in a tremendous improvement in limb salvage and survival. During the six-year study, major amputation was reduced from 68% to 20% and death from 75 to 50% (Figure 11.10). The single most independent factor for this prognosis improvement was immediate revascularization with an at that time heavily doubted odds ratio of 36 (Table 11.4).

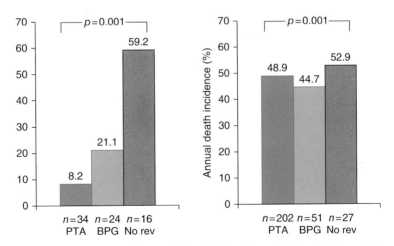

Figure 11.10 Major amputation rate (a) and deaths (b) are significantly lower in those with immediate revascularization and strict pharmacotherapy. (Source: Modified after Faglia E et al. 2009 [116].)

Table 11.4 Factors for prognosis improvement.

	Odds ratio (95% CI)	p
No revascularization	36 (13-100)	<0.001
Crural artery occlusion	8 (1-50)	0.022
Dialysis	5 (2-12)	0.001
Wound infection	2 (1-4)	0.004

Unpublished data from our group suggest that for limb salvage, immediate revascularization should be carried out, whereas for long-term survival, strict pharmacotherapy with achievement of treatment goals is necessary. In our 382 consecutive patients included in an ongoing prospective study, we can report after 4.2 years only 4 major and 12 minor amputations and 26 deaths (6.8%).

Thus, we recommend for all patients with diabetes and PAD:

- Immediate revascularization in highly qualified high-throughput centers for patients with stage III or IV (ischemia, ulcer, gangrene).
- Careful planning of interventions in patients with stage II (if only one vessel runoff is identified in preinterventional screening with CT angiography or MR angiography, an interdisplinary board should discuss the treatment options).
- No surgical procedures in the lower extremity in patients with PAD and diabetes prior to morphological (CT angiography or MR angiography) and hemodynamical (ABI, toe pressures) assessments.
- Primary amputations only in a leg-for-life situation, after consideration with the patient (bad prognosis after major amputations in patients especially above 80 years of age).
- A high cardiovascular morbidity and mortality rate requires intensified screening for coronary heart disease and cerebral ischemia.
- Strict multimodal pharmacotherapy (Table 11.1).

Case Study 1

A 61-year-old female patient with type 2 diabetes mellitus presents at the outpatient department with a reduced walking distance of 100 meters due to pain in the right calf, corresponding to PAD in stage IIb. The PAD of the patient was already treated in the past with two stents in the right proximal superficial femoral artery. The patient is obese, has hypertension and suffers from diabetic polyneuropathy and chronic venous insufficiency grade 1. The smoking anamnesis shows 80 pack-years of cigarettes. In addition to her PAD, the patient has undergone cardiac bypass grafting five years ago, had already had a minor stroke, and is on anticoagulant therapy for atrial fibrillation.

Multiple-Choice Questions

1 Should the patient receive additional anti-platelet aggregation therapy for her PAD?

   A No, she already has anticoagulant therapy

   B Yes, she would benefit in addition to her coronary heart disease

   C Yes, she would benefit in addition to her past stroke

   D Yes, she would benefit in addition to long-term patency for her femoralis stent

   E Yes, she would benefit in addition to her chronic venous insufficiency

2 What is the primary choice of treatment for this patient after assessment of vascular status morphologically and hemodynamically?

   A Stenting

   B Ballon dilatation

   C Peripheral bypass grafting

   D Walking exercise

   E Amputation of the lower leg to treat the pain

3 Later on, CT angiography reveals that the patient's walking pain is caused by in-stent restenosis. In addition, the CT images indicated that the patient has a two-vessel crural run-off. What is the treatment of choice now?

   A Additional anti-platelet medication

   B Ballon dilatation with stenting, if necessary

   C Peripheral bypass grafting

   D Walking exercise training

   E Amputation of the lower leg to treat the pain

4 What is the LDL goal for this elderly patient?

   A <50 mg/dl

   B <70 mg/dl

   C <100 mg/dl

   D <130 mg/dl

   E <160 mg/dl

5 What would be the antiplatelet/anticoagulant scheme if the patient were to require another peripheral stent?

   A Anticoagulant alone

   B Clopidogrel alone

   C Asprin alone

   D Aspirin, clopidogrel and anticoagulant (= triple therapy) for ever?

   E Aspirin, clopidogrel and low-molecular weight for six months, then stop all three and switch to anticoagulant therapy again

6 What is the blood pressure goal for this elderly patient?
  A <160/95 mmHg
  B <140/95 mmHg
  C <140/90 mmHg
  D <130/85 mmHg
  E <125/80 mmHg

Answers provided after the References

Guidelines

ACCF/AHA Focused Update of the Guideline for the management of patients with peripheral artery disease (Updating the 2005 Guideline): A report of the American College of Cardiology Foundation/American Heart Association Task Force on practice guidelines. *Circulation* 2011; 124: 2020–45.

Allard L, Cloutier G, Durand LG et al. Limitations of ultrasonic duplex scanning for diagnosing lower limb arterial stenoses in the presence of adjacent segment disease. *J Vasc Surg* 1994; 19: 650–57.

Dormandy JA, Rutherford RB. Management of peripheral arterial disease. TASC Working Group. *J Vasc Surg* 2000; 31: S1–S296.

Hiatt WR. Medical treatment of peripheral arterial disease and claudication. *N Engl J Med* 2001; 344: 1608–21.

Hirsch AT, Haskal ZJ, Hertzer NR et al. ACC/AHA 2005 guidelines for the management of patients with peripheral arterial disease. *J Am Coll Cardiol* 2006; 47: 1239–312.

Norgren L, Hiatt WR, Dormandy JA et al. Inter-society consensus for the management of peripheral arterial disease (TASC II). *Eur J Vasc Endovasc Surg* 2007; 33 Suppl 1: S1–75.

References

1 Boulton AJ, Vileikyte L, Ragnarsson-Tennvall G et al. The global burden of diabetic foot disease. *Lancet* 2005; 366: 1719–24.

2 Jeffcoate WJ, van Houtum WH. Amputation as a marker of the quality of foot care in diabetes. *Diabetologia* 2004; 47: 2051–8.

3 Prompers L, Schaper N, Apelqvist J et al. Prediction of outcome in individuals with diabetic foot ulcers: Focus on the differences between individuals with and without peripheral arterial disease. The EURODIALE Study. *Diabetologia* 2008; 51: 747–55.

4 Gershater MA, Löndahl M, Nyberg P et al. Complexity of factors related to outcome of neuropathic and neuroischaemic/ischaemic diabetic foot ulcers: A cohort study. *Diabetologia* 2009; 52: 398–407.

5 Bakker K, Apelqvist J, Schaper NC. Practical guidelines on the management and prevention of the diabetic foot 2011. *Diab Metab Res Rev* 2012; 28(Suppl 1): 225–31.

6 Adler AI, Boyko EJ, Ahroni JH et al. Lower-extremity amputation in diabetes: The independent effects of peripheral vascular disease, sensory neuropathy, and foot ulcers. *Diabetes Care* 1999; 22: 1029–35.

7 Adler AI, Erqou S, Lima TA et al. Association between glycated haemoglobin and the risk of lower extremity amputation in patients with diabetes mellitus-review and meta-analysis. *Diabetologia* 2010; 53: 840–49.

8 Escobar C, Blanes I, Ruiz A et al. Prevalence and clinical profile and management of peripheral arterial disease in elderly patients with diabetes. *Eur J Intern Med* 2011; 22: 275–81.

9 Apelqvist J, Elgzyri T, Larsson J et al. Factors related to outcome of neurois-chemic/ischemic foot ulcer in diabetic patients. *J Vasc Surg* 2011; 53: 1582–8.

10 Schofield CJ, Libby G, Brennan GM et al. DARTS/MEMO Collaboration. Mortality and hospitalization in patients after amputation: A comparison between patients with and without diabetes. *Diabetes Care* 2006; 29: 2252–6.

11 Morbach S, Furchert H, Gröblinghoff U et al. Long-term prognosis of diabetic foot patients and their limbs: Amputation and death over the course of a decade. *Diabetes Care* 2012; 35(10): 2021–7.

12 Schofield CJ, Yu N, Jain AS et al. Decreasing amputation rates in patients with dia-betes: A population-based study. *Diabet Med* 2009; 26: 773–7.

13 Tseng CL, Rajan M, Miller DR et al. Trends in initial lower extremity amputation rates among Veterans Health Administration health care system users from 2000 to 2004. *Diabetes Care* 2011; 34: 1157–63.

14 Li Y, Burrows NR, Gregg EW et al. Declining rates of hospitalization for nontrau-matic lower-extremity amputation in the diabetic population aged 40 years or older: U.S., 1988–2008. *Diabetes Care* 2012; 35: 273–7.

15 Dormandy JA, Charbonnel B, Eckland DJ et al. Secondary prevention of macrovas-cular events in patients with type 2 diabetes in the PROactive Study (PROspective pioglitAzone Clinical Trial In macroVascular Events): A randomised controlled trial. *Lancet* 2005; 366: 1279–89.

16 Dormandy JA, Betteridge DJ, Schernthaner G et al. Impact of peripheral arterial dis-ease in patients with diabetes: Results from PROactive (PROactive 11). *Atherosclerosis* 2009; 202: 272–81.

17 Althouse AD, Abbott JD, Sutton-Tyrrell K et al. for the BARI 2D Study Group. Favorable effects of insulin sensitizers pertinent to peripheral arterial disease in type 2 diabetes: Results from the Bypass Angioplasty Revascularization Investigation 2 Diabetes (BARI 2D) trial. *Diabetes Care* 2013; 36: 3269–75.

18 Bach RG, Brooks MM, Lombardero M et al. for the BARI 2D Investigators. Rosiglita-zone and outcomes for patients with diabetes mellitus and coronary artery disease in the Bypass Angioplasty Revascularization Investigation 2 Diabetes (BARI 2D) Trial. *Circulation* 2013; 12: 785–94.

19 Blinc A, Kozak M, Sabovic M et al. Prevention of ischemic events in patients with peripheral arterial disease design, baseline characteristics and 2-year results an observational study. *Int Angiol* 2011; 30: 555–66.

20 Heald CL, Fowkes FG, Murray GD et al. Ankle Brachial Index Collaboration. Risk of mortality and cardiovascular disease associated with the ankle-brachial index: Systematic review. *Atherosclerosis* 2006; 189: 61–9.

21 Dormandy JA, Rutherford RB. Management of peripheral arterial disease. TASC Working Group. *J Vasc Surg* 2000; 31: S1–S296.

22 Kallio M, Forsblom C, Groop PH et al. Development of new peripheral arterial occlu-sive disease in patients with type 2 diabetes during a mean follow-up of 11 years. *Diabetes Care* 2003; 26: 1241–5.

23 Jude EB, Oyibo SO, Chalmers N et al. Peripheral arterial disease in diabetic and nondiabetic patients: A comparison of severity and outcome. *Diabetes Care* 2001; 24: 1433–7.

24 Beach KW, Bedford GR, Bergelin RO et al. Progression of lower-extremity arterial occlusive disease in type II diabetes mellitus. *Diabetes Care* 1988; 11: 464–72.

25 Boyko EJ, Ahroni JH, Smith DG et al. Increased mortality associated with diabetic foot ulcer. *Diabet Med* 1996; 13: 967–72.

26 Leibson CL, Ransom JE, Olson W et al. Peripheral arterial disease, diabetes, and mortality. *Diabetes Care* 2004; 27: 2843–9.

27 Cavanagh PR, Lipsky BA, Bradbury AW et al. Treatment for diabetic foot ulcers. *Lancet* 2005; 366: 1725–35.

28 Sämann A, Tajiyeva O, Müller N et al. Prevalence of the diabetic foot syndrome at the primary care level in Germany: A cross-sectional study. *Diabet Med* 2008; 25: 557–63.

29 Diehm N, Shang A, Silvestro A et al. Association of cardiovascular risk factors with pattern of lower limb atherosclerosis in 2659 patients undergoing angioplasty. *Eur J Vasc Endovasc Surg* 2006; 31: 59–63.

30 Faglia E, Mantero M, Caminiti M et al. Extensive use of peripheral angioplasty, particularly infrapopliteal, in the treatment of ischaemic diabetic foot ulcers: Clinical results of a multicentric study of 221 consecutive diabetic subjects. *J Intern Med* 2002; 252: 225–32.

31 Jude EB, Eleftheriadou I, Tentolouris N. Peripheral arterial disease in diabetes: A review. *Diabet Med* 2009; 27: 4–14.

32 Johansson KE, Marklund BR, Fowelin JH. Evaluation of a new screening method for detecting peripheral arterial disease in a primary health care population of patients with diabetes mellitus. *Diabet Med* 2002; 19: 307–10.

33 Adler AI, Stevens RJ, Neil A et al. UKPDS 59: Hyperglycemia and other potentially modifiable risk factors for peripheral vascular disease in type 2 diabetes. *Diabetes Care* 2002; 25: 894–9.

34 Fowkes FG. The measurement of atherosclerotic peripheral arterial disease in epidemiological surveys. *Int J Epidemiol* 1988; 17: 248–54.

35 Hirsch AT, Haskal ZJ, Hertzer NR et al. ACC/AHA 2005 guidelines for the management of patients with peripheral arterial disease. *J Am Coll Cardiol* 2006; 47: 1239–312.

36 2011 ACCF/AHA Focused Update of the Guideline for the management of patients with peripheral artery disease (Updating the 2005 Guideline): A report of the American College of Cardiology Foundation/American Heart Association Task Force on practice guidelines. *Circulation* 2011; 124: 2020–45.

37 Hiatt WR. Medical treatment of peripheral arterial disease and claudication. *N Engl J Med* 2001; 344: 1608–21.

38 Norgren L, Hiatt WR, Dormandy JA et al. Inter-society consensus for the management of peripheral arterial disease (TASC II). *Eur J Vasc Endovasc Surg* 2007; 33 Suppl 1: S1–75.

39 Waugh JR, Sacharias N. Arteriographic complications in the DSA era. *Radiology* 1992; 182: 243–46.

40 Prokop M. CT angiography of the abdominal arteries. *Abdom Imaging* 1998; 23: 462–8.

41 Jager KA, Ricketts HJ, Strandness DE, Jr., Duplex scanning for the evaluation of lower limb arterial disease. In: Bernstein EF, ed. *Noninvasive Diagnostic Techniques in Vascular Disease*. St Louis, MO: CV Mosby; 1985: 619–31.

42 Kohler TR, Nance DR, Cramer MM et al. Duplex scanning for diagnosis of aortoiliac and femoropopliteal disease: A prospective study. *Circulation* 1987; 76: 1074–80.

43 Moneta GL, Yeager RA, Antonovic R et al. Accuracy of lower extremty arterial duplex mapping. *J Vasc Surg* 1992; 15: 275–83.

44 Whelan JF, Barry MH, Moir JD. Color flow Doppler ultrasonography: Comparison with peripheral arteriography for the investigation of peripheral vascular disease. *J Clin Ultrasound* 1992; 20: 369–74.

45 Allard L, Cloutier G, Durand LG et al. Limitations of ultrasonic duplex scanning for diagnosing lower limb arterial stenoses in the presence of adjacent segment disease. *J Vasc Surg* 1994; 19: 650–57.

46 Dyet JF, Nicholson AA, Ettles DF. Vascular imaging and intervention in peripheral arteries in the diabetic patient. *Diabetes Metab Res Rev* 2000; 16(Suppl 1): S16–S22.

47 Ho KY, Leiner T, de Haan MW et al. Peripheral vascular tree stenoses: Evaluation with moving-bed infusion-tracking MR angiography. *Radiology* 1998; 206: 683–92.

48 Rofsky NM, Adelman MA. MR angiography in the evaluation of atherosclerotic peripheral vascular disease. *Radiology* 2000; 214: 325–38.

49 Meaney JF, Ridgway JP, Chakraverty S et al. Stepping-table gadolinium-enhanced digital subtraction MR angiography of the aorta and lower extremity arteries: Preliminary experience. *Radiology* 1999; 211: 59–67.

50 Meissner OA, Rieger J, Weber C et al. Critical limb ischemia: Hybrid MR angiography compared with DSA. *Radiology* 2005; 235: 308–18.

51 Visser K, Hunink MG. Peripheral arterial disease: Gadolinium-enhanced MR angiography versus color-guided duplex US – a meta-analysis. *Radiology* 2000; 216: 67–77.

52 Grobner T. Gadolinium: A specific trigger for the development of nephrogenic fibrosing dermopathy and nephrogenic systemic fibrosis? *Nephrol Dial Transplant* 2006; 21: 1104–8.

53 Thomsen HS. ESUR guideline: Gadolinium-based contrast media and nephrogenic systemic fibrosis. *Eur Radiol* 2007; 17: 2692–6.

54 Hodnett PA, Ward EV, Davarpanah AH et al. Peripheral arterial disease in a symptomatic diabetic population: Prospective comparison of rapid unenhanced MR angiography (MRA) with contrast-enhanced MRA. *AJR Am J Roentgenol* 2011; 197: 1466–73.

55 Levine GN, Gomes AS, Arai AE et al. Safety of magnetic resonance imaging in patients with cardiovascular devices: An American Heart Association scientific statement from the Committee on Diagnostic and Interventional Cardiac Catheterization, Council on Clinical Cardiology, and the Council on Cardiovascular Radiology and Intervention: Endorsed by the American College of Cardiology Foundation, the North American Society for Cardiac Imaging, and the Society for Cardiovascular Magnetic Resonance. *Circulation* 2007; 116: 2878–91.

56 Lapeyre M, Kobeiter H, Desgranges P et al. Assessment of critical limb ischemia in patients with diabetes: Comparison of MR angiography and digital subtraction angiography. *AJR Am J Roentgenol* 2005; 185: 1641–50.

57 Olin JW, Kaufman JA, Bluemke DA et al. Atherosclerotic Vascular Disease Conference. American Heart Association, Imaging, Writing Group IV. *Circulation* 2004; 109: 2626–33.

58 Rubin GD, Schmidt AJ, Logan LJ et al. Multi-detector row CT angiography of lower extremity arterial inflow and runoff: Initial experience. *Radiology* 2001; 221: 146–58.

59 Met R, Bipat S, Legemate DA, et al. Diagnostic performance of computed tomography angiography in peripheral arterial disease: A systematic review and meta-analysis. *JAMA* 2009; 301: 415–24.

60 Willmann JK, Wildermuth S, Pfammatter T et al. Aortoiliac and renal arteries: Prospective intraindividual comparison of contrast-enhanced three-dimensional MR angiography and multi-detector row CT angiography. *Radiology* 2003; 226: 798–811.

61 Merlino G, Fratticci L, Valente M et al. Association of restless legs syndrome in type 2 diabetes: A case-control study. *Sleep* 2007; 30: 866–71.

62 Ouwendijk R, Kock MC, Visser K et al. Interobserver agreement for the interpretation of contrast-enhanced 3D MR angiography and MDCT angiography in peripheral arterial disease. *AJR Am J Roentgenol* 2005; 185: 1261–7.

63 Schernthaner MB, Edelhauser G, Berzaczy D et al. Perceptibility and quantification of in-stent stenosis with six peripheral arterial stent types in vitro: Comparison of 16-MDCT angiography, 64-MDCT angiography, and MR angiography. *AJR Am J Roentgenol* 2010; 194: 1346–51.

64 Plank CM, Wolf F, Langenberger H et al. Improved detection of in-stent restenosis by blood pool agent-enhanced, high-resolution, steady-state magnetic resonance angiography. *Eur Radiol* 2011; 21: 2158–65.

65 Ouwendijk R, Kock MC, van Dijk LC et al. Vessel wall calcifications at multi-detector row CT angiography in patients with peripheral arterial disease: Effect on clinical utility and clinical predictors. *Radiology* 2006; 241: 603–8.

66 Meyer BC, Werncke T, Hopfenmuller W et al. Dual energy CT of peripheral arteries: Effect of automatic bone and plaque removal on image quality and grading of stenoses. *Eur J Radiol* 2008; 68: 414–22.

67 Ouwendijk R, de Vries M, Pattynama PM et al. Imaging peripheral arterial disease: A randomized controlled trial comparing contrast-enhanced MR angiography and multi-detector row CT angiography. *Radiology* 2005; 236:1094–103.

68 Kock MC, Adriaensen ME, Pattynama PM et al. DSA versus multi-detector row CT angiography in peripheral arterial disease: Randomized controlled trial. *Radiology* 2005; 237: 727–37.

69 Rubin GD. Data explosion: The challenge of multidetector-row CT. *Eur J Radiol* 2000; 36: 74–80.

70 Roos JE, Fleischmann D, Koechl A et al. Multipath curved planar reformation of the peripheral arterial tree in CT angiography. *Radiology* 2007; 244: 281–90.

71 Beitzke D, Wolf F, Edelhauser G et al. Computed tomography angiography of the carotid arteries at low kV settings: A prospective randomised trial assessing radiation dose and diagnostic confidence. *Eur Radiol* 2011; 21: 2434–44.

72 Sun Z. Diagnostic accuracy of multislice CT angiography in peripheral arterial disease. *J Vasc Interv Radiol* 2006; 17: 1915–21.

73 Tsai JC, Chan P, Wang CH et al. The effects of exercise training on walking function and perception of health status in elderly patients with peripheral arterial occlusive disease. *J Intern Med* 2002; 252: 448–55.

74 Owens CD, Conte MS. Medical management of peripheral arterial disease: Bridging the "gap"? *Circulation* 2012; 126(11): 1319–21

75 Gasse C, Jacobsen J, Larsen AC et al. Secondary medical prevention among Danish patients hospitalised with either peripheral arterial disease or myocardial infarction. *Eur J Vasc Endovasc Surg* 2008; 35: 51–8.

76 Cacoub PP, Abola MT, Baumgartner I et al. Cardiovascular risk factor control and outcomes in peripheral artery disease patients in the Reduction of Atherothrombosis for Continued Health (REACH) Registry. *Atherosclerosis* 2009; 204: e86–e92.

77 Subherwal S, Patel MR, Kober L et al. Missed opportunities: Despite improvement in use of cardioprotective medications among patients with lower extremity peripheral artery disease, underutilization remains. *Circulation* 2012; ePub Aug 8.

78 Pande RL, Perlstein TS, Beckman JA et al. Secondary prevention and mortality in peripheral artery disease: National Health and Nutrition Examination Study, 1999 to 2004. *Circulation* 2011; 124: 17–23.

79 González-Clemente JM, Piniés JA, Calle-Pascual A et al. Cardiovascular risk factor management is poorer in diabetic patients with undiagnosed peripheral arterial disease than in those with known coronary heart disease or cerebrovascular disease: Results of a nationwide study in tertiary diabetes centres. *Diabet Med* 2008; 25: 427–34.

80 Mehler PS, Coll JR, Estacio R et al. Intensive blood pressure control reduces the risk of cardiovascular events in patients with peripheral arterial disease and type 2 diabetes. *Circulation* 2003; 107: 753–6.

81 Sohn MW, Meadows JL, Oh EH et al. Statin use and lower extremity amputation risk in nonelderly diabetic patients. *J Vasc Surg* 2013; pii: S0741–5214 (13)01253-6. doi:10.1016/j.jvs.2013.06.069. Epub Aug 7.

82 Bavry AA, Anderson RD, Gong Y et al. Outcomes among hypertensive patients with concomitant peripheral and coronary artery disease: Findings from the International VErapamil-SR/Trandolapril STudy. *Hypertension* 2010; 55: 48–53.

83 Rosendorff C, Black HR, Cannon CP et al. Treatment of hypertension in the prevention and management of ischemic heart disease: A scientific statement from the American Heart Association Council for High Blood Pressure Research and the Councils on Clinical Cardiology and Epidemiology and Prevention. *Circulation* 2007; 115: 2761–788.

84 O'Sullivan CJ, Hynes N, Mahendran B et al. Haemoglobin A1c (HbA1C) in non-diabetic and diabetic vascular patients: Is HbA1C an independent risk factor and predictor of adverse outcome? *Eur J Vasc Endovasc Surg* 2006; 32: 188–97.

85 Ishii H, Kumada Y, Takahashi H et al. Impact of diabetes and glycaemic control on peripheral artery disease in Japanese patients with end-stage renal disease: Long-term follow-up study from the beginning of haemodialysis. *Diabetologia* 2012; 55: 1304–9.

86 Conte MS, Bandyk DF, Clowes AW et al. Risk factors, medical therapies and perioperative events in limb salvage surgery: Observations from the PREVENT III multicenter trial. *J Vasc Surg* 2005; 42: 456–64.

87 Feringa HH, Karagiannis SE, van Waning VH et al. The effect of intensified lipid-lowering therapy on long term prognosis in patients with peripheral arterial disease. *J Vasc Surg* 2007; 45: 936–43.

88 Heart Protection Study Collaborative Group. Randomized trial of the effects of cholesterol-lowering with simvastatin on peripheral vascular and other major vascular outcomes in 20,536 people with peripheral arterial disease and other high-risk conditions. *J Vasc Surg* 2007; 45: 645–54.

89 Aung PP, Maxwell HG, Jepson RG et al. Lipid-lowering for peripheral arterial disease of the lower limb. *Cochrane Database Syst Rev* 2007; 17: CD000123.

90 Walldius G, Erikson U, Olsson AG et al. The effect of probucol on femoral atherosclerosis: The Probucol Quantitative Regression Swedish Trial (PQRST). *Am J Cardiol* 1994; 74: 875–83.

91 Johansson J, Olsson AG, Bergstrand L et al. Lowering of HDL2b by probucol partly explains the failure of the drug to affect femoral atherosclerosis in subjects with hypercholesterolemia: A Probucol Quantitative Regression Swedish Trial (PQRST) Report. *Arterioscler Thromb Vasc Biol* 1995; 15: 1049–56.

92 Ferrannini E, Cushman WC. Diabetes and hypertension: The bad companions. *Lancet* 2012; 380: 601–10.

93 Chobanian AV, Bakris GL, Black HR et al. Seventh report of the Joint National Committee on prevention, detection, evaluation, and treatment of high blood pressure. *Hypertension* 2003; 42: 1206–52.

94 Mancia G, De Backer G, Dominiczak A et al. 2007 guidelines for the management of arterial hypertension: The Task Force for the Management of Arterial Hypertension of the European Society of Hypertension (ESH) and of the European Society of Cardiology (ESC). *J Hypertens* 2007; 25: 1105–87.

95 Cushman WC, Evans GW, Byington RP et al. Effects of intensive blood-pressure control in type 2 diabetes mellitus. *N Engl J Med* 2010; 362: 1575–85.

96 Patel A, MacMahon S, Chalmers J et al. Effects of a fixed combination of perindopril and indapamide on macrovascular and microvascular outcomebin patients with type 2 diabetes mellitus (the ADVANCE trial): A randomised controlled trial. *Lancet* 2007; 370: 829–40.

97 Schiffrin EL. Hypertension: Treatments, diabetes, and developing regions. *Lancet* 2012; 380: 539–41.

98 Pohl MA, Blumenthal S, Cordonnier DJ et al. Independent and additive impact of blood pressure control and angiotensin II receptor blockade on renal outcomes in the irbesartan diabetic nephropathy trial: Clinical implications and limitations. *J Am Soc Nephrol* 2005; 16: 3027–37.

99 Cooper-DeHoff RM, Gong Y, Handberg EM et al. Tight blood pressure control and cardiovascular outcomes among hypertensive patients with diabetes and coronary artery disease. *JAMA* 2010; 304: 61–8.

100 Bangalore S, Kumar S, Lobach I et al. Blood pressure targets in subjects with type 2 diabetes mellitus/impaired fasting glucose: Observations from traditional and Bayesian random-effects meta-analyses of randomized trials. *Circulation* 2011; 123: 2799–810.

101 Antithrombotic Trialists' Collaboration. Collaborative meta-analyis of randomised trials of antiplatelet therapy for prevention of death, myocardial infarction, and stroke in high risk patients. *Brit Med J* 2002; 324: 71–86.

102 Cacoub PP, Bhatt DL, Steg PG et al. Patients with peripheral arterial disease in the CHARISMA trial. *Eur Heart J* 2009; 30: 192–201.

103 CAPRIE Steering Committee. A randomised, blinded, trial of clopidogrel versus aspirin in patients at risk of ischaemic events (CAPRIE). *Lancet* 1996; 348: 1329–39.

104 Fowkes FGR, Price JF, Stewart MCW et al. Aspirin for prevention of cardiovascular events in a general population screened for a low ankle brachial index: A randomized controlled trial. *JAMA* 2010; 303: 841–8.

105 Belch J, MacCuish A, Campbell I et al. The prevention of progression of arterial disease and diabetes (POPADAD) trial: Factorial randomised placebo controlled trial of aspirin and antioxidants in patients with diabetes and asymptomatic peripheral arterial disease. *Brit Med J* 2008; 337: a1840. doi:10.1136/bmj.a1840.

106 Robertson L, Ghouri MA, Kovacs F. Antiplatelet and anticoagulant drugs for prevention of restenosis/reocclusion following peripheral endovascular treatment. *Cochrane Database Syst Rev* 2012; 8: CD002071.

107 Hinchliffe RJ, Andros G, Apelqvist J et al. A systematic review of the effectiveness of revascularization of the ulcerated foot in patients with diabetes and peripheral arterial disease. *Diabetes Metab Res Rev* 2012; 28 Suppl 1: 179–217.

108 Imparato AM, Kim GE, Davidson T et al. Intermittent claudication: Its natural course. *Surgery* 1975; 78: 795–9.

109 Marston WA, Davies SW, Armstrong B et al. Natural history of limbs with arterial insufficiency and chronic ulceration treated without revascularization. *J Vasc Surg* 2006; 44: 108–14.

110 Dormandy J, Heeck L, Vig S. Predicting which patients will develop chronic critical leg ischemia. *Semin Vasc Surg* 1999; 12: 138–41.

111 DeRubertis BG, Pierce M, Ryer EJ et al. Reduced primary patency rate in diabetic patients after percutaneous intervention results from more frequent presentation with limb-threatening ischemia. *J Vasc Surg* 2008; 47: 101–8.

112 Dick F, Diehm N, Galimanis A et al. Surgical or endovascular revascularization in patients with critical limb ischemia: Influence of diabetes mellitus on clinical outcome. *J Vasc Surg* 2007; 45: 751–61.

113 Awad S, Karkos CD, Serrachino-Inglott F et al. The impact of diabetes on current revascularisation practice and clinical outcome in patients with critical lower limb ischaemia. *Eur J Vasc Endovasc Surg* 2006; 32: 51–9.

114 Reekers JA, Lammer J. Diabetic foot and PAD: The endovascular approach. *Diabetes Metab Res Rev* 2012; Suppl 1: 36–9.

115 Pedrajas FG, Cafasso DE, Schneider PA. Endovascular therapy: Is it effective in the diabetic limb? *Semin Vasc Surg* 2012; 25: 93–101.

116 Faglia E, Dalla Paola L, Clerici G et al. Peripheral angioplasty as the first-choice revascularization procedure in diabetic patients with critical limb ischemia: Prospective study of 993 consecutive patients hospitalized and followed between 1999 and 2003. *Eur J Vasc Endovasc Surg* 2005; 29: 620–27.

117 Giles KA, Pomposelli FB, Spence TL et al: Infrapopliteal angioplasty for critical limb ischemia: Relation of TransAtlantic InterSociety Consensus class to outcome in 176 limbs. *J Vasc Surg* 2008; 48: 128–36.

118 Conrad MF, Kang J, Cambria RP et al. Infrapopliteal balloon angioplasty for the treatment of chronic occlusive disease. *J Vasc Surg* 2009; 50: 799–805.

119 Faglia E, Clerici G, Clerissi J et al. When is a technically successful peripheral angioplasty effective in preventing above-the-ankle amputation in diabetic patients with critical limb ischaemia? *Diabet Med* 2007; 24: 823–9.

120 Haider SN, Kavanagh EG, Forlee M et al. Two-year outcome with preferential use of infrainguinal angioplasty for critical ischemia. *J Vasc Surg* 2006; 43: 504–12.

121 Dick F, Diehm N, Galimanis A et al. Surgical or endovascular revascularization in patients with critical limb ischemia: Influence of diabetes mellitus on clinical outcome. *J Vasc Surg* 2007; 45: 751–61.

122 Faglia E, Clerici G, Clerissi J et al. Long-term prognosis of diabetic patients with critical limb ischemia: A population-based cohort study. *Diabetes Care* 2009; 32: 822–7.

Answers to Multiple-Choice Questions for Case Study 1

1 A

2 D

3 B

4 B

5 E

6 C

Index

Managing Cardiovascular Complications in Diabetes, First Edition.
Edited by D. John Betteridge and Stephen Nicholls.
© 2014 John Wiley & Sons, Ltd. Published 2014 by John Wiley & Sons, Ltd.